Comprehensive Healthcare Simulation

Series Editors

Adam I. Levine
Department of Anesthesiology
Mount Sinai Medical Center
New York, USA

Samuel DeMaria Jr.
Department of Anesthesiology
Mount Sinai Medical Center
New York, USA

This new series focuses on the use of simulation in healthcare education, one of the most exciting and significant innovations in healthcare teaching since Halsted put forth the paradigm of "see one, do one, teach one." Each volume focuses either on the use of simulation in teaching in a specific specialty or on a cross-cutting topic of broad interest, such as the development of a simulation center. The volumes stand alone and are also designed to complement Levine, DeMaria, Schwartz, and Sim, eds., *The Comprehensive Textbook of Healthcare Simulation* by providing detailed and practical guidance beyond the scope of the larger book and presenting the most up-to-date information available. Series Editors Drs. Adam I. Levine and Samuel DeMaria Jr. are affiliated with the Icahn School of Medicine at Mount Sinai, New York, New York, USA, home to one of the foremost simulation centers in healthcare education. Dr. Levine is widely regarded as a pioneer in the use of simulation in healthcare education. Editors of individual series volumes and their contributors are all recognized leaders in simulation-based healthcare education.

More information about this series at http://www.springer.com/series/13029

William C. McGaghie • Jeffrey H. Barsuk
Diane B. Wayne
Editors

Comprehensive Healthcare Simulation: Mastery Learning in Health Professions Education

Springer

Editors
William C. McGaghie
Northwestern University
Feinberg School of Medicine
Departments of Medical Education and Preventive Medicine
Chicago, IL,
USA

Jeffrey H. Barsuk
Northwestern University
Feinberg School of Medicine
Departments of Medicine and Medical Education
Chicago, IL,
USA

Diane B. Wayne
Northwestern University
Feinberg School of Medicine
Departments of Medicine and Medical Education
Chicago, IL,
USA

ISSN 2366-4479 ISSN 2366-4487 (electronic)
Comprehensive Healthcare Simulation
ISBN 978-3-030-34810-6 ISBN 978-3-030-34811-3 (eBook)
https://doi.org/10.1007/978-3-030-34811-3

This Springer imprint is published by the registered company Springer Nature Switzerland AG
The registered company address is: Gewerbestrasse 11, 6330 Cham, Switzerland

This book is dedicated to our parents and spouses, key shapers of our lives, ambitions, and professional work. We are forever grateful for their influence on our thoughts and actions.

For my parents, William McGaghie and Vivian McGaghie, and for my wife, Pamela Wall McGaghie

William C. McGaghie, PhD

For my parents, Sidney Barsuk and Maxene Barsuk, and for my wife, Ranelle Barsuk

Jeffrey H. Barsuk, MD, MS

For my parents, Dr. Eugene Bronstein and Enid Bronstein, and for my husband, Dr. Jeffrey D. Wayne

Diane B. Wayne, MD

Foreword

To title a book *Comprehensive Healthcare Simulation: Mastery Learning in Health Professions Education* is to set high expectations. Fortunately, Dr. William McGaghie and his Northwestern University medical simulation and education research colleagues are up to the task. They pose the question: "How can we improve health professions education?" This is a humbling question for leaders in their field to ask and an even more daunting task to back it up. This is not the first time the Northwestern University team asked this question, and they are determined to provide an answer.

My professional relationship with William McGaghie extends over two decades originating from our collaboration with the "Miami Group" of medical simulation educators and researchers. This group, including McGaghie and other leading simulation educators, met at the University of Miami to conduct multicenter studies and use research findings to convince the health professions education community that held on to "time-honored," traditional beliefs to update instruction and assessment practices.

One of the most important, and highly cited, studies performed by the "Miami Group" was a systematic review undertaken under auspices of the Best Evidence Medical Education (BEME) collaboration that addressed the question: "What are the features and uses of high-fidelity medial simulations that lead to effective learning?" [1] We scoured hundreds of journal articles that span the range of healthcare professions and all levels of learners—from first-year nursing and medical students to practicing clinical providers. Individual research reports were coded, classified, evaluated for strength, and synthesized qualitatively. The research review results were telling and robust. The findings showed that the studies with the strongest effects shared several common traits: feedback, repetitive practice, defined outcomes, curriculum integration, individualized learning, progressive difficulty, and variety of practice [1].

The Northwestern Group used the results from the BEME review to rethink its medical education traditions. The "best evidence" confirmed what we had studied and experienced in medical education. However, Northwestern and Miami investigators were also surprised that while many of the simulation studies sought to recreate the conditions for patient findings and clinical environment, they also frequently adopted the apprenticeship model and applied it to their simulation training. Progress was being made, but it was limited by educational inertia. Positive results and statistically significant improvements in learner performance were produced, but overall, the level of skill achieved was far below a mastery standard we expected for trainees to be judged competent to apply clinical skills to real patients.

The most basic means of learning requires a language that everyone can understand. In our research, we also noted the lack of a unified approach that transcended professions, disciplines, and specialties. For example, surgeons did things differently than anesthesiologists, internists, and nurses. The Northwestern group saw early on that while much of the focus was on innovations in simulators, environment, and operations, this did not extend to the learning methodology. What medical education needed was a unifying approach to training and learning, one that would challenge the time-honored, nostalgic, yet obsolete Oslerian model that had not kept pace with changes in healthcare. There needed to be a complete disruption and reengineering of how we train clinicians to care for the lives of patients. That solution is *Comprehensive Healthcare Simulation: Mastery Learning in Health Professions Education.*

Over the past 15 years, the Northwestern University medical simulation and education research group has methodically and systematically developed, implemented, and rigorously evaluated the mastery learning model to a degree never before achieved in health sciences education. This has been a courageous journey because along the way, the Northwestern Group has held up a mirror to the traditions and limitations of their own program, using it as a springboard to challenge an antiquated system that allowed large numbers of trainees and practitioners to perform skills on patients without first demonstrating mastery. At each step along the journey, they meticulously documented and published their work so others could learn and adopt the mastery learning approach.

The Northwestern medical simulation and education research team has always emphasized that patient care and welfare should not just be the focus but indeed the ultimate outcome of a mastery learning program. Their goal is simple: better patient outcomes, reduced patient in-hospital stays and costs for the healthcare system, and a commitment to excellence in every aspect of a training program. This book is the result of a 15-year journey toward that goal. The volume has been carefully crafted to include rich insight, guidance, and models for all of us who are responsible for training students and providers in all disciplines and professions. The first half of the book provides a step-by-step guide on developing and implementing a comprehensive mastery learning program. This should be required reading for anyone involved in health sciences education. The next several chapters provide detailed guidance on specific skills that span all specialties and professions and demonstrate the universal applicability of the mastery learning model, including communication and teamwork skills. In the heart of this book, the readers will find guidance and examples for developing a training curriculum that will not only lead to immediate improvements in skills but also improvements that will be sustained over time and translate to better patient care practices and improved patient outcomes. These are goals to which many aspire but very few achieve. While many of the examples use some method of simulation as a means to replicate the clinical environment, the mastery learning model is useful for any teaching strategy and approach because it is grounded in the science of human learning.

The final section of the book provides a broader view of mastery learning, describing how it can provide the foundation for current and future competency-based models along the continuum of healthcare education. This is particularly well-suited for key stakeholders such as deans and program and clerkship directors who are tasked with providing the necessary resources for the success of a mastery learning program.

At the core of mastery learning are those willing to change: instructors, faculty, evaluators, technicians, administrative personnel, and learners. Mastery learning requires a team effort and involves hard work not only for trainees but also for those who make it happen. The lives and welfare of our patients and their families deserve no less. For too long, naysayers have hoisted obstacles to changing the status quo in medical education, providing excuses that tradition has always worked or that change is too resource-intensive or costly. I counter by asking: "What is the cost to our patients and the health system if we do not change?" Those of us familiar with the outdated, ineffective approaches to health professions education are saddened and frustrated, but not surprised, when health services researchers point out that medical errors could be the third largest cause of death in the United States. The system of healthcare is complex, constantly changing and adapting, influenced by innovation, new technologies, and scientific discoveries at a pace unparalleled in human history. The authors of this book embrace this transformation and have provided a path out of the dark ages of medical education. Together, we are empowered to change and improve how we prepare and train our learners to better care for the lives of patients. This is the objective of their work and the integrity of their purpose.

S. Barry Issenberg, MD, FACP
Professor of Medicine
University of Miami
Miller School of Medicine
Miami, FL
USA

Reference

1. Issenberg SB, McGaghie WC, Petrusa ER, et al. Features and uses of high-fidelity medical simulations that lead to effective learning: a BEME systematic review. Med Teach. 2005;27(1):10–28.

Preface

Innovators in health professions education are the only persons who are asked to present evidence about the value of new educational approaches. Defenders of the educational status quo are never expected to present data to support business as usual. Over three decades ago, Samuel Bloom wrote about the power of inertia in medical education and, by inference, about other health professions [1]. Bloom argued that despite many blue ribbon commissions, lofty foundation reports, policy statements by professional associations, and technological advancements, improvements in twentieth-century (now twenty-first-century) medical education have moved at a snail's pace. This is historical evidence of "reform without change" in medical and health professions education, the common situation where educational improvement is discussed from the podium and seen on paper but is not embraced in practice. Reform without change underscores the power of inertia in health professions education, the conservative impulse to assert "we have always taught our students this way;" I got great bedside teaching, so can you;" "our students pass board exams with flying colors;" or "our graduates are in great demand, they are scooped up in the marketplace."

This book challenges such complacent ideas. We know that better and more powerful approaches to educating doctors, nurses, dentists, physical therapists, midwives, social workers, and many other healthcare team members are now available. We believe it is time to move beyond the traditional, apprenticeship model of clinical education in the health professions. Historical approaches to clinical education—lectures, time-limited clinical rotations, nursing foundation courses, ward rounds with varied content—for doctors, nurses, and other health professionals are "time-honored" but obsolete in today's healthcare environment. These passive approaches yield uneven clinical skills and do not ensure the safety of graduates to practice independently. We must do better if the goal is learner acquisition of clinical skill and acumen. After decades of research and study, we believe that systematic education grounded in learning science principles—mastery learning—is needed, featuring clear expectations, rigorous assessment, high achievement standards, feedback, coaching, and constant opportunities for improvement.

This book aims to achieve seven key objectives:

1. Introduce the health professions education community to ideas, principles, and practices about mastery learning: theory, history, current status, and future prospects.

2. Review data that show the mastery learning model works and inspire others to adopt, adapt, and use the model locally.
3. Present practical details about introducing and using the mastery learning model in health professions education including curriculum development, instruction design and delivery, outcome assessment, standard setting, program implementation and management, feedback and debriefing, and faculty development.
4. Review how mastery learning is being used in the health professions to help learners acquire and hone key clinical competencies in a variety of domains: communication skills, teamwork, surgical skills, bedside procedures, clinical emergencies, and essential clinical skills.
5. Map transfer of training pathways from learning results achieved in classroom or laboratory settings to translational outcomes in terms of better patient care practices and improved patient outcomes. Transfer of training also involves maintenance and dissemination of mastery learning programs including cultural, historical, organizational, and interprofessional barriers in health professions education that stymie efforts to move beyond the status quo.
6. Address the impact and consequences of mastery learning in the contemporary context of health professions education: undergraduate entrustable professional activities (EPAs) and postgraduate milestones in medicine, continuing professional education (CPE) and maintenance of certification (MOC), financial and professional return on investment (ROI), and educational policy consequences of mastery learning.
7. Identify and discuss mastery learning research opportunities in health professions education in terms of theory, measurement, and program evaluation. This research should address its limitations and how to make the science stronger.

The scope of *Comprehensive Healthcare Simulation: Mastery Learning in Health Professions Education* reflects its seven specific aims. The book is organized as five sections, each containing from one to eight chapters. The five sections are *Clinical Education in the Health Professions*, *The Mastery Learning Model*, *Mastery Learning in Action*, *Transfer of Training from Mastery Learning*, and *The Road Ahead*. The book is structured to move from a critique of current practices used to educate and evaluate health professionals to a detailed description of the mastery learning model; a steady stream of practical ideas and examples of mastery learning at work in health professions education, extending the learner assessment endpoint from classroom and laboratory settings to the bedside and clinic; and finally new opportunities for mastery learning education and research in the health professions.

Planning and writing this book also achieved three aims unique to the Northwestern University Feinberg School of Medicine simulation education and research team. The first aim was to produce a practical yet scholarly book that is the seminal source of information about mastery learning in health professions education. The second aim addresses Northwestern faculty development. This meant providing our faculty, especially at junior ranks, opportunities to coauthor book chapters as a means of scholarly learning and expression. The editors are mentors in service of this aim. The third aim was to document the Northwestern simulation and education research team's impact as the founder, seat of inspiration, and source of dissemination of simulation-based mastery learning to other institutions, health professions, and countries.

Several unexpected collateral effects became clear to the Northwestern team as a consequence of writing *Comprehensive Healthcare Simulation: Mastery Learning in Health Professions Education*. First, the book project strengthened our ties as a professional team. Social psychological challenges from managing such a large team scholarly enterprise can be daunting, yet this was an enjoyable endeavor with lasting benefits. Second, engaging in the book project made the team more thoughtful, better writers. Ericsson and Pool explain from their experience writing *Peak: Secrets from the New Science of Expertise* [2]. "There was a steady interplay between the writing of the book and our conceptualization of the topic, and as we looked for ways to make our message clearer to the reader, we would come up with new ways to think about [the topic] ourselves. Researchers refer to this sort of writing as 'knowledge transforming,' as opposed to 'knowledge telling,' because the process of writing changes and adds to the knowledge that the writer had when starting out."

We anticipate that this book will be a valued educational resource for teachers and curriculum developers throughout the health professions worldwide. We also hope that publication of this book will inspire health professions education scholars to study mastery learning—applications, features, timing, measures, impact—to advance the technology, improve education for the learners we are privileged to serve, and enhance healthcare for individual patients and the public. No doubt subsequent editions of this book will amplify its current content and methods with new and better thinking and novel applications of mastery learning principles across the health professions.

Special acknowledgments are warranted due to the contributions to this book made by groups and key individuals. We recognize our patients who shape and drive the meaning of what we do. We are indebted to our students at all levels and participants in Northwestern University mastery learning courses and programs for the privilege to serve their needs and interests. We are indebted to Barry Issenberg and Matthew Lineberry for their critical comments about early chapter drafts. We especially thank Desmond G. Fenty for his organizational, clerical, and database wizardry at keeping the book project on track and Laura Seul for her excellence at preparing graphics and images.

Chicago, IL, USA William C. McGaghie
Chicago, IL, USA Jeffrey H. Barsuk
Chicago, IL, USA Diane B. Wayne

References

1. Bloom SW. Structure and ideology in medical education: an analysis of resistance to change. J Health Soc Behav. 1988;29(4):294–306.
2. Ericsson A, Pool R. Peak: secrets from the new science of expertise. Boston: Houghton, Mifflin, Harcourt; 2016.

Contents

Author Biography

Mark Adler, MD is a professor in the Departments of Pediatrics and Medical Education at Northwestern University Feinberg School of Medicine in Chicago. He is Founder and Director of the kidSTAR Medical Educational Program and is a pediatric emergency medicine physician at the Ann & Robert H. Lurie Children's Hospital of Chicago. He has developed and implemented numerous simulation-based medical education programs and programs of assessment. He has published more than 40 peer-reviewed articles and book chapters in the field of medical education. In 2018, he became a Fellow in the Society for Simulation in Healthcare Academy. Dr. Adler also serves as a member of the Board of the International Network for Simulation-Based Pediatric Innovation, Research, and Education.

Katherine A. Barsness, MD, MS is an associate professor in the Departments of Surgery and Medical Education at Northwestern University Feinberg School of Medicine in Chicago. She is a pediatric surgeon at the Ann & Robert H. Lurie Children's Hospital of Chicago, where she is also Director of the Pediatric Surgery Fellowship Training Program. She has devoted her career to surgical education and is a nationally and internationally recognized leader in training pediatric surgeons to master advanced minimally invasive skills for neonatal operations. She is also an inventor of 3-D printed models for neonatal surgery, which are recognized as the gold standard of educational tools for pediatric minimally invasive surgical skill acquisition.

Jeffrey H. Barsuk, MD, MS is a professor in the Departments of Medicine and Medical Education at Northwestern University Feinberg School of Medicine in Chicago. He completed a residency in Internal Medicine at the McGaw Medical Center of Northwestern University. He also completed a Master of Science degree in Clinical Investigation and a certificate program in Healthcare Quality and Patient Safety. Dr. Barsuk currently serves as a key clinical faculty member in the Internal Medicine Residency Program and the Medical Director of Northwestern Simulation. His research is focused on how simulation-based mastery learning can improve healthcare quality and safety while providing return on investment.

Sidney A. Barsuk, MBA received a Master of Business Administration degree in 1971 from Rochester Institute of Technology. He is a seasoned executive who spent over 25 years in hospital senior management. Mr. Barsuk has built and trained multiple boards and committees and has worked closely with corporate CEOs and political leaders at the national, state, and local levels. He taught organizational behavior focusing on change management at Northwestern University.

Kenzie A. Cameron, PhD, MPH, FACH is a research professor in the Departments of Medicine, Medical Education, Medical Social Sciences, and Preventive Medicine at Northwestern University Feinberg School of Medicine in Chicago. She has authored over 100 peer-reviewed publications and served as principal investigator, co-investigator, or mentor on over 45 funded grants and contracts ranging from improving colorectal cancer screening to promoting safe opioid use to simulation-based mastery learning. In 2016, she was named a Fellow of the Academy on Communication in Healthcare and was awarded the Feinberg School of Medicine 2016 Mentor of the Year Award.

Elaine R. Cohen, MEd is a research associate in the Department of Medicine at Northwestern University Feinberg School of Medicine in Chicago. She earned a Bachelor of Arts degree in Sociology from the University of Wisconsin-Madison and a Master of Education degree in *Measurement, Evaluation, Statistics, and Assessment* from the University of Illinois at Chicago. Her research interests include medical education, simulation, and competency assessment.

Aashish K. Didwania, MD is the Vice Chair for Education in the Department of Medicine, an associate professor in the Departments of Medicine and Medical Education, and Director of the Internal Medicine Residency Program at Northwestern University Feinberg School of Medicine in Chicago. He graduated from the University of Michigan Medical School in 2002, completed an Internal Medicine residency at the McGaw Medical Center of Northwestern University, and served as a chief medical resident. Dr. Didwania joined the Northwestern University Feinberg School of Medicine Division of General Internal Medicine and continues to serve as a primary care physician. In addition to serving as clinician, teacher, and administrator, Dr. Didwania has pursued research activities in simulation-based medical education, professionalism, and healthcare quality and safety.

Brigid M. Dolan, MD, MEd is an associate professor in the Departments of Medicine and Medical Education and Director of Workplace-Based Assessment for Undergraduate Medical Education at Northwestern University Feinberg School of Medicine in Chicago. She received a medical degree from the University of Pittsburgh and completed residency training at Brigham and Women's Hospital. In addition to her role in undergraduate medical education, she also serves as Director of the Internal Medicine Residency women's health track. She has published on medical education assessment and innovations in women's healthcare and training.

Walter J. Eppich, MD, PhD is an associate professor in the Departments of Pediatrics and Medical Education at Northwestern University Feinberg School of Medicine in Chicago. He practices pediatric emergency medicine at the Ann & Robert H. Lurie Children's Hospital of Chicago and is Director of the Northwestern University Feinberg Academy of Medical Educators. In 2018, he completed a PhD in Medical Education at Maastricht University in the Netherlands. Dr. Eppich speaks internationally about simulation, feedback, and debriefing. In 2017, he became an Inaugural Fellow in the Society for Simulation in Healthcare Academy. His research uses qualitative methodologies to study how talk within teams influences learning and performance in both simulated and clinical workplace settings.

Joe Feinglass, PhD is a research professor in the Departments of Medicine and Preventive Medicine at Northwestern University Feinberg School of Medicine in Chicago. He is a health services researcher with a degree in Public Policy Analysis. He has over 25 years of experience in health policy, medical education, quality improvement, health disparities, medical informatics, patient safety, and social epidemiology research and has co-authored more than 200 peer-reviewed publications.

Joshua L. Goldstein, MD is Associate Dean for Graduate Medical Education (GME), Designated Institutional Officer for the McGaw Medical Center of Northwestern University, and an associate professor in the Departments of Pediatrics, Medical Education, and Neurology at Northwestern University Feinberg School of Medicine in Chicago. His areas of scholarly interest include GME oversight and training. Clinically, he is a child neurologist specializing in neurocritical care and ICU EEG monitoring. His specific areas of clinical focus include the use of EEG in cases of non-accidental head injury, cardiac arrest, refractory status, and acute liver failure.

Marianne M. Green, MD is Senior Associate Dean for Medical Education, the Raymond H. Curry, MD, Professor of Medical Education, and a professor in the Departments of Medicine and Medical Education at Northwestern University Feinberg School of Medicine in Chicago. Her academic work has focused on the assessment of competence, with a specific interest in portfolio-based learning and assessment in competency-based medical education. She has held various leadership roles at the American Board of Internal Medicine (ABIM) and was recently named chair of the AIBM Board of Directors.

Heather L. Heiman, MD was Medical Director of the Clinical Education Center and was an associate professor in the Departments of Medicine and Medical Education at Northwestern University Feinberg School of Medicine in Chicago. She received a medical degree from Harvard Medical School and completed residency training at Brigham and Women's Hospital. Dr. Heiman is currently Associate Dean for Medical Education at the University of Illinois College of Medicine at Chicago.

Eric S. Holmboe, MD is Chief Research, Milestones Development, and Evaluation Officer at the Accreditation Council for Graduate Medical Education (ACGME). He is an adjunct professor in the Department of Medical Education at Northwestern University Feinberg School of Medicine in Chicago, and an adjunct professor at the Yale University School of Medicine and the Uniformed Services University of the Health Sciences. He is a graduate of Franklin and Marshall College and the University of Rochester School of Medicine. He completed an internal medicine residency and chief residency at Yale New Haven Hospital and was a Robert Wood Johnson Clinical Scholar at Yale University.

Eric S. Hungness, MD is a professor in the Departments of Surgery and Medical Education at Northwestern University Feinberg School of Medicine in Chicago and the S. David Stulberg professor of Advanced Surgical Education. His clinical interest in minimally invasive gastrointestinal surgery includes one of the highest volume clinical experiences worldwide in peroral esophageal myotomy for the treatment of achalasia. He is also the Surgical Director of Northwestern Simulation, focusing on the use of simulation-based mastery learning in the acquisition of minimally invasive surgical skills.

Nabil Issa, MD, MHPE is an associate professor in the Departments of Surgery and Medical Education at Northwestern University Feinberg School of Medicine in Chicago. He completed a medical degree from Almustansiriyah University College of Medicine in Baghdad, Iraq; surgical training at Cleveland Clinic Fairview Hospital; and a fellowship in Surgical Critical Care at the University of Michigan. He also completed a Master of Health Professions Education degree from the University of Illinois at Chicago. Dr. Issa is a trauma and critical care surgeon at Northwestern and is actively involved in the education of students, residents, and fellows. He is well published in educational research including curriculum development, learner assessment, and multimedia education.

William C. McGaghie, PhD is a professor in the Departments of Medical Education and Preventive Medicine at Northwestern University Feinberg School of Medicine in Chicago. He has been engaged in medical and health professions education research and scholarship for 45 years. He has authored or edited ten books, hundreds of journal articles and textbook chapters and is a frequent invited lecturer at medical schools in the United States and worldwide. In 2017, Dr. McGaghie became a Inaugural Fellow in the Society for Simulation in Healthcare Academy. He received the 2019 John P. Hubbard Award for excellence in medical education evaluation from the National Board of Medical Examiners.

Graham T. McMahon, MD, MMSc is the President and Chief Executive Officer of the Accreditation Council for Continuing Medical Education (ACCME®) and adjunct professor in the Departments of Medical Education and Medicine at Northwestern University Feinberg School of Medicine in Chicago. The ACCME assures and advances quality learning for healthcare professionals that drives improvements in patient care. He leads efforts to strengthen the role of accredited CME as a strategic resource to public health initiatives on the national and international level.

Debi L. Mitra, MD is an assistant professor in the Department of Medicine at Northwestern University Feinberg School of Medicine in Chicago. She is a practicing hospitalist who specializes in the inpatient care of oncology patients. She also serves as Co-Director of Simulation for the Internal Medicine Residency Program at Northwestern and leads procedural and team simulation training for residents. Her academic interests include mastery learning, teamwork, and communication.

Celia Laird O'Brien, PhD is an assistant professor in the Department of Medical Education and Director of Assessment and Program Evaluation in the Augusta Webster, MD, Office of Medical Education at Northwestern University Feinberg School of Medicine in Chicago. She completed a doctorate in Higher Education at the University of Arizona. Her research and most recent publications focus on student assessment, competency-based medical education, and related issues in the undergraduate medical education environment. At Northwestern, she is responsible for medical student assessment systems and evaluation of curricular outcomes.

David H. Salzman, MD, MEd is an associate professor in the Departments of Emergeny Medicine and Medical Education at Northwestern University Feinberg School of Medicine in Chicago and is Assistant Director of the Emergency Medicine Residency Program, Director of the Emergency Medicine Education Fellowship Program, and Director of Simulation for Undergraduate Medical Education at Northwestern. He is a graduate of Northwestern University Feinberg School of Medicine, where he also completed emergency medicine residency training. Following residency, Dr. Salzman completed a medical education and simulation fellowship at Northwestern University while concurrently obtaining a Master of Education degree from the University of Cincinnati. His research focuses on integration of simulation-based education into larger curricula, use of simulation-based mastery learning, and entrustable professional activities for medical students.

Clara Schroedl, MD, MS is an assistant professor in the Departments of Medicine and Medical Education and Medical Director of the Office of Continuing Medical Education at Northwestern University Feinberg School of Medicine in Chicago. She is also Associate Program Director of the Pulmonary and Critical Care Fellowship Program at Northwestern University. She is a member of the Accreditation Council for Continuing Medical Education's Accreditation Review Committee and serves as the Continuous Professional Development section chair for the central region of the Association of American Medical Colleges (AAMC) Group on Education Affairs. Her research interests include simulation-based mastery learning for trainees and advance practice providers in the intensive care unit.

Nahzinine Shakeri, MD is an assistant professor in the Department of Emergency Medicine at the Northwestern University Feinberg School of Medicine in Chicago and Assistant Program Director of the Emergency Medicine Residency Program at Northwestern. She completed a Medical Education Scholarship Fellowship at Northwestern University which focused on simulation, competency-based medical education, and medical education research. Her research uses simulation-based mastery learning to teach emergency medicine residents communication skills.

Ezra N. Teitelbaum, MD, MEd is an assistant professor in the Department of Surgery at Northwestern University Feinberg School of Medicine in Chicago and Associate Program Director of the General Surgery Residency Program at Northwestern. His clinical interests are minimally invasive foregut, bariatric and general surgery, and surgical endoscopy. His research interests include esophageal physiology and surgical education, with a focus on simulation-based mastery learning curricula and the use of operative video review in resident training.

Jennifer Trainor, MD is a professor in the Departments of Pediatrics and Medical Education at Northwestern University Feinberg School of Medicine in Chicago and Associate Chair for Education in the Department of Pediatrics at Ann & Robert H. Lurie Children's Hospital of Chicago. Her clinical background and board certification are in Pediatrics and Pediatric Emergency Medicine. Her primary academic interests involve the use of simulation to teach medical students, residents, and fellows clinical pediatrics and pediatric emergency medicine. She has a particular interest in interprofessional communication, residency preparation, and career mentoring.

Erin D. Unger, MD is an interventional cardiology fellow in the Department of Medicine at the McGaw Medical Center of Northwestern University. She earned a medical degree and completed her Internal Medicine residency training at Northwestern University where she was selected to serve as a chief medical resident. Her research interests include curriculum development, medical education, simulation, and point-of-care cardiac ultrasound.

Julia H. Vermylen, MD, MPH is an assistant professor in the Departments of Medicine and Medical Education at Northwestern University Feinberg School of Medicine in Chicago. Her academic work centers on educational research surrounding communication skills training for undergraduate and graduate medicine trainees and practicing clinicians. She has a particular focus applying concepts of mastery learning to improve outcomes for communication skills training. She attended medical school, completed a master's degree in Public Health, and completed both a residency in Internal Medicine and fellowship training in Palliative Medicine at the McGaw Medical Center of Northwestern University.

Diane B. Wayne, MD is Vice Dean for Education, Chair of the Department of Medical Education, and the Dr. John Sherman Appleman Professor of Medicine and Medical Education at Northwestern University Feinberg School of Medicine in Chicago. She is a graduate of Northwestern University Feinberg School of Medicine and is board-certified in internal medicine. In her professional career, Dr. Wayne has held many leadership roles at Northwestern's medical school and health system and has received multiple professional awards including the Teacher of the Year Award in the Department of Medicine and the Mentor of the Year Award at the Feinberg School of Medicine.

Gordon J. Wood, MD, MSCI, FAAHPM is an associate professor in the Departments of Medicine and Medical Education at Northwestern University Feinberg School of Medicine in Chicago. He is Associate Director of the Palliative Medicine Fellowship Program and serves as Associate Director of the Education in Palliative and End-of-Life Care Program at Northwestern. His academic work centers on communication skills, including the application of mastery learning principles to communication skills training. He attended medical school at the University of Chicago and finished an internal medicine residency at the University of California, San Francisco. He completed a palliative medicine fellowship and obtained a Master of Science in Clinical Investigation at Northwestern University.

Contributors

Mark Adler, MD Northwestern University Feinberg School of Medicine, Departments of Pediatrics and Medical Education, Chicago, IL, USA

Katherine A. Barsness, MD, MS Northwestern University Feinberg School of Medicine, Departments of Surgery and Medical Education, Chicago, IL, USA

Jeffrey H. Barsuk, MD, MS Northwestern University Feinberg School of Medicine, Departments of Medicine and Medical Education, Chicago, IL, USA

Sidney A. Barsuk, BS, MBA Northwestern University School of Professional Studies (retired), Chicago, IL, USA

Kenzie A. Cameron, PhD, MPH Northwestern University Feinberg School of Medicine, Departments of Medicine, Medical Education, Medical Social Sciences, and Preventive Medicine, Chicago, IL, USA

Elaine R. Cohen, MEd Northwestern University Feinberg School of Medicine, Department of Medicine, Chicago, IL, USA

Aashish K. Didwania, MD Northwestern University Feinberg School of Medicine, Departments of Medicine and Medical Education, Chicago, IL, USA

Brigid M. Dolan, MD, MEd Northwestern University Feinberg School of Medicine, Departments of Medicine and Medical Education, Chicago, IL, USA

Walter J. Eppich, MD, PhD Northwestern University Feinberg School of Medicine, Departments of Pediatrics and Medical Education, Chicago, IL, USA

Joe Feinglass, PhD Northwestern University Feinberg School of Medicine, Departments of Medicine and Preventive Medicine, Chicago, IL, USA

Joshua L. Goldstein, MD Northwestern University Feinberg School of Medicine, Departments of Pediatrics, Medical Education, and Neurology, Chicago, IL, USA

Marianne M. Green, MD Northwestern University Feinberg School of Medicine, Departments of Medicine and Medical Education, Chicago, IL, USA

Heather L. Heiman, MD Northwestern University Feinberg School of Medicine, Departments of Medicine and Medical Education, Chicago, IL, USA

Eric S. Holmboe, MD Accreditation Council for Graduate Medical Education, Chief Research, Milestone Development, and Evaluation Officer, Department of Milestones, Chicago, IL, USA

Northwestern University Feinberg School of Medicine, Adjunct Professor of Medical Education, Chicago, IL, USA

Eric S. Hungness, MD Northwestern University Feinberg School of Medicine, Departments of Surgery and Medical Education, Chicago, IL, USA

Nabil Issa, MD, MHPE Northwestern University Feinberg School of Medicine, Departments of Surgery and Medical Education, Chicago, IL, USA

William C. McGaghie, PhD Northwestern University Feinberg School of Medicine, Departments of Medical Education and Preventive Medicine, Chicago, IL, USA

Graham T. McMahon, MD, MMSc Accreditation Council for Continuing Medical Education, President and CEO, Chicago, IL, USA

Northwestern University Feinberg School of Medicine, Adjunct Professor, Departments of Medical Education and Medicine, Chicago, IL, USA

Debi L. Mitra, MD Northwestern University Feinberg School of Medicine, Department of Medicine, Chicago, IL, USA

Celia Laird O'Brien, PhD Northwestern University Feinberg School of Medicine, Department of Medical Education, Chicago, IL, USA

David H. Salzman, MD, MEd Northwestern University Feinberg School of Medicine, Departments of Emergency Medicine and Medical Education, Chicago, IL, USA

Clara Schroedl, MD, MS Northwestern University Feinberg School of Medicine, Departments of Medicine and Medical Education, Chicago, IL, USA

Nahzinine Shakeri, MD Northwestern University Feinberg School of Medicine, Department of Emergency Medicine, Chicago, IL, USA

Ezra N. Teitelbaum, MD, MEd Northwestern University Feinberg School of Medicine, Department of Surgery, Chicago, IL, USA

Jennifer Trainor, MD Northwestern University Feinberg School of Medicine, Departments of Pediatrics and Medical Education, Chicago, IL, USA

Erin D. Unger, MD Northwestern University Feinberg School of Medicine, Department of Medicine, Chicago, IL, USA

Julia H. Vermylen, MD, MPH Northwestern University Feinberg School of Medicine, Departments of Medicine and Medical Education, Chicago, IL, USA

Diane B. Wayne, MD Northwestern University Feinberg School of Medicine, Departments of Medicine and Medical Education, Chicago, IL, USA

Gordon J. Wood, MD, MSCI Northwestern University Feinberg School of Medicine, Departments of Medicine and Medical Education, Chicago, IL, USA

Part I

Clinical Education in the Health Professions

Clinical Education: Origins and Outcomes

1

William C. McGaghie, Jeffrey H. Barsuk, and Diane B. Wayne

What does the American public expect when accessing the healthcare system? While expectations vary between individuals, most Americans expect to receive high-quality medical care from well-trained physicians and other members of the healthcare team. US medical schools graduate nearly 19,000 students each year (https://www.aamc.org/download/321532/data/factstableb2-2pdf) and certify them fit for graduate medical education (GME) in core residency programs such as internal medicine, general surgery, neurology, and pediatrics. US nurse education programs produce over 105,000 graduates at the basic RN level annually (http://www.nln.org.newsroom/nursing-education-statistics/graduations-from-rn-programs). Can we say with confidence that all of these health professionals are ready to make the transition to graduate education or practice and provide skilled healthcare to their patients? Unfortunately, the answer is no. During a 15-year journey, our research group has rigorously assessed common clinical skills of hundreds of physicians-in-training and their supervisors. Despite receiving diplomas from prestigious medical schools and often having much clinical experience, we have consistently found weak performance of core clinical skills such as bedside procedures and patient and family communication. This book recounts our journey to understand the issues surrounding the development of health professions expertise and to develop a path forward that ensures that health professions graduates are competent to care for patients.

Medical education research data can tell a powerful story about the problem we aim to solve and the solution we propose—mastery learning. Figure 1.1 presents

W. C. McGaghie (✉)
Northwestern University Feinberg School of Medicine, Departments of Medical Education and Preventive Medicine, Chicago, IL, USA
e-mail: wcmc@northwestern.edu

J. H. Barsuk · D. B. Wayne
Northwestern University Feinberg School of Medicine, Departments of Medicine and Medical Education, Chicago, IL, USA
e-mail: dwayne@northwestern.edu

W. C. McGaghie et al. (eds.), *Comprehensive Healthcare Simulation: Mastery Learning in Health Professions Education*, Comprehensive Healthcare Simulation, https://doi.org/10.1007/978-3-030-34811-3_1

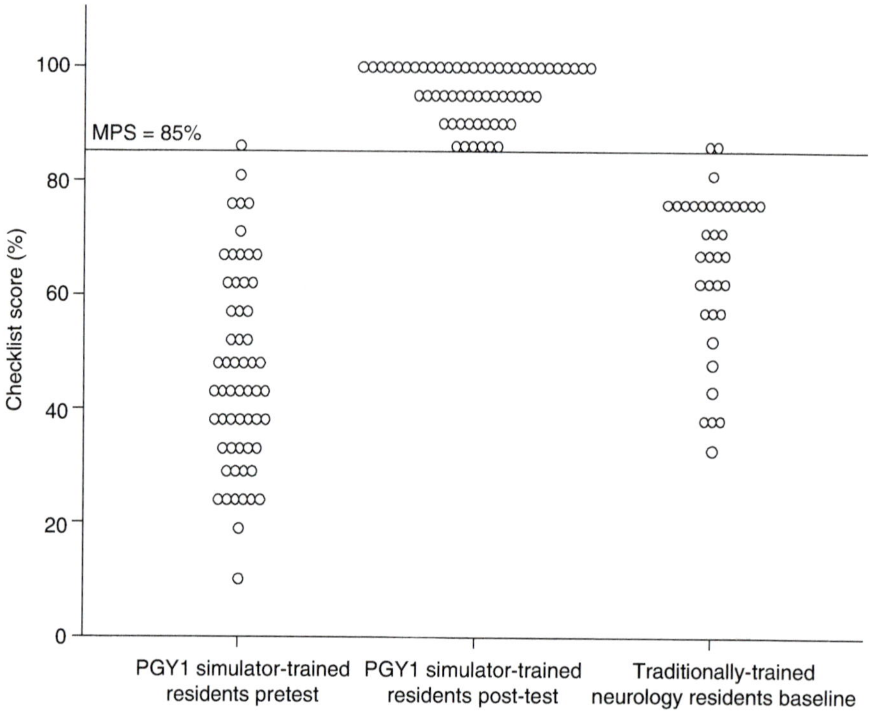

Fig. 1.1 Clinical skills examination (checklist) pre- and final posttest performance of 58 first-year simulator-trained internal medicine residents and baseline performance of 36 traditionally trained neurology residents. Three internal medicine residents failed to meet the minimum passing score (MPS) at initial posttesting. PGY = postgraduate year. (Source: Barsuk et al. [1]. Reprinted with permission of Wolters Kluwer Health)

data from a mastery learning skill acquisition study involving 58 internal medicine (IM) residents and 36 neurology residents learning to perform lumbar puncture (LP) [1]. Lumbar punctures are bedside procedures performed by medical professionals to obtain cerebrospinal fluid (CSF) and evaluate patients for central nervous system conditions such as life-threatening infections or spread of cancerous tumors. The IM residents were all in the first postgraduate year (PGY-1) of training at the McGaw Medical Center of Northwestern University in Chicago after earning MD degrees from medical schools across the United States. The neurology residents were PGY-2, PGY-3, and PGY-4 volunteers for this cohort study drawn from three other academic medical centers in metropolitan Chicago. All of the neurology residents had experience with the LP procedure that they learned using traditional, learn-by-doing, bedside methods practicing on real patients.

The IM residents had little or no LP experience. The IM residents started LP learning with a pretest on a mannequin using a 21-item LP skills checklist. The IM residents then experienced a systematic LP mastery learning skill acquisition curriculum involving feedback about pretest performance, deliberate practice (DP) of LP skills, formative assessments, frequent actionable feedback, and coaching and more practice for at least 3 hours in a simulation laboratory. The IM residents were assessed to see if they met or surpassed a minimum passing standard (MPS) on the skills checklist set earlier by an expert panel. Posttest scores (after training completion) from the PGY-1 IM residents were compared to scores of the neurology residents.

The research report shows that one of the 58 IM residents met the MPS at pretest and 55 of the 58 (95%) met the MPS at posttest after the 3-hour simulation-based curriculum. The three IM residents who did not reach the MPS at immediate posttest later reached the goal with less than 1 hour of more practice. This is a 107% improvement from pretest to posttest measured as LP checklist performance by the IM residents.

Figure 1.1 also shows that by contrast, only 2 of 36 (6%) of the traditionally trained PGY-2, PGY-3, and PGY-4 neurology residents met the MPS despite years of experience and performing multiple LPs on real patients. This study also revealed two surprising findings about the traditionally trained neurology residents not shown in Fig. 1.1. First, nearly 50% of the PGY-2, PGY-3, and PGY-4 neurology residents could not report the correct anatomical location for the procedure. They did not know where to stick the needle. Second, over 40% of the neurology residents could not list routine tests (glucose, cell count, protein, Gram stain, culture) to be ordered for the CSF after the fluid sample was drawn. They did not know about basic laboratory medicine.

Publication of the educational findings from this cohort study in the journal *Neurology* prompted a strong statement from a journal editorial which stated that these findings were a clear "wake-up call" regarding traditional methods of medical education and questioned whether these methods are "enough to ensure the best education, and thus the best care for patients" [2].

This research example is one short chapter in a long story about today's approaches to clinical education in the health professions. As the LP example illustrates, traditional clinical health professions education grounded in clinical experience produces uneven results that do not meet the expectations of the profession or the public. Other examples address the now well-known finding that clinical experience alone—expressed as either years of medical practice or number of performed clinical procedures—is not a proxy for medical competence [3, 4].

A recent report from the National Academies of Science, Engineering, and Medicine titled, *Improving Diagnosis in Health Care* [5], demonstrates that traditional experiential health professions education produces many clinicians with variable diagnostic acuity. The report makes recommendations about improving diagnostic education for healthcare providers and also identifies a number of areas of performance that could be improved including:

- Clinical reasoning
- Teamwork
- Communication with patients, their families, and other healthcare professionals
- Appropriate use of diagnostic tests and the application of these results on subsequent decision making
- Use of health information technology

These areas of performance improvement make up the majority of the daily tasks done by healthcare providers in clinical practice.

The idea of "excellence for all," a foundation principle of mastery learning, is a far cry from the expectations and measured outcomes that are now achieved in most settings of health professions education. Student nurses, physicians, pharmacists, occupational therapists, and many other health professions advance through clinical education programs where training time is fixed and learning outcomes vary widely. This is despite ambitious goals to educate students, residents, and fellows to deliver uniformly safe and effective healthcare under supervision and when working autonomously as individuals and teams.

The times are changing in health professions education. Awareness is growing that traditional, experienced-based models of clinical education are antiquated and ineffective [6, 7]. There are at least three reasons for this awakening. First, technological advances in the biomedical, engineering, and behavioral sciences are growing exponentially every year. New education models are needed to realistically prepare clinicians for the future of the professions [8]. Second, there is a growing emphasis across the health professions on using rigorously measured learning outcomes as benchmarks for student curriculum progress. The nursing profession is moving toward outcomes and competencies as education targets for graduates at several levels [9]. Undergraduate medical education is now focused on *Core Entrustable Professional Activities [EPAs] for Entering Residency* as a set of minimum outcome expectations [10]. Analogous "milestones" for graduate medical education aim to bring greater uniformity to specialty curricula and rigor to educational outcome measurement [11, 12]. These innovations are a big step toward improved accountability in health professions education which has been diffuse or lacking historically. Third, health professions education has become increasingly reliant on simulation technology with deliberate practice as a method of instruction and a platform for research [13, 14]. This is due to a growing body of evidence that simulation is superior to traditional clinical education on grounds of effectiveness [15], cost [16] (Chap. 19), and patient safety [17] (Chap. 16).

This opening chapter has three sections. The first section traces the historical origins of clinical medical education from antiquity through the middle ages to the early twentieth century. Other health professions such as dentistry, nursing, midwifery, and pharmacy emerged during that time. The new health professions expanded, matured, and experienced educational evolutions similar to medicine. The second section describes the current state-of-affairs in clinical health professions education starting with its origins in Sir William Osler's ideas about the *natural method of teaching* (i.e., experiential learning). The section proceeds to address problems with the status quo in clinical education including (a) uneven educational opportunities, (b) lack of rigorous learner evaluation and feedback, and (c) poor clinical practice outcomes. The third chapter section presents a call to action and advances new directions for clinical education in the health professions.

Historical Origins of Clinical Education

The history of clinical education in medicine has been traced from antiquity to the middle ages in the writings of Theodor Puschmann [18] and other scholars such as Henry Sigerist [19, 20]. These authors teach that clinical medicine in the ancient world in such places as Egypt, Mesopotamia, and India was taught using an apprenticeship model. Boys in early adolescence were selected and trained to be physicians often due to family tradition and primogeniture. The advent of European universities in the fourteenth- and fifteenth-century Berlin, London, Padua, Paris, Prague, Zurich, and other cities began to embed medical education in academic settings yet still relied on the apprenticeship for clinical training. Learning by doing was the medical education principle at that time despite the absence of a scientific foundation for medical practice.

The modern era of clinical medical education in North America and Western Europe has been chronicled by Kenneth Ludmerer [21, 22] and many other writers including James Cassedy [23], Paul Starr [24], and Molly Cooke and colleagues [25]. This historical scholarship addresses medical education events and trends from the mid-nineteenth century, including the US War between the States, to the early twentieth century. This work speaks to medical curricula and student evaluation acknowledging the primitive technologies that were available, judged by today's standards. Historical medical education scholarship by Molly Cooke and colleagues [25] also attributes the importance of the Flexner Report [26], *Medical Education in the United States and Canada*, as a turning point to improve medical education standards by grounding professional education in university settings, enforcing rigorous admissions standards, emphasizing clinical science, and weeding out fly-by-night proprietary medical schools. By contrast, medical sociologist Paul Starr [24] downplays the watershed status of the Flexner Report. Starr argues that economic conditions, state licensing requirements, and other secular trends before and after publication of the Flexner report were the real reasons for medical education reform in the early twentieth century.

Similar historical conditions in clinical care and education were underway for other healthcare professions including nursing [9], dentistry [27], pharmacy [28], and physical therapy [29]. In the early twentieth century, all US healthcare professions were afloat on the same river—after classroom and laboratory instruction in the basic health sciences, clinical education was wholly experiential and based on chance encounters. At that time, little or nothing was said or known about novel clinical education technologies including systematic curriculum planning, formative and summative assessment, psychometric testing, problem-based learning (PBL), objective structured clinical examinations (OSCEs), standardized patients (SPs), simulation-based exercises, and DP that are now in widespread use.

Current State-of-Affairs in Clinical Education

The clinical education legacy of physician Sir William Osler and his Johns Hopkins School of Medicine colleagues has been described in detail elsewhere [6, 7]. In brief, Osler expressed his ideas about the best approach to clinical education for US doctors in a 1903 address to the New York Academy of Medicine titled, "The hospital as a college." The talk was published later in *Aequanimitas* [30], a collection of his essays. Osler's ideas about clinical education were shaped by his prior experience in Europe where he considered medical education to be far more advanced. Osler writes, "The radical reform needed is in the introduction into this country of the system of clinical clerks…." He continues, "In what may be called the *natural method of teaching* the student begins with the patient, continues with the patient, and ends his studies with the patient [emphasis added]. Teach him how to observe, give him plenty of facts to observe, and the lessons will come out of the facts themselves" [30].

William Halsted, a Johns Hopkins surgeon colleague, echoed Osler's principles in a 1904 essay, "The training of the surgeon" [31]. Osler and Halsted argued that the clinical medical curriculum is embodied in patients. Medical historian Kenneth Ludmerer elaborates this position, "… house officers admitted patients by what might be termed the 'laissez faire method of learning.' Interns and residents received patients randomly … Medical educators presumed that, over time, on a large and active teaching service, house officers would be exposed to a sufficient volume and variety of patients to emerge as experienced clinicians" [22].

Drs. Osler and Halsted were considered visionary medical educators in their day. However, the clinical education model they championed is chiefly passive, active only in the sense that students encountered many patients. The Osler model has no place for today's science of learning or science of instruction: structured, graded educational requirements; deliberate skills practice; objective formative and summative assessment with feedback; multimedia learning; accountability; and supervised reflection for novice doctors to master their craft [6, 7, 32, 33]. The Osler clinical curriculum tradition dominated twentieth-century medical education and continues into the twenty-first century.

The nineteenth-century model of clinical medical education is seen in 2020 as undergraduate clinical clerkships, postgraduate medical residency rotations, and subspecialty medical and nursing fellowships. Clinical learners participate in patient care without adequate supervision and with random clinical experiences as they advance in the curriculum. Clinical learners rarely receive feedback. Educational experiences are structured by time (days, weeks, or months) and location (clinical sites) [34]. Because of the reliance on this time-based model, learners are rarely engaged in planned and rigorous educational activities that address measured learning outcomes. There are few tests that really matter beyond multiple-choice licensure and specialty board examinations. Structural and operational expressions of Osler's *natural method of teaching* are seen every day at medical schools, nursing schools, and residency and fellowship programs where traditional, "time-honored" educational practices like morning report (daily group discussions about a select patient's diagnosis and treatment) and professor rounds (informal rounds where a senior clinician sees "interesting" patients with a group of residents and medical students) are routine, sustained, and valued. Foundation courses in nursing education fulfill a similar role. Yet these clinical education experiences designed over a century ago now operate in a complex healthcare environment where health professions education is often subordinate to patient care needs and financial incentives.

Osler's *natural method of teaching* has been in place for over a century in clinical education among the health professions. The model worked well in the early twentieth century, especially at prestigious medical and health professions schools where patients were hospitalized for extended lengths of stay, medical and educational technology were very simple, and the faculty focus was solely on patient care and clinical service. However, the Osler model has limited utility today due to many competing clinical priorities, financial disincentives, and at least three educational flaws: (a) uneven educational opportunities, (b) lack of rigorous learner evaluation and feedback, and (c) poor clinical practice outcomes.

Uneven Educational Opportunities

Experiential medical education, a synonym for Osler's *natural method of teaching* [30] and Ludmerer's [22] *laissez faire method of learning*, is not a good way to structure and manage a medical student's or resident's educational agenda. On grounds of educational experience alone, student exposure to patient problems needs to be broad, deep, and engaging. It needs to be controlled, with evaluation and feedback, not left to chance.

A telling example of uneven educational opportunities is a surgical education study reported by Richard Bell and colleagues [35] that documented the operative experience of residents in US general surgery residency education programs. Surgery residency program directors graded 300 operative procedures A, B, or C using these criteria: A, graduating general surgery residents should be competent to perform the procedure independently; B, graduating residents should be familiar with the procedure, but not necessarily competent to perform it; and C, graduating residents neither need to be familiar with nor competent to perform the procedure. The actual operative experience of all US residents completing general surgery training in June 2005 was compiled, reviewed, and compared with the three procedural criteria.

The study results enlighten, inform, and address Osler's *natural method of teaching* directly. Bell et al. [35] report:

> One hundred twenty-one of the 300 operations were considered A level procedures by a majority of program directors (PDs). Graduating 2005 US residents (n = 1022) performed only 18 of the 121 A procedures, an average of more than 10 times during residency; 83 of the 121 procedures were performed on average less than 5 times and 31 procedures less than once. For 63 of the 121 procedures, the mode (most commonly reported) experience level was 0. In addition, there was significant variation between residents in operative experience for specific procedures.

The investigators conclude:

> Methods will have to be developed to allow surgeons to reach a basic level of competence in procedures which they are likely to experience only rarely during residency. Even for more commonly performed procedures, the numbers of repetitions are not very robust, stressing the need to determine objectively whether residents are actually achieving basic competency in these operations.

These findings are reinforced by a nearly identical follow-up study published 4 years later by Malangoni and colleagues [36] that documented an increase in total operations performed by surgical residents. However, the operative logs of graduating surgery residents still showed a wide and uneven variation in practical experience with clinical cases. Many essential surgical procedures were neither performed nor practiced during residency education. This is strong evidence that Osler's *natural method of teaching*, grounded solely in patient care experience, is insufficient to ensure the procedural competence of new surgeons. The authors conclude "…alternate methods for teaching infrequently performed procedures are needed" [36].

The Bell et al. [35] and Malangoni et al. [36] findings of very uneven, frequently nonexistent, clinical learning opportunities for surgeons in training are neither restricted to surgery nor unique to the present. Nearly four decades ago, Bucher and Stelling [37] documented via qualitative research the "randomness of rotation assignments for internal medicine residents." Another 1970s observation was made by McGlynn and colleagues [38] that, "If left to chance alone, many residents do not in fact have an opportunity to manage patients with common problems such as coronary artery disease or to use common primary care medications such as insulin in their primary care practice…. The wide variety of clinical situations needed to catalyze the residents' development of clinical judgment for primary care situations does not occur in many residents' practices" [38].

Many other medical education research reports reinforce the idea that irregular clinical experience alone is not the pathway to clinical competence. A sample of three journal articles, beginning in the late 1970s, starts with "Physician profiles in training the graduate internist" [39]. This observational study of house-staff clinical practice found, "There was a fourfold difference in the total number of patient encounters, a twelvefold variation in average cost of ancillary services per patient visit, and more than a twofold variation in the average time spent per patient. …Range of variation was equally great in each year of training." A contemporary expression of poor educational opportunities due to traditional clinical education is seen in the work of Peets and Stelfox [40] where "…over a 9-year period, the opportunities offered to residents to admit patients and perform procedures during ICU [intensive care unit] rotations decreased by 32% and 34%, respectively." Other indictments of traditional clinical education in medicine report reduced resident "code blue" experience over a 6-year time span [41], "underexposure" of students at 17 US medical schools to essential bedside procedures and comfort in performing them [42], and a wide variation in the clinical and educational experience among pulmonary and critical care fellows due to the lack of a "common core" [43]. These and many other medical education studies document the power of inertia in today's clinical education.

Unfortunately, these uneven educational opportunities lead to unsafe patient care when doctors graduate from residency or fellowship and are in clinical practice as attending physicians. For example, Birkmeyer and colleagues [44] rigorously evaluated the video-recorded surgeries of 20 attending bariatric surgeons in Michigan performing laparoscopic gastric bypass. This study showed significant variation in the surgical skills of these physicians with less skilled surgeons causing more operative complications. Barsuk and colleagues [45] evaluated the simulated central venous catheter (CVC) insertion skills of 108 attending emergency medicine, IM, and critical care physicians with significant CVC insertion experience. Less than 20% of these doctors were able to demonstrate competent skills measured by their ability to meet or exceed a MPS on a 29-item CVC insertion skills checklist. However, these senior attending physicians were supervising residents and inserting CVCs frequently in their hospitals.

This problem of uneven educational opportunities for learners in clinical settings due to patient encounters governed by chance is not unique to the medical profession. Leaders in nursing education are sounding a similar alarm by pointing out that despite its longevity, the traditional apprenticeship model of clinical education in nursing is now obsolete [46–49].

Traditional clinical education in the health professions, grounded in Osler's *natural method of teaching*, provides variable and insufficient opportunities for learners to acquire knowledge, skills, and attributes of professionalism needed for competent practice. A much more systematic, carefully managed, and accountable approach to clinical education is needed.

Learner Evaluation and Feedback

Health professions students are typically evaluated in three ways after classroom and laboratory instruction in the basic sciences and advancement to clinical education settings: (a) objective tests of acquired knowledge, (b) objective structured clinical examinations (OSCEs) in several formats, and (c) subjective evaluations of clinical performance.

Objective tests of acquired knowledge are ubiquitous in the health professions. They have a long history, dating to the formation of the National Board of Medical Examiners in the United States in 1915 [50] and the rise of psychometric science in the early twentieth century [51]. These evaluations are usually administered via multiple-choice questions, may cover hundreds of test items, require many hours of testing time, and yield highly reliable data, whose scores are used to render high-stakes decisions about learner educational achievement and professional certification. The United States Medical Licensing Examinations (USMLE) Steps (except for the clinical skills section) fulfill these purposes for the US medical profession [52]. Similar examinations are now in place in the United States. for other health professions including nursing [53], dentistry [54], pharmacy [55], physical therapy [56], physician assistants [57], osteopathic medicine [58], and many other specialties.

Today's tests of acquired knowledge in the health professions, now delivered in controlled, computer-based settings, are very sophisticated. The tests provide precise estimates of theoretical and factual learning among students, residents, and fellows in a variety of health sciences. Psychometric science has produced measurement methods and analytic technologies that are far ahead of other evaluation approaches used in health professions education [59].

Health professions learners receive norm-referenced feedback from objective tests of acquired knowledge often as a percentile rank in comparison with peers. This feedback is usually nonspecific. It does not pinpoint one's knowledge-based strengths or weaknesses, only one's relative standing among similar learners. Thus, norm-referenced feedback from acquired knowledge measurements cannot usually be used as a roadmap for improvement or as a pathway to boost one's fund of knowledge in needed directions. In fact, Neely and colleagues [60] reported that USMLE scores had a negative association with the level of performance of PGY-3 IM residents measured by summative evaluations from faculty, peers, and patients. Another study showed USMLE test scores are not correlated with reliable measures of medical students', residents', and fellows' skills in clinical examination, communication, and medical procedures [61].

The OSCE originated from the work of Ronald Harden at the University of Dundee in the United Kingdom in the 1970s [62]. Briefly, an OSCE is a measure of clinical skill acquisition and performance now used in a wide variety of health professions including medicine, nursing, and other specialties [63, 64]. The goal of an OSCE is to perform a rigorous, standardized assessment of a health professions student's clinical skills, and sometimes theoretical knowledge, as a benchmark for professional school advancement or certification [65].

Health sciences students taking an OSCE rotate through a series of examination stations, usually of short duration (5–15 minutes). Each station probes student skill or knowledge at specific clinical competencies such as physical examination; history taking; communication with patients and their families; medical procedures; health promotion counseling; radiographic, telemetry, or other image interpretation; clinical reasoning; prescription writing; medication reconciliation; and many other challenges. OSCE assessments may involve SPs who play out scripted roles, simulations, analyses of biomedical specimens including blood and tissue samples, or entries and verification of record keeping systems like electronic health records. Learners respond to realistic clinical problems in an OSCE, either skill-based (e.g., suturing, chest compressions) or case-based (e.g., infant seizures). Performance is scored objectively using checklists or other measures that yield reliable data.

OSCEs in many variations, e.g., the mini-clinical evaluation exercise (mini-CEX) [66–69], are now almost everywhere among the health professions. Their focus on measuring clinical skill acquisition and providing feedback to clinicians in training has had a palpable impact on health professions education. The Association of American Medical Colleges [70], for example, reports that the percentage of US medical schools that require students to undergo a final SP/OSCE examination before graduation has increased from 87% in academic year 2006–2007 to 91% in 2014–2015. In the same 9-year time span, the percentage of US medical schools that require passing a final SP/OSCE examination increased from 58% to 74%. Thus, while nearly all US medical students *experience* a summative OSCE, a much smaller percentage of students must *perform to a high standard* on a summative OSCE.

Creation and management of OSCEs in health professions education settings is labor intensive. An OSCE must have a sufficient number of stations (usually about 12), trained and calibrated raters, meaningful MPSs for individual stations and the total test, and consistent SPs to yield reliable data that are useful for making educational decisions [71]. Such conditions require dedication and hard work but can be reached in most educational settings.

Subjective student and resident evaluations are also ubiquitous in the health professions but address learning processes and outcomes that are different from knowledge acquisition [72]. Learning processes and outcomes evaluated subjectively typically involve faculty perceptions of clinical skills and attributes of professionalism that include interpersonal and communication skills, teamwork, procedural competence, altruism, clinical judgment, and efficiency. These subjective evaluations of clinical learners are made by experienced, but not necessarily trained, educational supervisors. The supervisor's evaluations of students are usually recorded on rating scales ranging from poor to excellent performance. Subjective learner evaluations in the health professions are intended to complement objective measures of knowledge acquisition, and clinical skills assessment via OSCEs, to present a broad picture of student readiness to practice professionally.

There is a downside to subjective faculty evaluations of student clinical fitness. The problem is that decades of research shows that faculty ratings of student clinical performance are subject to many sources of bias and error that reduce the utility of the assessments [73]. Examples are plentiful. To illustrate, nearly four decades ago sociologist Charles Bosk [74] wrote in *Forgive and Remember: Managing Medical Failure* that senior surgeons' subjective evaluations of junior trainees were highly intuitive, impressionistic, and focused more on learner character than on technical skill. Jack Haas and William Shaffir [75] cited many years ago the "ritual evaluation of competence" embodied in clinical evaluation schemes where learners engage in active "impression management" to influence supervisors' evaluations. These and many other studies reported over the past 40 years point out that the quality, utility, and validity of clinical ratings of health professions students, residents, and fellows are in doubt. Rigorous, standardized, and generalizable measures of clinical competence are needed.

Contemporary writing about subjective evaluations of health professions learners by faculty in clinical settings continue to testify about flaws in this approach. Physician Eric Holmboe is an outspoken critic of faculty observations as an approach to evaluate clinical skills among medical trainees. There are two reasons for Holmboe's criticism: (a) "the biggest problem in the evaluation of clinical skills is simply getting faculty to observe trainees" [76] and (b) "current evidence suggests significant deficiencies in faculty direct observation evaluation skills" [77]. A similar situation has been reported about clinical evaluations of nursing students where "questioning students to assess their grasp of their assigned patients' clinical status" occurs rarely [47]. Thus, subjective observational evaluations of learner clinical skills in the health professions are flawed due to sins of omission and sins of commission.

In summary, current approaches used to evaluate achievement among learners in the health professions—tests of acquired knowledge, OSCEs, and subjective evaluations of clinical performance—provide an incomplete record of readiness for clinical practice among learners. Evaluation data are also used infrequently to give learners specific, actionable feedback for clinical skill improvement. Standardized knowledge tests typically yield very reliable data that can contribute to a narrow range of decisions about learner clinical fitness. Evaluation data derived from OSCEs and especially subjective observations tend to be much less reliable and have low or little utility for reaching educational decisions. Consequently, many programs of health professions education fall short of Holmboe's admonition, "Medical educators have a moral and professional obligation to ensure that any trainee leaving their training program has attained a minimum level of clinical skills to care for patients safely, effectively, and compassionately" [77].

Clinical Practice Outcomes

Osler's *natural method of teaching*, expressed as experiential clinical learning in the health professions, has been the educational mainstay for over a century. The problem is that longitudinal clinical education without a competency focus, rigorous evaluation, detailed feedback, tight management, and accountability does not work very well.

Published evaluation studies about clinical skill acquisition among medical learners who were educated traditionally reveal consistent, concerning results. There are many examples.

To illustrate, a 3-year study conducted in the 1990s involved objective evaluations of 126 pediatric residents. The residents failed to meet faculty expectations about learning basic skills such as physical examination, history taking, laboratory use, and telephone patient management as a consequence of education based solely on clinical experience [78]. Other studies report that residents and students who only receive experiential learning acquire very weak ECG interpretation skills [79–81] and are not ready for professional practice. Another line of medical education research documents skill and knowledge deficits among medical school graduates about to start postgraduate residency education at the University of Michigan. These studies report that skill and knowledge deficits include such basic competencies as interpreting critical laboratory values, cross-cultural communication, evidence-based medicine, radiographic image interpretation, aseptic technique, advanced cardiac life support, and cardiac auscultation [82, 83].

A recent study conducted under auspices of the American Medical Association reports, "One hundred fifty-nine students from medical schools in 37 states attending the American Medical Association's House of Delegates Meeting in June 2015 were assessed on an 11-element skillset on BP measurement. Only one student demonstrated proficiency on all 11 skills. The mean number of elements performed properly was 4.1. The findings suggest that changes in medical school curriculum emphasizing BP measurement are needed for medical students to become, and remain, proficient in BP measurement. Measuring BP correctly should be taught and reinforced throughout medical school, residency, and the entire career of clinicians" [84].

Traditional undergraduate clinical education in medicine, grounded chiefly in patient care experience, has failed to produce young doctors who are ready for postgraduate education in a medical specialty. A recent survey of medicine residency program directors shows that, "a significant proportion of [new] residents were not adequately prepared in order filling, forming clinical questions, handoffs, informed consent, and promoting a culture of patient safety" [85]. Survey research results in surgical education paint a similar picture. A 2017 multi-institution surgical education study under auspices of the Procedural Learning and Safety Collaboration (PLSC) concluded that "US GS (general surgery) residents are not universally ready to independently perform the most common core procedures by the time they complete residency training. Significant gaps remain for less common core and non-core procedures" [86]. Other reports have spawned the growth of "boot camp" clinical education crash courses designed to better prepare new physicians for patient care responsibilities they will face as residents [87–94].

The weight of evidence is now very clear that traditional clinical education in medicine and other health professions, mostly based on clinical experience, is simply not effective at producing competent practitioners. The conclusion is evident: there is an acute need to modernize health professions education to match expectations expressed by the National Academy of Sciences, Engineering, and Medicine [5], "… [health professions] educators should ensure that curricula and training programs across the career trajectory employ educational approaches that are aligned with evidence from the learning sciences."

New Directions for Clinical Education

The premise of this chapter is that clinical education in the health professions is not standardized and is ineffective. It is based on an obsolete model about the acquisition of knowledge, skill, and professionalism attributes grounded chiefly in clinical experience that has not kept up with the rapidly changing healthcare environment. Today, unmanaged clinical experience alone is insufficient to ensure that nurses, physicians, physical therapists, pharmacists, dentists, midwives, and other health professionals are fit to care for patients.

The weakness of traditional clinical education is especially evident in comparison to new education approaches like simulation-based education with deliberate practice. In medicine, for example, this has been demonstrated in a systematic, meta-analytic, head-to-head comparison of traditional clinical education versus simulation-based medical education (SBME) with DP [15]. Quantitative aggregation and analysis of 14 studies involving 633 medical learners shows that without exception SBME with DP produces much better education results than clinical

Research Design and Study	Statistics for Each Study: Correlation	Lower Limit	Upper Limit	*P*-Value
Randomized Trials				
1. Wayne et al, 2005	0.81	0.70	0.88	0.000
2. Ahlberg et al, 2007	0.80	0.56	0.91	0.000
3. Andreatta et al, 2006	0.67	0.40	0.84	0.000
4. Korndorffer et al, 2005	0.62	0.29	0.82	0.001
5. Korndorffer et al, 2005	0.52	0.17	0.75	0.006
6. Van Sickle et al, 2008	0.51	0.17	0.74	0.005
Cohort Studies				
7. Issenberg et al, 2001	0.78	0.73	0.82	0.000
8. Barsuk et al, 2009	0.61	0.29	0.81	0.001
9. Butter et al 2010	0.59	0.47	0.69	0.000
Case-Control Studies				
10. Wayne et al, 2008	0.51	0.29	0.68	0.000
Pre-Post Baseline Studies				
11. Wayne et al, 2008	0.80	0.72	0.86	0.000
12. Barsuk et al, 2009	0.79	0.70	0.86	0.000
13. Barsuk et al, 2009	0.77	0.71	0.82	0.000
14. Stefanidis et al, 2006	0.71	0.55	0.83	0.000
Overall Effect Size d = 2.00	0.71	0.65	0.76	0.000

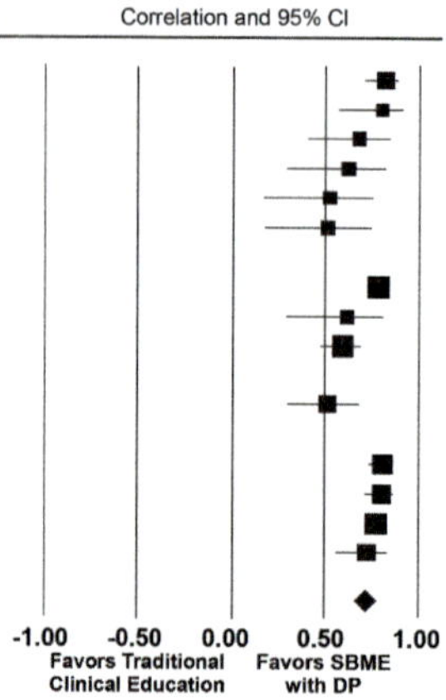

Fig. 1.2 Random-effects meta-analysis of traditional clinical education compared with simulation-based medical education (SBME) with deliberate practice (DP). Effect size correlations with 95% confidence intervals (95% CIs) represent the 14 studies included in the meta-analysis. The diamond represents the pooled overall effect size. (Source: McGaghie et al. [15]. Reprinted with permission of Wolters Kluwer Health)

experience alone (Fig. 1.2). The effect size for the overall difference between SBME with DP and traditional clinical education is expressed as a Cohen's *d* coefficient = 2.00 [7]. This is a huge difference, a magnitude never before reported in health professions education comparative research.

There are at least five new directions for clinical education in the health professions that warrant attention: (a) focus on the learning sciences; (b) active learning; (c) deliberate practice, (d) rigorous, reliable measurement with feedback; and (e) mastery learning.

Learning Sciences

Psychologist Richard Mayer [32] separates the science of learning from the science of instruction. The science of learning seeks to understand how people learn from words, pictures, observation, and experience—and how cognitive operations mediate learning. The science of learning is about acquisition and maintenance of knowledge, skill, professionalism, and other dispositions needed for clinical practice. The science of instruction, by contrast, "is the scientific study of how to help people learn" [32]. Health professions educators need to be conversant with both the science of learning and the science of instruction to plan and deliver educational programs that produce competent and compassionate clinicians.

There are, in fact, a variety of learning sciences that find homes for application in health professions education. A detailed description of the various learning theories is beyond the scope of this chapter (but see Chap. 2). Many scientists too numerous to fully name or credit here have sought to deepen our understanding of human learning in the health professions via empirical and synthetic scholarship. Several select, yet prominent, examples of learning sciences include behaviorism [95], cognitive load theory [96], constructivism [97], problem-based learning [98], and social cognitive theory [99]. Many other illustrations addressing different scientific perspectives could be identified.

The important point is that health professions educators need to make better use of current learning sciences knowledge, in addition to advancing the learning sciences research agenda, as education programs in the health professions are designed and maintained.

Active Learning

A meta-analysis of 225 science education research studies published in the *Proceedings of the National Academy of Science* [33] shows unequivocally that active learning—in-class problem-solving, worksheets, personal response systems, and peer tutorials—is far superior than passive learning from lectures to achieve student learning goals. The authors assert, "The results raise questions about the continued use of traditional lecturing as a control in research studies, and support active learning as the preferred, empirically validated teaching practice in regular classrooms." The lesson is that health science learners need to be actively engaged in professionally relevant tasks to grow and strengthen their competence. Passive learning strategies such as listening to lectures or watching videos are much less effective.

Deliberate Practice

Deliberate practice is a construct coined and advanced by psychologist K. Anders Ericsson and his colleagues [95, 100–104]. The Ericsson team sought to study and explain the acquisition of expertise in a variety of skill domains including sports, music, writing, science, and the learned professions including medicine and surgery [102]. Rousmaniere [105] has extended this work to education for professional psychotherapists. The Ericsson team's research goal was to isolate and explain the variables responsible for the acquisition and maintenance of superior reproducible (expert) performance. Ericsson and his colleagues found consistently that the origins of expert performance across skill domains do not reside in measured intelligence, scholastic aptitude, academic pedigree, or longitudinal experience. Instead, acquisition of expertise stems from about 10,000 hours of DP depending on each specific skill domain.

Ericsson writes that his research group:

> ...identified a set of conditions where practice had been uniformly associated with improved performance. Significant improvements in performance were realized when individuals were (1) given a task with a well-defined goal, (2) motivated to improve, (3) provided with feedback, (4) provided with ample opportunities for repetition and gradual refinements of their performance. Deliberate efforts to improve one's performance beyond its current level demands full concentration and often requires problem-solving and better methods of performing the tasks [101].

Deliberate practice in health professions education means that learners are engaged in planned, difficult, and goal-oriented work, supervised and coached by teachers, who provide feedback and correction, under conditions of high achievement expectations, with revision and improvement to existing mental representations. Deliberate practice is the polar opposite of the *natural method of teaching* favored in Osler's [30] day or even the more recent "laissez faire method of learning" described by Kenneth Ludmerer [22].

Rigorous, Reliable Measurement with Feedback

The use of quality measures that yield highly reliable data is essential to provide learners with specific, actionable feedback to promote their improvement in knowledge, skill, and professionalism. Highly reliable assessment data have a strong "signal" with very little "noise" or error [106]. Reliable data are also needed to make accurate decisions about learner advancement decisions in educational programs. Educational quality improvement (QI) requires that the reliability of data derived from measurements and assessments should be checked regularly and improved as needed to ensure the accuracy and fairness of learner evaluations.

Over the past decade, a Northwestern University team of researchers completed a series of simulation-based (S-B) clinical skill acquisition programs that feature attention to learning science, active learning, deliberate practice, and mastery learning. A key to the success of these programs is constant QI attention to the reliability of outcome measurement data. A visible example of one such program, led by physician Jeffrey Barsuk, concerns training IM and emergency medicine residents on proper insertion of CVCs in a medical intensive care unit (MICU) with subsequent training of ICU nurses on CVC maintenance skills. In brief, the research program results demonstrate reliable measurement of CVC skills acquired in the simulation laboratory [107]. Downstream translational measured outcomes [108] also show that residents who received S-B training inserted CVCs in the MICU with significantly fewer patient complications than traditionally trained residents [109]. A before-after study in the MICU showed that the simulation-based educational intervention also produced a reliably measured 85% reduction in central line-associated bloodstream infections over 39 months [17]. S-B training also produced large improvements in ICU nurses' CVC maintenance skills to a median score of 100% measured with high reliability [110].

There is no doubt about the importance of rigorous, reliable measurement with feedback to boost health professions education and translate into meaningful clinical outcomes.

Mastery Learning

Mastery learning, the theme of this book, aims to achieve "excellence for all" in health professions education. The basic idea is that any health professions curriculum—medicine, nursing, pharmacy, dentistry, etc.—is a sample of professional practice. Tests, evaluations, and examinations are a sample of the curriculum. The educational aim is to align learner evaluations with curriculum and professional practice goals, an alignment that will never be flawless.

Mastery learning requires that all learners achieve all curriculum learning objectives to high performance standards without exception. Educational outcomes are uniform among learners, while the time needed to reach the outcomes may vary. This is a radical departure from the traditional model of health professions education where learning time is fixed and measured learning outcomes vary, often distributed as a normal curve. The idea of mastery learning conforms with a medical education recommendation proposed by Cooke, Irby, and O'Brien in their book, *Educating Physicians: A Call for Reform of Medical School and Residency* [25], "Standardize learning outcomes and individualize learning processes."

The time has come for a new model of clinical education in the health professions. We have relied for too long on time-based rotations for learners to acquire clinical skills and multiple-choice tests as proxy measures of clinical learning outcomes. The new model will complement, sometimes replace, traditional clinical education and will link classroom and learning laboratory measurements with downstream clinical impacts. Mastery learning will be the cornerstone of this new model of clinical education.

Coda

For all the reasons discussed in this chapter, current healthcare provider education simply does not work very well. The current model needs to be augmented by a new and improved training model that will complement clinical training and enhance education and downstream patient outcomes. We must move from time-based rotations and multiple-choice tests to routine and continuous assessments of actual clinical skills [111]. Chapter 2 of this book describes the mastery learning model in detail and provides examples of its utility in health professions education.

References

1. Barsuk JH, Cohen ER, Caprio T, McGaghie WC, Simuni T, Wayne DB. Simulation-based education with mastery learning improves residents' lumbar puncture skills. Neurology. 2012;79(2):132–7.
2. Nathan BR, Kincaid O. Does experience doing lumbar punctures result in expertise? A medical maxim bites the dust. Neurology. 2012;79(2):115–6.

3. Choudhry NK, Fletcher RH, Soumerai SB. Systematic review: the relationship between clinical experience and quality of health care. Ann Intern Med. 2005;142:260–73.
4. Barsuk JH, Cohen ER, Feinglass J, McGaghie WC, Wayne DB. Experience with clinical procedures does not ensure competence: a research synthesis. J Grad Med Educ. 2017;9:201–8.
5. National Academy of Sciences, Engineering, and Medicine. Improving diagnosis in healthcare. Washington, DC: The National Academies Press; 2015.
6. Issenberg SB, McGaghie WC. Looking to the future. In: McGaghie WC, editor. International best practices for evaluation in the health professions. London: Radcliffe Publishing, Ltd.; 2013. p. 341–59.
7. McGaghie WC, Kristopaitis T. Deliberate practice and mastery learning: origins of expert medical performance. In: Cleland J, Durning SJ, editors. Researching medical education. New York: John Wiley & Sons; 2015. p. 219–30.
8. Susskind R, Susskind D. The future of the professions: how technology will transform the work of human experts. New York: Oxford University Press; 2015.
9. National League for Nursing. Outcomes and competencies for graduates of practical/vocational, diploma, baccalaureate, master's practice, doctorate, and research. Washington, DC: National League for Nursing; 2012.
10. Association of American Medical Colleges. Core entrustable professional activities for entering residency. Curriculum developer's guide. Washington, DC: AAMC; 2014.
11. Holmboe ES, Edgar L, Hamstra S. The milestones guidebook. Chicago: Accreditation Council on Graduate Medical Education; 2016.
12. Nasca TJ, Philibert I, Brigham T, Flynn TC. The next GME accreditation system—rationale and benefits. N Engl J Med. 2012;366(11):1051–6.
13. Levine AI, DeMaria S Jr, Schwartz AD, Sim AJ, editors. The comprehensive textbook of healthcare simulation. New York: Springer; 2013.
14. Fincher R-ME, White CB, Huang G, Schwartzstein R. Toward hypothesis-driven medical education research: task force report from the Millennium Conference 2007 on educational research. Acad Med. 2010;85:821–8.
15. McGaghie WC, Issenberg SB, Cohen ER, Barsuk JH, Wayne DB. Does simulation-based medical education with deliberate practice yield better results than traditional clinical education? A meta-analytic comparative review of the evidence. Acad Med. 2011;86:706–11.
16. Cohen ER, Feinglass J, Barsuk JH, Barnard C, O'Donnell A, McGaghie WC, Wayne DB. Cost savings from reduced catheter-related bloodstream infection after simulation-based education for residents in a medical intensive care unit. Simul Healthc. 2010;5:98–102.
17. Barsuk JH, Cohen ER, Feinglass J, McGaghie WC, Wayne DB. Use of simulation-based education to reduce catheter-related bloodstream infections. Arch Intern Med. 2009;169:1420–3.
18. Puschmann T. A history of medical education. New York: Hafner Publishing Co.; 1966. (Originally published 1891).
19. Siegerist HE. A history of medicine, vol. I: primitive and archaic medicine. New York: Oxford University Press; 1951.
20. Siegerist HE. A history of medicine, vol. II: early Greek, Hindu, and Persian medicine. New York: Oxford University Press; 1961.
21. Ludmerer KM. Learning to heal: the development of American medical education. Baltimore: Johns Hopkins University Press; 1985.
22. Ludmerer KM. Let me heal: the opportunity to preserve excellence in American medicine. New York: Oxford University Press; 2015.
23. Cassedy JL. Medicine in America: a short history. Baltimore: Johns Hopkins University Press; 1991.
24. Starr P. The social transformation of American medicine. New York: Basic Books; 1982.
25. Cooke M, Irby DM, O'Brien BC. Educating physicians: a call for reform of medical school and residency. Stanford: Carnegie Foundation for the Advancement of Teaching; 2010.

26. Flexner A. Medical education in the United States and Canada. Bulletin no. 4 of the Carnegie Foundation for the Advancement of Teaching. New York: Carnegie Foundation for the Advancement of Teaching; 1910.
27. Committee on the Future of Dental Education, Division of Healthcare Services, Institute of Medicine, Field MS, editor. Dental education at the crossroads: challenges and change. Washington, DC: National Academy Press; 1995.
28. Buerki RA, editor. Teaching the history of pharmacy today. Madison: American Institute of the History of Pharmacy; 1999. Retrieved from https://pharmacy.wisc.edu/sites/default/files/content/american-institute-history-pharmacy/resources-teaching/teachinghistpharm.pdf.
29. Murphy W. Healing the generations: a history of physical therapy and the American Physical Therapy Association. Alexandria: American Physical Therapy Association; 1995.
30. Osler W. The hospital as a college. In: Osler W, editor. Aequanimitas. Philadelphia: P. Blakiston's Son & Co.; 1932. p. 313–25.
31. Halsted WS. The training of the surgeon. Bull Johns Hopkins Hosp. 1904;15:267–75.
32. Mayer RE. Applying the science of learning to medical education. Med Educ. 2010;44:543–9.
33. Freeman S, Eddy SI, McDonough M, Smith MK, Okoraoafor N, Jordt H, Wenderoth MP. Active learning increases student performance in science, engineering, and mathematics. PNAS. 2014;111(23):8410–5.
34. Holmboe E, Ginsburg S, Bernabeo E. The rotational approach to medical education: time to confront our assumptions? Med Educ. 2011;45:69–80.
35. Bell RH Jr, Biester TW, Tabuenca A, Rhodes RS, Cofer JB, Britt D, Lewis FR Jr. Operative experience of residents in U.S. general surgery programs: a gap between expectation and experience. Ann Surg. 2009;249:719–24.
36. Malangoni MA, Biester TW, Jones AT, Klingensmith ME, Lewis FA Jr. Operative experience of surgery residents: trends and challenges. J Surg Educ. 2013;70(6):783–8.
37. Bucher R, Stelling JG. Becoming professional. Beverly Hills: Sage Publications; 1977.
38. McGlynn TJ Jr, Munzenrider RF, Zizzo J. A resident's internal medicine practice. Eval Health Prof. 1979;2(4):463–76.
39. Reid RA, Lantz KH. Physician profiles in training the graduate internist. J Med Educ. 1977;52:301–7.
40. Peets AD, Stelfox HT. Changes in residents' opportunities for experiential learning over time. Med Educ. 2012;46:1189–93.
41. Mickelsen S, McNeil R, Parikh P, Persoff J. Reduced patient "code blue" experience in the era of quality improvement. New challenges in physician training. Acad Med. 2011;86(6):726–30.
42. Barr J, Graffeo CS. Procedural experience and confidence among graduating medical students. J Surg Educ. 2016;73(3):46–7.
43. Shah NG, Seam N, Woods CJ, Fessler HE, Goyal M, McAreavey D, Lee B. A longitudinal regional educational model for pulmonary and critical care fellows emphasizing small group and simulation-based learning. Ann Am Thorac Soc. 2016;13(4):469–74.
44. Birkmeyer JD, Finks JF, O'Reilly A, Oerline M, Carlin AM, Nunn AR, Dimick J, Banerjee M, Birkmeyer NJO. Surgical skill and complication rates after bariatric surgery. N Engl J Med. 2013;369(15):1434–42.
45. Barsuk JH, Cohen ER, Nguyen D, Mitra D, O'Hara K, Okuda Y, Feinglass J, Cameron K, McGaghie WC, Wayne DB. Attending physician adherence to a 29 component central venous catheter bundle checklist during simulated procedures. Crit Care Med. 2016;44:1871–81.
46. Gubrud-Howe P, Schoessler M. From random access opportunity to a clinical education curriculum. J Nurs Educ. 2008;47(1):3–4.
47. Ironside PM, McNelis AM. Clinical education in prelicensure nursing programs: findings from a national survey. Nurs Educ Perspect. 2010;31(4):264–5.
48. Niederhauser V, Schoessler M, Gubrud-Howe PM, Magnussen L, Codier E. Creating innovative models of clinical nursing education. J Nurs Educ. 2012;51(11):603–8.
49. Ironside PM, McNelis AM, Ebrigret P. Clinical education in nursing: rethinking learning in practice settings. Nurs Outlook. 2014;62(3):185–91.

50. Hubbard JP. Measuring medical education: the tests and the experience of the National Board of Medical Examiners. 2nd ed. Philadelphia: Lea & Febiger; 1978.
51. Monroe WS. An introduction to the theory of educational measurements. Boston: Houghton Mifflin; 1923.
52. Federation of State Medical Boards of the United States, Inc., and the National Board of Medical Examiners. Bulletin of information; 2016. Retrieved from http://usmle.org.
53. National Council of State Boards of Nursing. NCLEX examination candidate bulletin; 2016. Retrieved from https://www.ncsbn.org/1213.htm.
54. American Dental Association. Report of the ADA-recognized dental specialty certifying boards; 2015. Retrieved from http://www.ada.org/.
55. American College of Clinical Pharmacy. Board certification and recertification; 2016. Retrieved from http://www.accp.com/careers/certification.aspx.
56. American Physical Therapy Association. About the national physical therapy examination; 2016. Retrieved from http://www.apta.org/Licensure/NPTE?.
57. National Commission on Certification of Physician Assistants. Initial certification for physician assistants, PANCE Exam; 2016. Retrieved from http://www.nccpa.net/become-certified.
58. American Osteopathic Association. AOA board certification; 2016. Retrieved from https://www.osteopathic.org/inside-aoa/development/aoa-board-certification.
59. Clauser BE, Margolis MJ, Case SM. Testing for licensure and certification. In: Brennan RL, editor. Educational measurement. 4th ed. Westport: American Council on Education and Praeger Publishers; 2006. p. 701–31.
60. Neely D, Feinglass J, Wallace WH. Developing a predictive model to assess applicants to an internal medicine residency. J Grad Med Educ. 2010;2(1):129–32.
61. McGaghie WC, Cohen ER, Wayne DB. Are United States Medical Licensing Exam Step 1 and 2 scores valid measures for postgraduate medical residency selection decisions? Acad Med. 2011;86(1):48–52.
62. Harden RM, Stevenson M, Downie WW, Wilson GM. Assessment of clinical competence using objective structured examination. BMJ. 1975;1:447–51.
63. Rushforth HE. Objective structured clinical examination (OSCE): review of literature and implications for nursing education. Nurse Educ Today. 2007;27(5):481–90.
64. Sloan DA, Donnelly MB, Schwartz RW, Strodel WE. The objective structured clinical examination: the new gold standard for evaluating postgraduate clinical performance. Ann Surg. 1995;222(6):735–42.
65. Yudkowsky R. Performance tests. In: Downing SM, Yudkowsky R, editors. Assessment in health professions education. New York: Routledge; 2009. p. 217–43.
66. Norcini JJ, Blank LL, Arnold GK, Kimball HR. The mini-CEX (clinical evaluation exercise): a preliminary investigation. Ann Intern Med. 1995;123(10):795–9.
67. Behere R. Introduction of mini-CEX in undergraduate dental education in India. Educ Health. 2014;27(3):262–8.
68. Milner KA, Watson SM, Steward JG, NeNisco S. Use of mini-CEX tool to assess clinical competence in family nurse practitioner students using undergraduate students as patients and doctoral students as evaluators. J Nurs Educ. 2014;53(12):718–20.
69. Weijs CA, Coe JB, Hecker KG. Final-year students' and clinical instructors' experience of workplace-based assessments used in a small-animal primary-veterinary-care clinical rotation. J Vet Med Educ. 2015;42(4):382–92.
70. Association of American Medical Colleges. Number of medical schools requiring final SP/OSCE examination: 2006–2007 through 2010–2011; 2016. Retrieved from https://www.aamc.org/initiatives/cir/406426/9.html.
71. Brannick MT, Erol-Korkmaz HT, Prewett M. A systematic review of the reliability of objective structured clinical examination scores. Med Educ. 2011;45:1181–9.
72. McGaghie WC, Butter J, Kaye M. Observational assessment. In: Downing SM, Yudkowsky R, editors. Assessment in health professions education. New York: Routledge; 2009. p. 185–215.
73. Williams RG, Klamen DA, McGaghie WC. Cognitive, social, and environmental sources of bias in clinical performance ratings. Teach Learn Med. 2003;15(4):270–92.

74. Bosk CL. Forgive and remember: managing medical failure. 2nd ed. Chicago: University of Chicago Press; 2003.
75. Haas J, Shaffir W. Becoming doctors: the adoption of a cloak of competence. Greenwich: JAI Press; 1987.
76. Holmboe ES. Direct observation by faculty. In: Holmboe ES, Hawkins RE, editors. Practical guide to the evaluation of competence. Philadelphia: Mosby Elsevier; 2008. p. 119–29.
77. Holmboe ES. Faculty and the observation of trainees' clinical skills: problems and opportunities. Acad Med. 2004;79(1):16–22.
78. Joorabchi B, Devries JM. Evaluation of clinical competence: the gap between expectation and performance. Pediatrics. 1996;97(2):179–84.
79. Pinkerton RE, Francis CK, Ljungquist KA, Howe GW. Electrocardiographic training in primary care residency programs. JAMA. 1981;246:148–50.
80. Boltri JM, Hash RB, Vogel RL. Are family practice residents able to interpret electrocardiograms? Adv Health Sci Educ. 2003;8:149–53.
81. Wilcox JE, Raval Z, Patel AB, Didwania A, Wayne DB. Imperfect beginnings: incoming residents vary in their ability to interpret basic electrocardiogram findings. J Hosp Med. 2014;9(3):197–8.
82. Lypson ML, Frohna JG, Gruppen LD, Woolliscroft JO. Assessing residents' competencies at baseline: identifying the gaps. Acad Med. 2004;79(6):564–70.
83. Wagner D, Lypson ML. Centralized assessment in graduate medical education: cents and sensibilities. J Grad Med Educ. 2009;1:21–7.
84. Rakotz MK, Townsend RR, Yang J, et al. Medical students and measuring blood pressure: results from the American Medical Association blood pressure check challenge. J Clin Hypertens. 2017;19:614–9.
85. Perlmen RE, Pawelczak M, Yacht AC, et al. Program director perceptions of proficiency of the core entrustable professional activities. J Grad Med Educ. 2017;9(5):588–92.
86. George BC, Bohnan JD, Williams RG, Procedural Learning and Safety Collaborative (PLSC), et al. Readiness of US general surgery residents for independent practice. Ann Surg. 2017;266(4):582–94.
87. Laack TA, Newman JS, Goyal DG, Torsher LC. A 1-week simulated internship course helps prepare medical students for transition to residency. Simul Healthc. 2010;5:127–32.
88. Antonoff MB, Swanson JA, Green CA, Mann BD, Maddaus MA, D'Cunha J. The significant impact of a competency-based preparatory course for senior medical students entering surgical residency. Acad Med. 2012;87(3):308–19.
89. Cohen ER, Barsuk JH, Moazed F, Caprio T, Didwania A, McGaghie WC, Wayne DB. Making July safer: simulation-based mastery learning during intern boot camp. Acad Med. 2013;88:233–9.
90. Naylor RA, Hollett LA, Castellvi A, Valentine RJ, Scott DJ. Preparing medical students to enter surgical residencies. Am J Surg. 2010;199(1):105–9.
91. Nishisake A, Hales R, Bigas K, Cheifetz I, Corriveau C, Garber N, Hunt E, Jarrah R, McCloskey J, Morrison W, Nelson K, Niles D, Smith S, Thomas S, Tuttle S, Helfaer M, Nadkarni V. A multi-institutional high-fidelity simulation "boot camp" orientation and training program for first year pediatric critical care fellows. Pediatr Crit Care Med. 2009;10:157–62.
92. Reed T, Pirotte M, McHugh M, Oh L, Lovett S, Hoyt AE, Quinones D, Adams W, Gruener G, McGaghie WC. Simulation-based mastery learning improves medical student performance and retention of core clinical skills. Simul Healthc. 2016;11:173–80.
93. Salzman DH, McGaghie WC, Caprio T, Even E, Hufmeyer K, Issa N, Schaefer E, Trainor J, Wayne DB. Use of simulation-based capstone course to teach and assess entrustable professional activities to graduating medical students. Med Sci Educ. 2016;26:453–6.
94. Salzman DH, McGaghie WC, Caprio TW, et al. A mastery learning capstone course to teach and assess components of three entrustable professional activities to graduating medical students. Teach Learn Med. 2019;31(2):186–94.

95. Ericsson KA, Krampe RT, Tesch-Römer C. The role of deliberate practice in the acquisition of expert performance. Psychol Rev. 1993;100:363–406.
96. Leppink J, van Gog T, Paas F, Sweller J. Cognitive load theory: researching and planning teaching to maximize learning. In: Cleland J, Durning SJ, editors. Researching medical education. Oxford: Wiley Blackwell; 2015. p. 207–18.
97. Mann K, MacLeod A. Constructivism: learning theories and approaches to research. In: Cleland J, Durning SJ, editors. Researching medical education. Oxford: Wiley Blackwell; 2015. p. 51–65.
98. Norman GR, Schmidt HG. The psychological basis of problem-based learning: a review of the evidence. Acad Med. 1992;67(9):557–65.
99. Torre D, Durning SJ. Social cognitive theory: thinking and learning in social settings. In: Cleland J, Durning SJ, editors. Researching medical education. Oxford: Wiley Blackwell; 2015. p. 105–16.
100. Ericsson KA. Deliberate practice and the acquisition and maintenance of expert performance in medicine and related domains. Acad Med. 2004;79(10, Suppl):S70–81.
101. Ericsson KA. Deliberate practice and the acquisition of expert performance: a general overview. Acad Emerg Med. 2008;15:988–94.
102. Ericsson KA, Charness N, Feltovich PJ, Hoffman RR, editors. The Cambridge handbook of expertise and expert performance. New York: Cambridge University Press; 2006.
103. Ericsson K, Pool R. Peak: secrets from the new science of expertise. Boston: Houghton Mifflin Harcourt; 2016.
104. Ericsson KA, Shyte J, Ward P. Expert performance in nursing: reviewing research on expertise in nursing within the framework of the expert performance approach. Adv Nurs Sci. 2007;30(1):E58–71.
105. Rousmaniere T. Deliberate practice for psychotherapists: a guide to improving clinical effectiveness. New York: Routledge; 2017.
106. Axelson RD, Kreiter CD. Reliability. In: Downing SM, Yudkowsky R, editors. Assessment in health professions education. New York: Routledge; 2009. p. 57–73.
107. Barsuk JH, McGaghie WC, Cohen ER, Balachandran JS, Wayne DB. Use of simulation-based mastery learning to improve the quality of central venous catheter placement in a medical intensive care unit. J Hosp Med. 2009;4:397–403.
108. McGaghie WC. Medical education research as translational science. Sci Transl Med. 2010;2:19cm8.
109. Barsuk JH, McGaghie WC, Cohen ER, O'Leary KJ, Wayne DB. Simulation-based mastery learning reduces complications during central venous catheter insertion in a medical intensive care unit. Crit Care Med. 2009;37:2697–701.
110. Barsuk JH, Cohen ER, Mikolajczak A, Seburn S, Slade M, Wayne DB. Simulation-based mastery learning improves central line maintenance skills of ICU nurses. J Nurs Adm. 2015;45(10):511–7.
111. van der Vleuten CPM, Schuwirth LWT. Assessing professional competence: from methods to programmes. Med Educ. 2005;39:309–17.

Part II

The Mastery Learning Model

2 Mastery Learning: Origins, Features, and Evidence from the Health Professions

William C. McGaghie

This chapter starts with an anecdote about a mastery learning experience from long ago that was published in a 2015 article in the journal *Medical Education* [1]. The story is about my involvement in a sophomore-level college course in statistics taught in 1968, over 50 years ago. The statistics course was presented as 16 weekly sequential units ordered by difficulty. Students engaged in several types of active study and practice opportunities including reading, problem sets, group discussion, peer comment, and teacher coaching. We were focused, practiced statistical problems deliberately, and worked very hard. Brief, formative unit quizzes gauged our progress and provided feedback for improvement. The story continues,

> After teaching and practice, we reported for unit testing at 10:00 A.M. every Tuesday on a pass-the-test, see-you-next-week basis. Retests, as needed, were scheduled for Fridays at 5:00 P.M. (party time for U.S. college students) or, as a last resort, at 7:00 A.M. on Sunday mornings (doomsday option: never needed).

The final outcome was that, "All 30 students passed the course with an A grade, with no differences among us. We all felt great about this success experience. The only downside was that the Professor, Dr. Jack Michael, was reprimanded by the dean for grading too leniently. "'How can everyone be a high achiever?' groused the dean. 'Someone must fail!'"

The mastery learning experience in the undergraduate statistics course affected me forever. The course laid an intellectual foundation in quantitative statistical methods that made it possible for me to endure and succeed in advanced statistics courses (e.g., correlation and regression, multivariate analysis) that were taught poorly. I advanced where other graduate students struggled. The early statistics

W. C. McGaghie (✉)
Northwestern University Feinberg School of Medicine, Departments of Medical Education and Preventive Medicine, Chicago, IL, USA
e-mail: wcmc@northwestern.edu

W. C. McGaghie et al. (eds.), *Comprehensive Healthcare Simulation: Mastery Learning in Health Professions Education*, Comprehensive Healthcare Simulation, https://doi.org/10.1007/978-3-030-34811-3_2

course that was presented using mastery learning principles made it possible for me to move forward in a Ph.D. program despite bad teaching. The undergraduate statistics course also gave me pause to ask, “Why is the mastery learning model not used in other college courses?” “Why is mastery learning so unusual?”

What Is Mastery Learning?

Mastery learning, an especially stringent variety of competency-based education [2], means that all learners acquire essential knowledge and skill, measured rigorously against fixed achievement standards, without regard to the time needed to reach the outcome. Mastery learning indicates a much higher level of performance than competence alone. In mastery learning, educational *results* are uniform, with little or no variation, while educational *time* may vary among trainees.

An example from a postgraduate, pediatric medical education program illuminates the mastery learning approach using simulation technology.

Northwestern University Lurie Children’s Hospital pediatrician Marcelo Malakooti observed that new US postgraduate pediatric residents struggle with caring for children experiencing seizures, especially when seizures progress to status epilepticus (SE) where patient management is highly time-sensitive [3]. This observation was reinforced by a needs assessment among the pediatric residents which revealed they were uncomfortable managing SE patients and had difficulty recalling and using a standard treatment protocol. Dr. Malakooti and his colleagues framed the situation as both a medical education and a patient safety problem. They resolved to develop a simulation-based mastery learning (SBML) curriculum for inpatient management of SE to help the residents become better doctors and reduce risks to children [3].

The SBML curriculum was derived from a SE management algorithm based on the standard of care [4, 5] that was developed at Lurie Children’s Hospital, Chicago (Fig. 2.1). The curriculum was embodied in a scripted simulation scenario involving “a 2-year old child [who] develops tonic-clonic seizures requiring recall and practical application of the SE algorithm” [3]. The scenario allowed the residents to engage in deliberate practice [6–8] of SE management in a fully equipped, high-fidelity, standardized environment including nursing staff. The SE algorithm was also used to create a 22-item checklist to evaluate resident skill acquisition and to provide feedback. A minimum passing standard (MPS) was established for the checklist by an expert panel of pediatric neurologists.

> Each resident was scheduled individually for the simulation, allowing sufficient time for a pretest to assess baseline knowledge, and to provide individualized education in a separate debriefing room. Without knowing the case content, the participant first performed the simulation (pretest), and after scoring, returned for debriefing. During each debriefing, participants were taught each step of the algorithm and checklist in detail, received individualized feedback on performance, and were provided feedback on how to perform each step correctly.

The simulation scenario, checklist evaluation, debriefing, and feedback were repeated for each resident until the MPS was reached. “All participants achieved

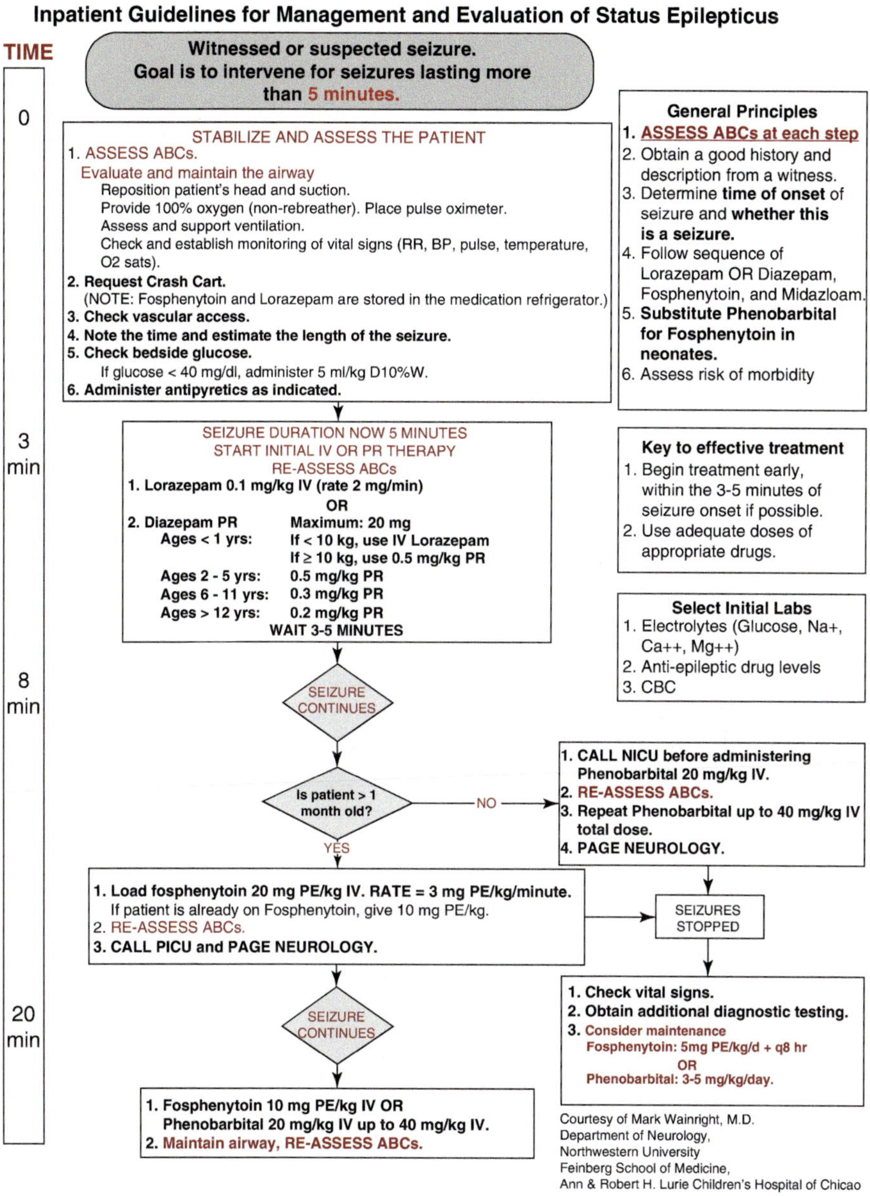

Fig. 2.1 Inpatient guidelines for management and evaluation of status epilepticus. (Source: Malakooti et al. [3]. Reprinted with permission from the Accreditation Council on Graduate Medical Education)

mastery of the algorithm after debriefing and deliberate practice; the majority of participants required 2 simulation and debriefing sessions." Finally, "All participants highly rated the educational intervention (median grade 8 of 10). All reported a preference for simulation-based learning with debriefing over other didactic models, and reported feeling that it had better prepared them to manage SE" [3].

A mastery learning curriculum like the SE program must be planned carefully and in detail, implemented and managed with skill and care, with a focus on the achievement of every learner. Chapter 3 in this volume on developing a mastery learning curriculum teaches how to address these educational goals. This is in sharp contrast with uncontrolled clinical learning environments described in Chap. 1 where the curriculum is embodied in random patients.

Mastery Learning Origins

The idea and practice of mastery learning are not new. The earliest expressions are seen in Carleton Washburne's Winnetka plan for elementary education in suburban Chicago [9] and in writing about secondary education from Professor Henry C. Morrison at the University of Chicago's Laboratory School [10]. Seminal scholarship by Harvard University professor John B. Carroll described educational mastery as "A model of school learning" in a formative journal article [11]. The Carroll model of school learning was grounded, in part, on behavioral psychology principles articulated by B.F. Skinner a decade earlier [12, 13].

Mastery learning and its variations, e.g., Keller's [14] and Keller and Sherman's [15] personalized system of instruction, gained traction in elementary, secondary, and higher education in the 1970s and 1980s. Scholarship about mastery learning also grew in that time period with major contributions by Benjamin Bloom [16, 17]; James Block [18, 19]; Block and Burns [20]; Block and Anderson [21]; Thomas Guskey [22]; and Kay Pomerance Torshen [23]. Several meta-analyses [24, 25] and narrative reviews [26, 27] and an empirical report [28] present strong evidence that mastery learning programs have positive effects on student cognitive, affective, communication, and skill learning in the biological and social sciences, mathematics and statistics, medicine, languages, business, library science, and other fields. In short, the mastery learning legacy is one of great effectiveness with learners at all educational levels in a wide variety of academic disciplines.

The Carroll [11] "model of school learning" extensions by Bloom [16, 17] and more recent writings [29] set the intellectual foundation for mastery learning for the last 50 years. The mastery learning idea is very plain and rests on four assumptions:

1. Educational excellence is expected and can be achieved by all learners who are able and motivated and work hard. Nearly all health professions learners have these attributes due to rigorous screening, careful selection, and strong achievement motives.
2. Little or no variation in measured outcome among learners will be seen in a mastery environment.
3. Learning in any domain, no matter how complex, depends on learning a sequence of less complex components. By dissecting a complex domain into a chain of elements, and ensuring learner mastery of each link in the chain, it should be possible for any learner to master even complex skills.

4. If students are distributed normally regarding aptitude or readiness to learn a subject and then receive uniform instruction in terms of educational quality and learning time, then student achievement will also be distributed normally. "However, if students are normally distributed on aptitude but each learner received optimal quality of instruction and the learning time required, then a majority of students could be expected to attain mastery" [18].

Psychological Foundations

Mastery learning is grounded in three psychological traditions. The traditions are complementary theoretical frameworks that together provide a foundation for curriculum design; instruction, deliberate practice, and faculty coaching; formative and summative evaluation; feedback and its interpretation; and short-run and downstream learning outcomes. The three psychological foundations, illustrated in Fig. 2.2, are behavioral, constructivist, and social cognitive.

Behavioral

The behavioral framework has roots in a positivist philosophy governed by the principle of objectivity with specific, discoverable, natural laws. In education, its focus is on behavior change and improvement. Behaviorism originated in early scientific psychology and found its peak in the science and writing of B. F. Skinner [12, 13] in the mid-twentieth century. Practical expressions of behaviorism in health professions education include behavioral learning objectives; deliberate practice with supervision and coaching; rigorous, reliable measurement of observable behavior; and immediate, specific, and actionable feedback in service of performance improvement. Behavior

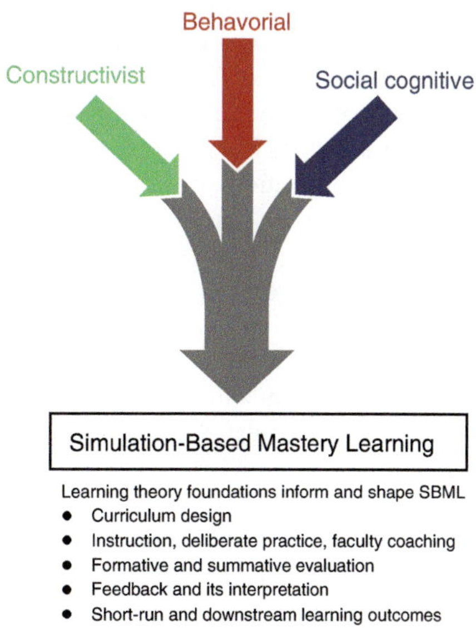

Fig. 2.2 Theoretical foundations of mastery learning. (Source: McGaghie and Harris [30]. Reprinted with permission from the Society for Simulation in Healthcare)

change, testing, teaching, and coaching in this framework are complementary educational activities that not only boost clinical competence among learners but also enhance memory—the mnemonic effect of testing [31]. For example, citing a learning retention study of advanced cardiac life support (ACLS) published by Wayne et al. [32], Larsen, Butler, and Roediger [31] state, "... teaching cardiac life support through a simulation prevents forgetting of this knowledge over time. This finding could be interpreted as a testing effect because the simulations serve as hands-on tests."

Constructivist

Professional competence is far more complicated than responding correctly to serial order checklist items. Knowledge, understanding, service, and professionalism are in many ways socially constructed realities mediated by language and shared meaning that are open to multiple interpretations. Medical experts, for example, may disagree about the best approach and solution to many clinical problems because most clinical problems have more than one correct answer. Learning from the constructivist perspective is an active process of constructing meaning, motivated by authentic problems. Constructivist learning goals not only include knowledge and skill acquisition and interpretation but also self-direction and mindfulness. The constructivist perspective sees teachers as facilitators rather than coaches [33–35].

Cheung et al. [36] recently reported a mastery learning study that included an observational practice component before hands-on deliberate practice of central venous catheter (CVC) skills. The observational practice feature was intended to help learners acquire a mental model of the clinical task to prime skill learning and enhance learner motivation. Observational practice greatly improved the efficiency and effectiveness of the CVC mastery learning curriculum. This conforms with recent writing by Ericsson and Pool [37], "The purpose of deliberate practice [a core principle of mastery learning] is to develop effective mental representations … mental representations in turn play a key role in deliberate practice." Ericsson and Pool [37] continue, "The more effective the mental representation is, the better the performance will be." Finally, "In any area, the relationship between skill and mental representations is a *virtuous circle*: the more skilled you become, the better your mental representations are, and the better your mental representations are, the more effectively you can practice to hone your skill."

Social Cognitive

The social cognitive theoretical perspective frames learning and professional development as situated events because learning and behavior occur in context. A substantial proportion of learning in the health professions, including professional socialization, is situated in the clinical workplace in addition to controlled laboratory settings. This makes the social cognitive framework a useful model for curriculum development and especially for outcome evaluation [38].

A key concept in the social cognitive model is the formation and maintenance of self-efficacy (S-E), the belief in one's capabilities to organize and execute the courses of action needed to manage prospective situations. Self-efficacy is believing in oneself to take action.

Albert Bandura is a thought leader in the social cognitive realm. Two of Bandura's seminal books *Social Foundations of Thought and Action: A Social Cognitive Theory* [39] and *Self-Efficacy: The Exercise of Control* [40] provide detailed accounts of the social cognitive perspective in general and S-E in particular. Bandura and other social cognitive scholars view people as self-organizing, proactive, self-regulating, and self-reflecting, not just reactive organisms shaped by environmental forces or driven by inner impulses.

In health professions education S-E is a *product* of mastery, not a *source* of mastery. As an educational outcome, S-E refers to a student's confidence to participate in activities that will help achieve clear goals. Self-regulation helps individuals set future goals and manage behavior and plans to reach them: goal setting, self-monitoring, and self-influence. Research shows there is an in-kind rise in clinical S-E as learners acquire clinical skills and sharpen their mental representations in a mastery learning environment. Behavioral, cognitive, and affective growth occur simultaneously [3, 41, 42].

The three theoretical frameworks capture the dynamic interplay of behavioral, cognitive, and affective features of competence in the health professions which are often separated in educational settings but are unified in practice.

Mastery Learning Model

John Carroll's [11] "model of school learning" is expressed as a simple formula shown in Fig. 2.3 from Block [18] that postulates the degree of learning in educational settings is shaped by five variables. Two variables that address time spent are in the numerator: (a) time allowed and (b) perseverance. Three are denominator variables that address time needed: (a) aptitude, (b) quality of instruction, and (c) ability to understand instruction. The mastery learning model states in its most basic form that the degree of learning is expressed as a ratio of time spent on learning/ time needed for learning.

Time Allowed

The time allowed for learning is an index of opportunity, a measure of the temporal distance from the start of instruction in any form to its conclusion. Time allowed is fixed, uniform, in most educational settings. Examples include hourly class

Mastery learning

$$\text{Degree of learning} = f\left(\frac{\text{1. Time allowed 2. Perseverance}}{\begin{array}{l}\text{3. Aptitude 4. Quality of instruction}\\ \text{5. Ability to understand instruction}\end{array}}\right) = \frac{\text{Time spent}}{\text{Time needed}}$$

Fig. 2.3 Formula for the mastery learning model. (From Block [18]. Reprinted with permission from the publisher)

schedules, curriculum blocks, semesters, and academic years. Clocks and calendars govern educational time allowed and usually produce wide variation in measured educational achievement. The mastery learning model, by contrast, is not governed by clock or calendar time. Instead, it permits learning time to vary among students.

Perseverance

John Carroll [11] defines perseverance as "... the time the learner is willing to spend on learning." Motivation, the desire to learn, is a synonym for perseverance. Perseverance is captured by K. Anders Ericsson's [43] concept of deliberate practice which embodies goal orientation, full concentration, and repetitive practice toward a target performance supervised by a coach or teacher that produces or depends on effective mental representations, formative measurement, feedback from faculty in service of improvement, and continued hard work to achieve a (mastery) MPS. Reaching a MPS is a powerful reinforcement for learners that goes far beyond pleasing one's teachers, peers, or friends or to achieve external rewards like academic honors or making the Dean's List.

Aptitude

Aptitudes are current capabilities. They are expressed as measures of readiness to do, or learn to do, academic, social, vocational, professional, or other tasks easily and quickly. Aptitudes are an ability baseline. Aptitudes are prospective indexes of capacity to acquire and refine a broader and deeper set of skills, knowledge, dispositions, and competencies needed for life and work.

Aptitudes are multidimensional, not unitary. Scholars have pointed out for decades that, like intelligence, measures of aptitude have many faces—verbal, numerical, mechanical, spatial visualization, motor control, social and interpersonal, practical—and a host of others [44, 45]. Some aptitudes are clear and can be measured objectively, but many—especially for professional practice—are tacit [46]. Our success at incorporating indices of aptitude into the mastery learning model stems from research and experience at recognizing reliable markers of professional readiness.

John Carroll's [11] notion about educational readiness was much more basic and did not reside in test assessment batteries or psychometric detail. He wrote, instead, that

> ... the amount of time the pupil will need to learn the task under these conditions is the primary measure of a variable which we shall call his *aptitude for learning this task.* In ordinary parlance, learners who need only a small amount of time are said to have high aptitude; learners who need a large amount of time are said to have low aptitude.

In short, Carroll's argument is that for most students learning is governed chiefly by quality time-on-task rather than innate ability.

Quality of Instruction

Instructional quality refers to a set of conditions controlled by a teacher or an instructional designer who prepares materials for teaching or other educational experiences. The conditions include clear learning expectations expressed as objectives; systematic and coherent organization of concepts and skills to be learned; learning tasks presented in an order that uses them as cumulative building blocks; and rigorous assessments that provide reliable data for feedback and improvement. John Carroll [11] states, "This variable applies not only to the performance of a teacher but also to the characteristics of textbooks, workbooks, films, teaching-machine programs, etc."

If instructional quality is imperfect—a fair assumption in most educational settings—then most learners will need more time than needed under ideal conditions. According to Carroll [11] "Some learners will be more handicapped by poor instruction than others."

Ability to Understand Instruction

One's ability to understand instruction derives from a combination of general intelligence; verbal ability; prior experience in the learning domain; and the ability to comprehend, sort out, conceptualize, and solve problems with learning material that may be complicated, such as renal physiology, or presented with low instructional quality. Carroll [11] notes, "Learners with high ability in this respect will be able to figure out for themselves what the learning task is and how they can go about learning it; they will be able to overcome the difficulties presented by poor quality of instruction by perceiving concepts and relationships in the teaching materials which will not be grasped by those with lesser abilities."

Features of Mastery Learning

The discussion about the origins of mastery learning and components of the mastery model cast as a ratio or formula (Fig. 2.3) are insufficient to tell how it works in practice. Nurses, physical therapists, physicians, and other health professions educators ask, "How can we create or revise curricula to incorporate mastery learning? What does it take?"

The mastery learning model is a bundle of seven complementary features:

1. Baseline or diagnostic testing
2. Clear learning objectives
3. Educational activities
4. MPSs
5. Formative testing with actionable feedback
6. Evidence-based advancement
7. Continued practice and assessment until the MPS is reached [47–49]

Baseline, Diagnostic Testing

Baseline testing, assessment of learner knowledge, skill, acumen, or disposition before instruction, is a key feature of mastery learning. It is the first mastery learning educational intervention. Baseline testing is a cardinal example of "test enhanced learning" [31] that gives learners performance feedback. It tells learners where they stand on measures of professional fitness before instruction begins. Baseline test data must have high reliability to be useful, i.e., the data must have high "signal" and low "noise" [50]. Baseline data set a foundation, a point-of-departure, to start progress toward mastery. This is the first milestone on the mastery learning roadmap.

Clear Learning Objectives

Educational objectives set expectations. Objectives tell learners what needs to get done. Objectives inform learners about the knowledge, skills, dispositions, or signs of professionalism that need to be acquired and suggest how these achievements will be measured. Medical students, for example, are expected to acquire textbook knowledge about glucose metabolism to understand the pathophysiology of Type 2 diabetes: Glycosylated hemoglobin (HbA1c), anion gap, and other markers. Medical students are also expected to learn the communication skills needed to counsel diabetic patients about diet, exercise, and lifestyle for health promotion. The timing and order of these learning expectations may vary across medical school curricula but their presence is certain. These and many other educational objectives address core learning outcomes that most medical educators agree all physicians must master.

Learning objectives in a mastery environment are usually packaged as instructional units. The units are sequential building blocks from, say, A to Z, which move learners from simple to relatively more complex learning material. Fulfillment of unit A learning objectives is a sign of readiness to engage unit B objectives. The list continues in sequence and may move at a varied pace. Instructional units may be broad (e.g., pulmonary physiology) or discrete (e.g., inserting a urinary catheter), yet the principle is simple and straightforward—master each step on the staircase and then move ahead.

Educational Activities

Educational activities in a mastery learning setting are driven by demand. The activities focus on what is needed to reach stated educational objectives—reading, discussion, video observation, problem-based learning groups, calculations, deliberate practice of essential skills, feedback, and reflection. All educational approaches are valued and have a place. Psychologist and Nobel Laureate Daniel Kahneman [51] has it right:

> The acquisition of skills requires a regular environment, an adequate opportunity to practice, and rapid and unequivocal feedback about the correctness of thoughts and actions. When these conditions are fulfilled, skill eventually develops, and the intuitive judgments and choices that quickly come to mind will mostly be accurate.

Consider, for example, the five educational activities used to help Northwestern Memorial Hospital second year internal medicine residents achieve mastery of ACLS skills [42]. First, the residents must pass an American Heart Association 1-day provider course that has for decades been considered the "gold standard" of ACLS education, although its educational utility is in doubt [42]. Second, the residents read about in-hospital "code blue" events that trigger an ACLS response. Third, the residents undergo pretests on a high-fidelity simulator of six in-hospital "code blue" scenarios (e.g., asystole, ventricular tachycardia) that warrant an ACLS response. Fourth, the residents engage in rigorous deliberate practice [43] of ACLS patient care skills using the simulator (e.g., problem recognition, patient evaluation, obtaining patient consent, chest compressions, bag valve mask (BVM) oxygenation, drug administration, team leadership) needed for life-saving maneuvers. Fifth, the learners take a posttest, receive performance feedback, reflect about their work, continue with practice until the MPS is reached, enjoy ACLS mastery status and recognition, and feel ready to respond to a real "code blue" on the hospital floors. Chapter 11 in this volume, "Mastery Learning of Team Skills," amplifies the discussion of Northwestern ACLS education and offers more examples of powerful educational activities.

These educational activities are planned, scheduled, organized, and required—there are no exceptions. The ACLS education is mandatory, not left to chance, and does not follow the obsolete "see one, do one, teach one" educational routine still prevalent in clinical education settings across the health professions [43]. Learners and teachers are very engaged in these ACLS mastery education sessions—both groups work very hard.

The educational activities needed to help medical learners master ACLS knowledge and skills are not much different from those needed to educate and evaluate health professionals in a wide range of competencies, for example, engaging patients and their families about end-of-life discussions (Chap. 10); teamwork for patient safety at clinical "handoffs" and medication reconciliation (Chap. 11); mastering surgical skills (Chap. 12); and performance of invasive clinical procedures (Chap. 13). Educational events and engagements must be targeted to learning objectives. In health professions education these activities usually involve some type of planned and organized deliberate practice with reliable outcome evaluation.

Minimum Passing Standards

How much learning is enough? How can health professions educators be assured that students are ready to advance in the curriculum or care for patients with or without supervision? These are questions of mastery learning standards.

Classroom education passing standards in the health professions have been set historically "on the curve," in a competitive, normative way. Educational achievement has been defined as topping one's peers, on a written academic examination, usually expressed in standard deviation units, using the Gaussian normal curve. Scoring in the top 10% or 15% of test achievement has been the source of honors, academic recognition, and future career opportunities such as competitive postgraduate medical residency slots and advancements in other health professions.

Passing standards in clinical education settings have been clouded historically. Evaluations in medical clerkships, residency rotations, fellowship experiences, and similar activities in other health professions are usually done via fallible supervisor ratings that neither distinguish learner individual differences nor judge learner achievement against a competency standard [52]. Student failure in clinical settings rarely happens due to a lack of attention and rigorous assessments. False-positive advancement decisions about clinical learners are likely common but are documented rarely.

The situation is very different in a mastery learning environment. A MPS is set for each educational unit, ideally by an expert faculty panel, using state-of-the-art methods. See Chap. 6 of this volume for a detailed and practical account of standard setting for mastery learning. Until recently, mastery learning MPSs for evaluating clinical learning in the health professions have been set using procedures best suited to written tests of classroom performance: Angoff, Hofstee, and several others [53, 54]. However, the work of Rachel Yudkowsky and her colleagues at the University of Illinois College of Medicine in Chicago has improved traditional standard setting methods by introducing an approach grounded in patient safety [55, 56]. The patient safety approach to setting mastery learning standards usually sets a very "high bar" that learners must reach (Chap. 6).

Formative Testing with Feedback

Formative testing, i.e., "assessment for learning," is an essential part of the mastery learning model because it gives learners knowledge about their learning results as they move through educational material. Formative testing in a mastery learning environment uses reliable assessment data as a tool, not as a weapon [31]. Learners are measured frequently beginning with a pretest; learning gaps are identified; trainees receive performance feedback, practice deliberately with faculty coaching, and undergo more testing until the MPS is reached. The line between education and evaluation (testing) is no longer distinct because instruction and assessment coalesce as complementary partners in a dynamic training environment [57].

The role of feedback to learners in clinical education is essential, yet is frequently ignored. Several research reviews spanning decades of medical education research [58, 59] document the importance of performance feedback that is timely, focused, and actionable, for the acquisition of mastery learning clinical education goals. The importance of feedback in clinical medical education is addressed in Chaps. 8 and 9 in this volume.

Evidence-Based Advancement

Learner achievement in a mastery learning curriculum is based on objective measures of knowledge and skill acquisition that yield reliable performance data. Lineberry and colleagues teach that "... adopting a mastery learning system requires clear specification about how assessment scores will be interpreted and used" [60]. Lineberry et al. also state, "... the most important relationship to evaluate in a mastery learning system is whether assessment scores relate to learners' success in their subsequent educational unit(s), including their eventual transition to practice" [60]. The key issue is the reliability of the decision, based on assessment data, to allow a learner to advance in the curriculum.

Evidence-based advancement also suggests that the mastery learning model has promise not only for undergraduate and graduate degree programs in the health professions but also for continuing education and lifelong learning [47] (Chap. 18).

Continued Practice and Assessment

Learners in a mastery learning system will not reach the "finish line" at the same time. Instructional quality inefficiencies and learner variation in aptitude and perseverance will conspire to produce differences in the time needed to reach the MPS. Most students will progress without delay while a handful, usually about 10–20%, need more time for knowledge and skill acquisition beyond usual curriculum allocations [3, 42]. Most educational settings can find flexibility to accommodate variation in student time needed to reach the MPS including repeated study, deliberate practice, and testing. Trainees in nursing, medicine, pharmacy, physical therapy, and other health professions are also driven and eager to do well. Motivation to learn and perform is rarely an issue.

In the statistics course described at the start of this chapter, students who finished unit tests early served as tutors for others who needed more time. Peer tutoring had valuable academic and social consequences because all students eventually passed the unit tests and also formed lasting friendships. Learning, teaching, and social bonds coalesced.

Examples from the Health Professions

The power and utility of the mastery learning model are evident from descriptions of three successful educational programs in the health professions: (a) undergraduate nursing, (b) undergraduate medicine, and (c) postgraduate surgery. Each program uses the mastery model to educate learners to high and uniform performance standards.

Undergraduate Nursing

Melanie Cason and her colleagues at HealthCare Simulation of the Medical University of South Carolina in Charleston, SC, created a curriculum involving cooperative learning and simulation technology to help associate degree and baccalaureate nursing students achieve mastery of nasogastric tube insertion [61]. Their program employed "cooperative learning simulation skills training (CLSST) in the context of nasogastric tube insertion using a deliberate practice-to-mastery learning model." Cason et al. report that "Student dyads served as operator and student learner." "Student pairs alternated roles until they achieved mastery, after which they were assessed individually." Flawless checklist scores were achieved by the students due to hard work and rigorous feedback regarding this educational innovation. "CLSST in a deliberate practice-to-mastery learning paradigm offers a novel way to teach psychomotor skills in nursing curricula and decreases the instructor-to-student ratio" [61].

Undergraduate Medicine

Emergency Medicine (EM) physician Trent Reed and his colleagues at the Loyola University Chicago Stritch School of Medicine created a simulation-based, standardized evaluation to assess senior (fourth year) medical student acquisition and retention of six core clinical skills: (a) ultrasound-guided peripheral IV placement, (b) basic skin laceration repair, (c) chest compressions, (d) BVM ventilation, (e) defibrillator management, and (f) code leadership [62]. The student evaluation plan is embedded in a larger "readiness for residency" program under development at Loyola to better prepare all fourth year medical students for the rigors of postgraduate medical education.

Dr. Reed and other EM physicians developed the six procedural skills curricula, created and pilot tested measurement checklists, and derived MPS to test mastery of the six skills. Reed et al. report, "One hundred thirty five students on an emergency medicine clerkship were pretested on all six skills, viewed online videos asynchronously followed by a multiple choice computer-based skill-related quiz, received one-on-one hands-on skill training using deliberate practice with feedback, and were post-tested until MPS was met" [62]. The investigators compared pretest and posttest performances among the medical students. They also re-tested a sample of the students 1–9 months later to assess skill retention.

The results show that all students passed all six skill examinations, without exception, with slight variation in time-to-MPS. In addition, "Ninety eight percent of the students scored at or above the MPS when retested 1–9 months later" [62]. These data are presented in Fig. 2.4. The medical students rated the mastery learning education and evaluation experience very high. The investigators conclude, "Simulation-based mastery learning using a substantial asynchronous component is an effective way for senior medical students to learn and retain emergency medicine clinical skills" [62].

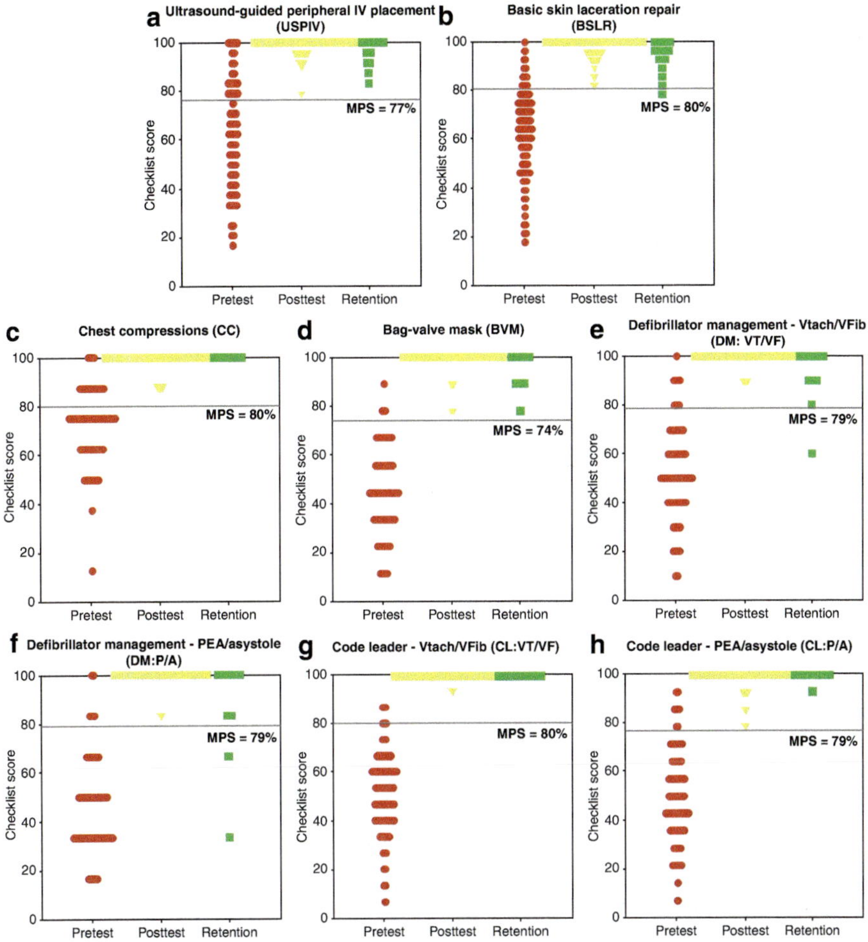

Fig. 2.4 (**a**) Ultrasound-guided peripheral IV. (**b**) Basic skin laceration repair. (**c**) Chest compressions. (**d**) Bag-valve mask ventilation. (**e**) Defibrillator management VT/VF. (**f**) Defibrillator management PEA/A. (**g**) Code leadership: VT/VF. (**h**) Code leadership: P/A. MPS, minimum passing standard. (Source: Reed et al. [62]. Reprinted with permission from the Society for Simulation in Healthcare)

Postgraduate Surgery

Northwestern University surgeon Dr. Ezra Teitelbaum and his colleagues developed and tested, "A simulator-based resident curriculum for laporascopic common bile duct exploration [LCBDE]" [63]. The LCBDE surgical procedure is considered an underused treatment for symptomatic gallstone disease chiefly because surgical residents are rarely exposed to the procedure during clinical training.

The project began by designing, fabricating, and testing a novel procedural simulator for LCBDE [64]. "The simulator allows for performance of both transcystic and transcholedochal LCBDE via the use of real instruments and a choledochoscope, while reproducing the three imaging modalities (laparoscopic, choledochoscopic, and fluoroscopic) necessary for the procedure" [63].

The residents participated in a pretest-posttest mastery learning skill acquisition study using the LCBDE simulator with deliberate practice and feedback. As expected, all ten residents did not meet the MPS set for the transcystic LCBDE pretest. However, given a powerful educational intervention involving reading, observing surgical videos, and deliberate practice in the simulation laboratory, all residents passed the transcystic LCBDE posttest at the first attempt. Training procedures and testing results were similar for transcholedochal LCBDE except that two residents did not meet the MPS on the first posttest yet reached the MPS after more deliberate practice and retesting. Resident confidence about performing both LCBDE surgeries improved significantly as a consequence of simulation-based training to mastery learning standards.

Coda

This chapter has described the origins and features of the mastery learning model and has provided evidence about its utility in health professions education. Much more powerful evidence favoring technology-enhanced mastery learning vs. traditional clinical education in the health professions derives from a recent meta-analytic literature review of 82 eligible studies [65]. The results show that mastery learning programs are associated with large effects on skills and moderate effects on patient outcomes compared to no intervention. Large benefits for mastery learning were also demonstrated compared to traditional education but required a little more time. The authors conclude, "The mastery model may be particularly relevant to competency-based education, given the shared emphasis on defined objectives rather than defined learning time" [65].

Figure 2.5 is an infographic published previously in *Academic Medicine* that gives a thumbnail summary of the mastery learning model including its features, procedures, and intended outcomes [66]. Subsequent chapters in this book will describe how to build, deliver, and evaluate mastery learning educational programs in the health professions.

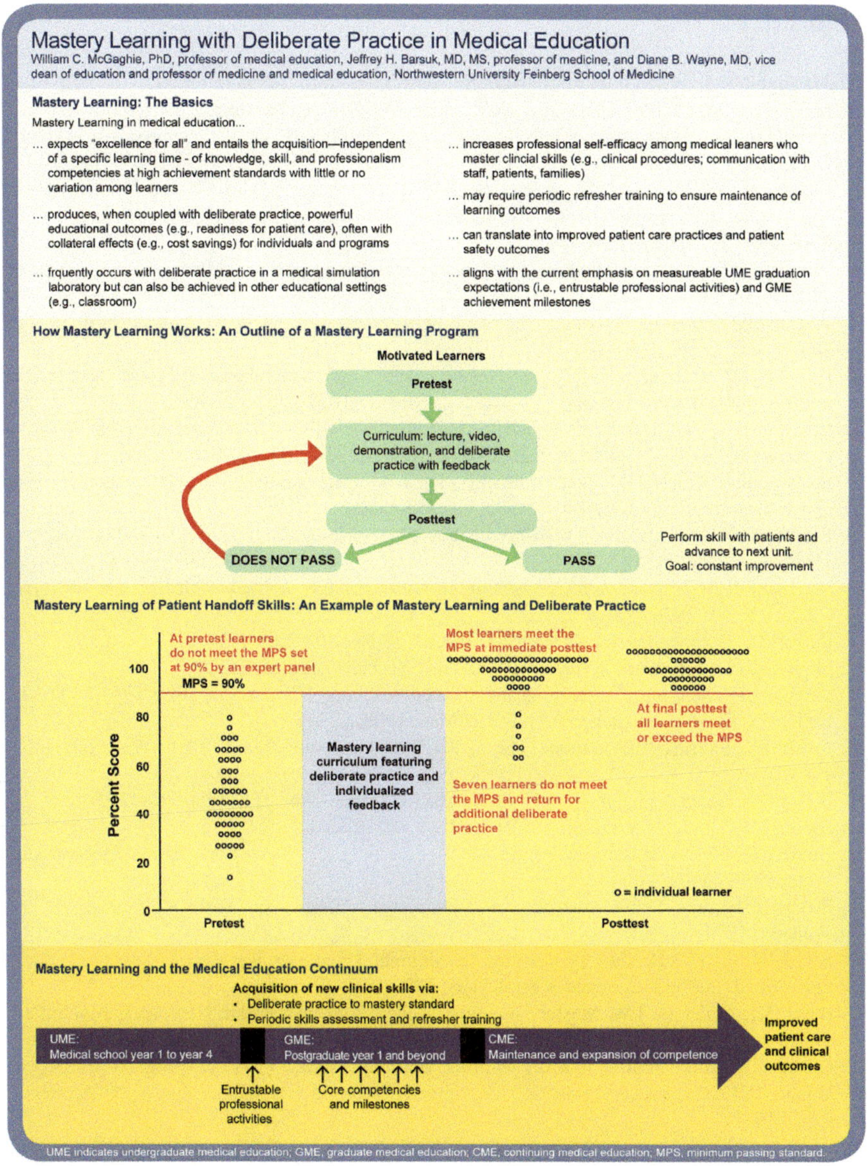

Fig. 2.5 Mastery learning with deliberate practice in medical education. (Source: McGaghie et al. [66]. Reprinted with permission from the Association of American Medical Colleges)

References

1. McGaghie WC. When I say … mastery learning. Med Educ. 2015;49:558–9.
2. McGaghie WC, Miller GE, Sajid AW, Telder TV. Competency-based curriculum development in medical education: an introduction. Public health paper no. 68. Geneva: World Health Organization; 1978.
3. Malakooti MR, McBride ME, Mobley B, Goldstein JL, Adler MD, McGaghie WC. Mastery of status epilepticus management via simulation-based learning for pediatrics residents. J Grad Med Educ. 2015;7(2):181–6.
4. Mitchell WG. Status epilepticus and acute serial seizures in children. J Clin Neurol. 2002;17(Suppl. 1):36–43.
5. Walker DM, Teach SJ. Update on the acute management of status epilepticus in children. Curr Opin Ped. 2006;18(3):239–44.
6. Ericsson KA. Deliberate practice and the acquisition and maintenance of expert performance in medicine and related domains. Acad Med. 2004;79(10, Suppl):S70–81.
7. Ericsson KA, Charness N, Feltovich PJ, Hoffman RR, editors. The Cambridge handbook of expertise and expert performance. New York: Cambridge University Press; 2006.
8. Ericsson KA, Krampe RT, Tesch-Römer C. The role of deliberate practice in the acquisition of expert performance. Psychol Rev. 1993;100:363–406.
9. Washburne CW. Educational measurement as a key to individual instruction and promotions. J Educ Res. 1922;5(3):195–206.
10. Morrison HC. The practice of teaching in the secondary school. Chicago: University of Chicago Press; 1926.
11. Carroll JB. A model of school learning. Teach Coll Rec. 1963;64:723–33.
12. Skinner BF. Science and human behavior. New York: Macmillan; 1953.
13. Skinner BF. The science of learning and the art of teaching. Harvard Educ Rev. 1954;24:86–97.
14. Keller FS. Good-bye, teacher. J Appl Beh Anal. 1968;1:79–89.
15. Keller FS, Sherman JG, editors. The Keller Plan handbook. Menlo Park: W.A. Benjamin; 1974.
16. Bloom BS. Learning for mastery. UCLA Eval Comment. 1968;1(2, Whole No. 2):1–12.
17. Bloom BS. Time and learning. Am Psychol. 1974;29:682–8.
18. Block JH, editor. Mastery learning: theory and practice. New York: Holt, Rinehart and Winston; 1971.
19. Block JH, editor. Schools, society, and mastery learning. New York: Holt, Rinehart and Winston; 1974.
20. Block JH, Burns RB. Mastery learning. In: Shulman LS, editor. Review of research in education. 4th ed. Itasca: F.E. Peacock Publishers; 1974. p. 3–49.
21. Block JH, Anderson LW. Mastery learning in classroom instruction. New York: Macmillan; 1975.
22. Guskey TR. Implementing mastery learning. Belmont: Wadsworth Publishing Co.; 1985.
23. Torshen KP. The mastery approach to competency-based education. New York: Academic Press; 1977.
24. Kulik C-L, Kulik JA, Bangert-Downs RL. Effectiveness of mastery learning programs: a meta-analysis. Rev Educ Res. 1990;60(2):265–99.
25. Kulik JA, Kulik C-L, Cohen PA. A meta-analysis of outcome studies of Keller's personalized system of instruction. Am Psychol. 1979;34(4):307–18.
26. Guskey TR. Closing achievements gaps: revisiting Benjamin S. Bloom's learning for mastery. J Advan Acad. 2007;19(1):8–31.
27. Kulik JA, Kulik C-L, Carmichael K. The Keller Plan in science. Science. 1974;183(4123):379–83.
28. Schwartz PL. A controlled trial of teaching clinical biochemistry by the Keller Plan. J Med Educ. 1980;55(12):1013–20.
29. McGaghie WC. Mastery learning: it is time for medical education to join the 21st century. Acad Med. 2015;90(11):1438–41.

30. McGaghie WC, Harris IB. Learning theory foundations of simulation-based mastery learning. Simul Healthc. 2018;13(3, Suppl):S15–20.
31. Larsen DP, Butler A, Roediger HL. Test-enhanced learning in medical education. Med Educ. 2008;42(10):959–66.
32. Wayne DB, Siddall VJ, Butter J, Fudala MJ, Wade LD, Feinglass J, McGaghie WC. A longitudinal study of internal medicine residents' retention of advanced cardiac life support skills. Acad Med. 2006;81(10, Suppl):S9–S12.
33. Harris I. Conceptions and theories of learning for workplace education. In: Hafler J, editor. Extraordinary learning in the workplace. New York: Springer; 2011. p. 39–62.
34. Schön DA. Educating the reflective practitioner: toward a new design for teaching and learning in the professions. San Francisco: Jossey-Bass; 1987.
35. Sternberg RJ, Forsythe GB, Hedlund J, Horvath JA, Wagner RK, Williams WM, Snook SA, Grigorenko EL. Practical intelligence in everyday life. New York: Cambridge University Press; 2000.
36. Cheung JJH, Koh J, Brett C, Bägli DJ, Kapralos B, Dubrowski A. Preparation with web-based observational practice improves efficiency of simulation-based mastery learning. Simul Healthc. 2016;11(5):316–22.
37. Ericsson A, Pool R. Peak: secrets from the new science of expertise. Boston: Houghton Mifflin Harcourt; 2016.
38. Singh T, Norcini JJ. Workplace-based assessment. In: McGaghie WC, editor. International best practices for evaluation in the health professions. London: Radcliffe Publishing, Ltd; 2013. p. 257–79.
39. Bandura A. Social foundations of thought and action: a social cognitive theory. Englewood Cliffs: Prentice-Hall; 1986.
40. Bandura A. Self-efficacy: the exercise of control. New York: W.H. Freeman; 1997.
41. Barsuk JH, Cohen ER, Mikolajczak A, Seburn S, Slade M, Wayne DB. Simulation-based mastery learning improves central line maintenance skills of ICU nurses. J Nurs Adm. 2015;45(10):511–7.
42. Wayne DB, Butter J, Siddall VJ, Fudala MJ, Wade LD, Feinglass J, McGaghie WC. Mastery learning of advanced cardiac life support skills by internal medicine residents using simulation technology and deliberate practice. J Gen Intern Med. 2006;21:251–6.
43. Ericsson KA. Acquisition and maintenance of medical expertise: a perspective from the expert performance approach with deliberate practice. Acad Med. 2015;90(11):1471–86.
44. Cronbach LJ, Snow RE. Aptitudes and instructional methods: a handbook for research on interactions. New York: Irvington Publishers; 1981.
45. Sternberg RJ, editor. Handbook of intelligence. New York: Cambridge University Press; 2000.
46. Sternberg RJ, Horvath JA, editors. Tacit knowledge in professional practice: researcher and practitioner perspectives. Mahwah: Lawrence Erlbaum Associates; 1999.
47. McGaghie WC, Siddall VJ, Mazmanian PE, Myers J. Lessons for continuing medical education from simulation research in undergraduate and graduate medical education: effectiveness of continuing medical education: American College of Chest Physicians evidence-based educational guidelines. Chest. 2009;135(3, Suppl):62S–8S.
48. McGaghie WC, Kristopaitis T. Deliberate practice and mastery learning: origins of expert medical performance. In: Cleland J, Durning SJ, editors. Researching medical education. Oxford, UK: Wiley-Blackwell; 2015. p. 219–30.
49. Issenberg SB, McGaghie WC. Looking to the future. In: McGaghie WC, editor. International best practices for evaluation in the health professions. London: Radcliffe Publishing, Ltd; 2013. p. 341–59.
50. Axelson RD, Kreiter CD. Reliability. In: Downing SM, Yudkowsky R, editors. Assessment in health professions education. New York: Routledge; 2009. p. 57–73.
51. Kahneman D. Thinking, fast and slow. New York: Farrar, Straus and Giroux; 2011.
52. Williams RG, Klamen DA, McGaghie WC. Cognitive, social, and environmental sources of bias in clinical competence ratings. Teach Learn Med. 2003;15(4):270–92.

53. Wayne DB, Fudala MJ, Butter J, Siddall VJ, Feinglass J, Wade LD, McGaghie WC. Comparison of two standard-setting methods for advanced cardiac life support training. Acad Med. 2005;80(10, Suppl):S63–6.
54. Yudkowsky R, Downing SM, Tekian A. Standard setting. In: Downing SM, Yudkowsky R, editors. Assessment in health professions education. New York: Routledge; 2009. p. 119–48.
55. Yudkowsky R, Tumuluru S, Casey P, Herlich N, Ledonne C. A patient safety approach to setting pass/fail standards for basic procedural skills checklists. Simul Healthc. 2014;9:277–82.
56. Yudkowsky R, Park YS, Lineberry M, Knox A, Ritter EM. Setting mastery learning standards. Acad Med. 2015;90(11):1495–500.
57. Grigorenko EL, Sternberg RJ. Dynamic testing. Psychol Bull. 1998;124(1):75–111.
58. Issenberg SB, McGaghie WC, Petrusa ER, Gordon DJ, Scalese RJ. Features and uses of high-fidelity medical simulations that lead to effective learning: a BEME systematic review. Med Teach. 2005;27(1):10–25.
59. van de Ridder JMM, Stokking KM, McGaghie WC, ten Cate OT. What is feedback in clinical education? Med Educ. 2008;42:189–97.
60. Lineberry M, Park YS, Cook DA, Yudkowsky R. Making the case for mastery learning assessments: key issues in validation and justification. Acad Med. 2015;90(11):1445–50.
61. Cason ML, Gilbert GE, Schmoll HH, Dolinar SM, Anderson J, Nickles BM, Pufpaff LA, Henderson R, Lee FW, Schaefer JJ. Cooperative learning using simulation to achieve mastery of nasogastric tube insertion. J Nurs Educ. 2015;54(3 Suppl):S47–51.
62. Reed T, Pirotte M, McHugh M, Oh L, Lovett S, Hoyt AE, Quinones D, Adams W, Gruener G, McGaghie WC. Simulation-based mastery learning improves medical student performance and retention of core clinical skills. Simul Healthc. 2016;11(3):173–80.
63. Teitelbaum EN, Soper NJ, Santos BF, Rooney DM, Patel P, Nagle AP, Hungness ES. A simulator-based resident curriculum for laparoscopic common bile duct exploration. Surgery. 2014;156:880–93.
64. Santos BF, Reif TJ, Soper NJ, Nagle AP, Rooney DM, Hungness ES. Development and evaluation of a laparoscopic common bile duct exploration simulator and procedural rating scale. Surg Endosc. 2012;26:2403–15.
65. Cook DA, Brydges R, Zendejas B, Hamstra SJ, Hatala R. Mastery learning for health professionals using technology-enhanced simulation: a systematic review and meta-analysis. Acad Med. 2013;88:1178–86.
66. McGaghie WC, Barsuk JH, Wayne DB. Mastery learning with deliberate practice in medical education (Last Page). Acad Med. 2015;90(11):1575.

Developing a Mastery Learning Curriculum

3

Jeffrey H. Barsuk and David H. Salzman

A 64-year-old male with a history of high blood pressure and diabetes arrived at the Emergency Department with atypical chest pain. His physical examination, laboratory tests, electrocardiogram, and chest x-ray were normal. He was admitted to the hospital telemetry unit for a stress test the next morning. At 11 PM, when the night doctors were covering, the patient developed a slow, but dangerous heart rhythm. The nurses called a doctor immediately. Then the patient's heart rhythm went into asystole (absence of electrical activity—flat line). A "code blue" was called, the cardiac arrest team answered, and cardiopulmonary resuscitation (CPR) was started. The scene was chaotic because the team seemed unfamiliar with the equipment, team leadership was unclear, and a nurse voiced concern about patient safety because the wrong medications were given. The clinical situation unraveled fast.

Fortunately, this was just a simulation. The healthcare providers in the simulation recently completed an American Heart Association (AHA) Advanced Cardiac Life Support (ACLS) provider course and should have been ready to treat the simulated patient. Research evidence suggests that the ACLS team responses prompted by the simulated case would likely be replicated when caring for a real patient [1].

Healthcare providers traditionally graduate and advance in training based on dated evaluation models. Many health professions schools still evaluate trainees using a normal distribution to determine passing standards where a standard deviation (or two) below the mean sets the passing score. This permits wide variation in graduates' skills and potentially substandard patient care. Clinical experiences,

J. H. Barsuk (✉)
Northwestern University Feinberg School of Medicine, Departments of Medicine and Medical Education, Chicago, IL, USA
e-mail: jbarsuk@northwestern.edu

D. H. Salzman
Northwestern University Feinberg School of Medicine, Departments of Emergency Medicine and Medical Education, Chicago, IL, USA

W. C. McGaghie et al. (eds.), *Comprehensive Healthcare Simulation: Mastery Learning in Health Professions Education*, Comprehensive Healthcare Simulation, https://doi.org/10.1007/978-3-030-34811-3_3

where learners participate in actual patient care with a supervisor, continue to rely on the classic Oslerian "see one, do one, teach one" apprenticeship model. These clinical experiences are often short and learners are not able to "see" many cases that represent healthcare practice. The apprenticeship model is especially illogical for rare or uncommon events because trainees often do not encounter these events during training [2]. In addition, many seasoned clinical teachers are not current with new procedures or were trained incorrectly [3]. This creates a situation where inaccurate skills and information are handed down from one generation of healthcare professionals to the next. These and other indictments of current clinical education are discussed in Chap. 1.

Mastery learning, described in Chap. 2, can contribute to the solution of this healthcare education problem. The Association of American Medical Colleges Entrustable Professional Activities (EPAs) project [4] and the Accreditation Council for Graduate Medical Education Milestones [5] are first steps toward certifying medical student and resident competence before graduation. Simulation-based mastery curricula conform with these frameworks. Chapter 17 provides a detailed discussion about undergraduate EPAs and postgraduate milestones in the context of mastery learning. Strong evidence shows that simulation-based mastery learning (SBML) produces better clinicians, improved patient care practices, and superior patient outcomes than traditional educational methods [6–10].

This chapter describes how to develop a SBML curriculum. First, we provide an overview about health professions curriculum development using a model created by Thomas, Kern and colleagues [11]. Second, we discuss the steps of mastery learning and demonstrate how the Thomas model can be augmented by mastery learning principles. Third, we provide an example of how we used these principles to develop a SBML curriculum for ACLS skills and convert it from a basic simulation experience to a mastery learning curriculum. Finally, we conclude with some challenges encountered when creating SBML curricula.

Curriculum Development

The word "curriculum" has Latin roots meaning "the course of a race." A curriculum is defined simply as a planned educational experience involving instruction and assessment. Health professions curricula have been developed using a variety of models ranging from subject centered to integrated and competency-based. However, the foundation that underlies all health professions curricula is that educators are preparing future healthcare workers to care for patients with skill and safety. A standardized approach simplifies curriculum development. Thomas and colleagues present a standardized model of health professions curriculum development that uses a six-step approach [11]. The six steps are:

1. Problem identification and general needs assessment
2. Targeted needs assessment
3. Goals and objectives

4. Educational strategies
5. Implementation
6. Evaluation and feedback

The Thomas curriculum development team proposes two more items to round out the stepwise approach: curriculum maintenance and enhancement, and dissemination. The Thomas model has been used to create and evaluate simulation-based medical education curricula to address a variety of clinical specialties including essential resuscitation skills for medical students [11], general surgery [12], and pediatrics [13].

Problem Identification and General Needs Assessment

A healthcare curriculum developer must first identify the specific problem the curriculum will address. Defining the problem is a critical step. Consider the example of the simulated cardiac arrest presented earlier. Is this a problem with team adherence to an ACLS algorithm? What about team communication skills? Could it be that team knowledge of ACLS is strong but teamwork and leadership are weak? Identifying and defining the education problem creates a roadmap that ensures all the subsequent curriculum development steps are focused.

Health professions curriculum developers should then perform a general needs assessment. The general needs assessment asks broad questions, such as the following: (a) How widespread is the healthcare problem that needs to be solved? (b) Is the current approach to this healthcare problem by patients, providers, hospitals, and social agencies appropriate? Do new healthcare approaches need to be created? The general needs assessment can be informed by many sources. Informed sources include health professions faculty observations that a procedural skill is not being performed effectively in the clinical environment, poor performance at meeting a local or national healthcare metric, critical incident reports, or regulatory agencies that require teaching core clinical competencies. General needs may also be informed by published studies that indicate better training is needed due to variability in physician performance of skills such as laparoscopic bariatric surgery [14].

Targeted Needs Assessment

The next step is to formulate a local or targeted needs assessment. The targeted needs assessment addresses what the students, school, patients, or local healthcare organization need to improve. The point of this step is to shape and refine the ground-level information that was learned from the general needs assessment. This allows application of knowledge learned from the general needs assessment to local learners and their learning environment. Discussions with key organizational stakeholders will inform the local needs assessment. Do our local surgeons, for example, have wide variation in laparoscopic bariatric skills,

Table 3.1 Questions asked during needs assessments

Who are the targeted learners?
What training is already planned?
What are expectations of scope of knowledge for this level of trainee?
What are existing proficiencies?
What are perceived deficiencies and needs?
What are reasons for past poor performance?
What are the learners' motivations to improve performance?
What are the attitudes about the current topic?
What are the preferred learning methods?
What is the learning environment and will it match?

reflecting the national problem? The targeted needs assessment should also include a decision about the intended learners—health professionals—most likely to contribute to solving the problem. Curriculum developers not only need to consider the intended learners, but also the focused learning environment (e.g., existing curriculum, stakeholders). The bariatric surgeons may need to participate in a simulation-based exercise because no other training opportunities exist. The local needs assessment prevents duplication of what is already underway, what is already known, or teaching above the level of the targeted learners. Questions that may be asked are seen in Table 3.1. These questions are answered by looking at local quality metrics through chart reviews; focus groups, surveys, or interviews; making observations during clinical care; or conducting formal assessments.

Goals and Objectives

Learning goals and objectives are written after general and targeted needs are established. The curriculum goal is a broad definition of the overall curriculum purpose. Objectives are specific learning outcomes. Objectives must be measurable and should include a noun and a verb that describe learner performance and a minimum standard to gauge learner achievement. Curriculum goals and objectives must be aligned with the needs assessment to ensure education success.

Health professions educators who write specific measureable learning objectives should use verbs that are discrete, measurable, and unambiguous. Verbs such as "describe," "perform," or "indicate" are specific and measurable. Objectives must tell what learners can do after training compared to what they could not do before training. The specifics of "*who will do how much (how well) of what*, by *when*" must be answered [11].

Objectives have several levels expressed by Bloom's Taxonomy (Fig. 3.1) [15]. Recognition and recall lie at the base of the pyramid. The pyramid ascends as learning objectives grow in complexity. The ability to evaluate or judge the quality of a skill or topic is at the apex. Healthcare providers aspire to reach this level but not every curriculum or curricular element needs to reach the summit. Descriptive verbs shown in Bloom's Taxonomy can be used to write learning objectives (e.g., know,

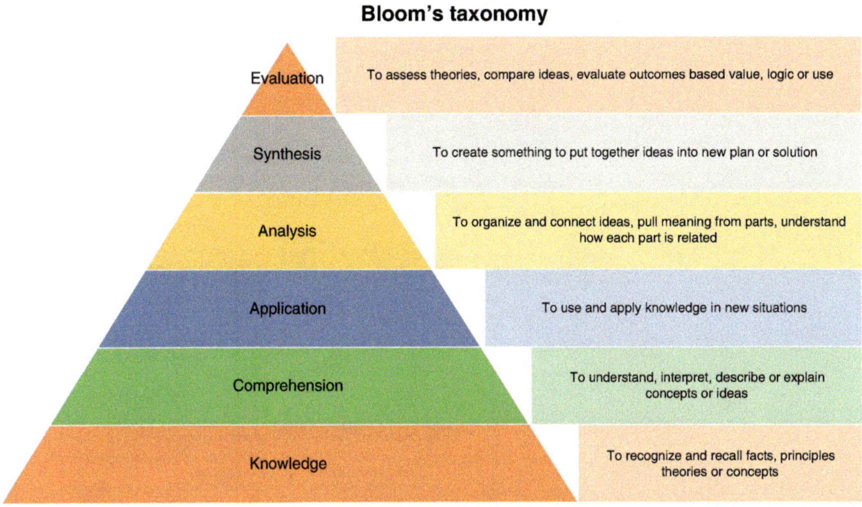

Fig. 3.1 Bloom's taxonomy of verbs that can be used during objective writing. As the pyramid ascends expectations of the learner increase and measurement becomes more complex

apply, evaluate). However, the verbs must be measurable. Verbs expressed as "knows" are easily measured by a written or oral examination. By contrast, "understands" is more difficult to evaluate objectively.

There are varieties of learning objectives. Objectives can be about the learner, the learning process, or educational outcomes. Objectives about the learner address cognitive, affective, and psychomotor outcomes. Levels of cognitive learning objectives (knowledge) are presented in Fig. 3.2. Affective learner objectives describe attitudes, values, beliefs, biases, emotions, and role expectations that influence a learner's achievement. Psychomotor learner objectives include skills such as hand or body movements, vision, speech, communication, or procedures. An example of a learning objective for the learner is, "All nursing students will perform a complete patient assessment before graduation."

Process learning objectives address curriculum implementation. These objectives describe the degree of participation, expected learner or faculty satisfaction with the curriculum, or success of the curriculum implementation. "Ninety percent of second year internal medicine residents will complete simulation training for central venous cathet (CVC) insertion successfully during the current academic year" is a process learning objective.

Outcome learning objectives include healthcare and patient outcomes or the curriculum impact beyond results stated in learner or process objectives. Outcome learning objectives change behaviors of patients and their health status or have a positive effect on healthcare in other ways. Outcome objectives are the key to sustained curriculum implementation. "Over 50 percent of our residency program graduates will pursue careers in academic medicine" is an outcome learning objective.

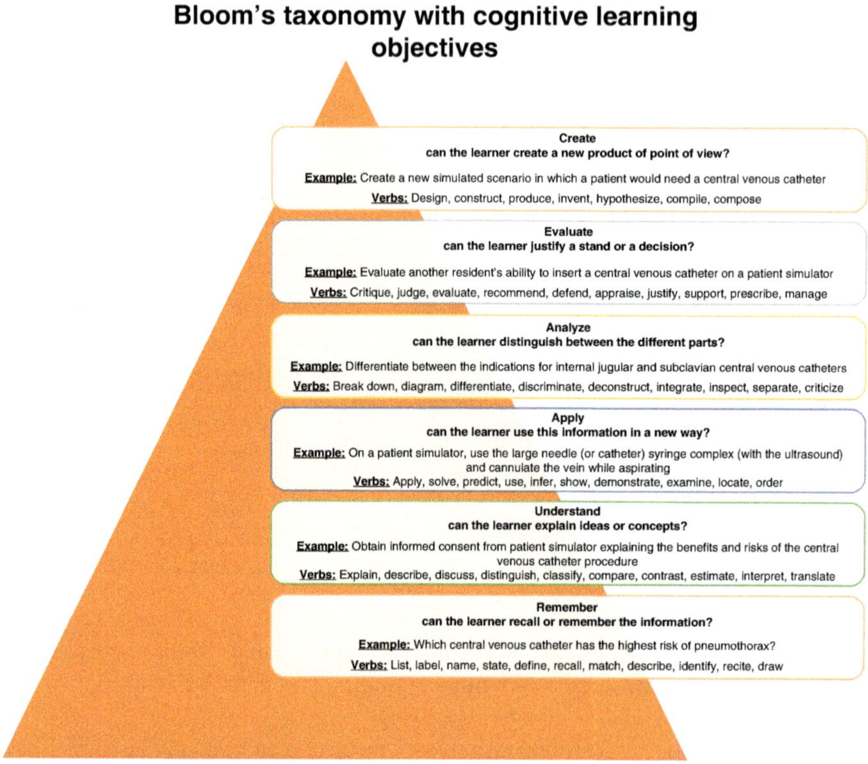

Fig. 3.2 Application of Bloom's taxonomy of cognitive learning objectives using central venous catheter insertion as an example

Education Strategies

Education strategies are addressed after goals and objectives are set. The education strategies are selected to address the learning objectives. Education strategies are the teaching and assessment methods that will be employed. Readings, lectures, online learning resources, discussions, tutorials, reflections on experience, feedback on performance, small group learning, problem-based learning, case-based learning, team-based learning, individualized learning projects, role modeling, demonstrations, role plays, simulations, standardized patients, clinical experiences, audio or video review, flipped classrooms, and mastery learning with deliberate practice are all examples of learning strategies (see Chap. 4). Using multiple educational strategies helps address different learning styles among trainees. Hands-on adult learning approaches are usually the most effective in healthcare education. While choosing education and assessment strategies, the curriculum developer must make sure that the assessments are aligned with learning methods. For instance, it is a mismatch to use a simulation-based assessment as a post course examination after a lecture series if leaners never experienced hands on simulation practice. A multiple-choice examination is better in this situation. Health professions educators also know that assessments are a key feature of the education intervention and that feedback must be provided after assessments.

Implementation

Implementation is the fifth step in curriculum development. Chapters 7 and 19 provide detailed discussions of implementation science and business principles to consider when implementing and sustaining an educational curriculum. A good implementation plan must consider how the curriculum will affect all stakeholders, a plan for communication to the stakeholders, financial support and resources, faculty and staff time, administrative support, a timeline, and a strategy to address curriculum barriers and supports. Chapter 7 also discusses long-term curriculum maintenance and dissemination.

Evaluation and Feedback

Program evaluation must be performed to determine if the curriculum is robust and accomplishes its training goals. Feedback is used for curriculum improvement. These are the final steps in curriculum development. Evaluation and feedback help those who have a stake in the curriculum make decisions or judgments about the curriculum and answer the central question, "Were the goals and objectives of the curriculum achieved?" Evaluation is intended to answer questions presented in Table 3.2. Specifically, evaluation should address whether the education problems isolated in steps 1 and 2 have been resolved or improved.

Evaluation in education refers to curriculum success. Did the learners achieve the curriculum goals and objectives? Was the curriculum implemented successfully? Did the learners [and teachers] enjoy the educational experience? Feedback from evaluations informs curriculum improvements in future iterations. Curriculum evaluation may also ask if the curriculum affected patient care practices or healthcare outcomes.

Table 3.2 Questions answered by evaluation and feedback

Are the learners motivated/did their attitudes change?
Did the individual student learn?
Was the curriculum able to be implemented as intended?
What needs to change to make the curriculum more effective?
How will formative feedback be delivered to encourage individual improvement?
Did the curriculum improve patient care or outcomes?
Is there justification for allocation of resources?
Can the learner be promoted/graduate or move on to the next stage of training?
What presentations, publications are necessary to allow adoption of curricular components by others?

Assessments demonstrate whether learning occurred and in what ways. Assessments must produce reliable and valid data. Assessments can be formative (*for learning*) or summative (*of* learning) to guide advancement decisions. Assessments must be integrated into every learning intervention. They are a key part of the education intervention and are important to guide learners. Additionally, baseline assessments (pretests) heighten learner awareness as they move through a curriculum and focus and guide subsequent learning. Assessments tell learners if their achievements match curriculum expectations. Learner assessments also give education program directors data to inform trainee promotion decisions. In healthcare, assessments provide critical information about learner readiness for independent and safe patient care. Chapter 5 discusses the process of creating assessments that produce reliable data which contribute to valid decisions.

The six steps of the Thomas curriculum development scheme are iterative. Decisions made at each step inform and impact other curriculum development components. The order of steps presents a structured way of thinking, because the curriculum development process is nonlinear and may move out of order, back and forth. For instance, objectives are refined based on evaluation and feedback. Educational strategies and various steps are revisited after new information is obtained. Health professions curricula should be reviewed and improved periodically based on evaluation and feedback.

Mastery Learning

The idea of simulation-based mastery learning in medical education is congruent with the Thomas six-step approach to curriculum development. Mastery learning takes the Thomas model as a point-of-departure and adds high expectations about education objectives, achievement standards, education strategies, and evaluation and feedback. Mastery learning begins with the mantra of "excellence for all." The goal is to ensure that clinical learners acquire information and skills to very high achievement standards, patient care practices improve, and patients are safer and better due to outstanding care.

McGaghie and colleagues outlined seven principles of a mastery learning curriculum bundle in health professions education [16]. The seven mastery learning principles are:

1. Baseline, i.e., diagnostic testing
2. Clear learning objectives, sequenced as units in increasing difficulty
3. Engagement in educational activities
4. A set minimum passing standard (MPS) for each educational unit
5. Formative or summative testing to gauge unit completion at a preset MPS for mastery
6. Advancement to the next education unit given measured achievement at or above the mastery standard
7. Continued practice or study on an educational unit until the mastery standard is reached

An additional step that was recently added pertains to performing follow-up testing to ensure learners maintain their high level of skills over time for tasks that are rare or can put patients at risk.

The mastery model of health professions education ensures that all learners achieve all education objectives to a very high standard with little or no outcome variation. In contrast with traditional time-based medical curricula, mastery learning permits the time needed to reach a unit's educational objectives to vary among learners. Research shows that about 10–20% of health professions learners are unable to meet or exceed the mastery standard at initial posttest and need more training time. For medical tasks including such clinical procedures as lumbar puncture and thoracentesis, the additional training usually takes less than 1 or 2 hours.

The pretest (baseline) assessment is one of the most important components of mastery learning. The baseline assessment is part of the educational intervention for at least five reasons. First, self-assessments of skill and knowledge are frequently inaccurate [17]. Therefore, a baseline assessment often serves as a revelation to learners who believe they are masters of a skill, when in fact they are not. To illustrate, when attending physicians were tested rigorously on simulated CVC skills, many did not know how to use an ultrasound or about the need for full sterile barriers [3]. These skills are new innovations, may not have been common practice during medical training, and not all physicians have adopted the practices.

Second, baseline assessment motivates learners and heightens awareness during training. Healthcare providers are well intentioned and want to provide great patient care. Unpublished interviews of participants in CVC simulation-based mastery learning (SBML) training reveal that most learners recognize the value of the baseline test and the focus baseline data provide during didactic and hands-on training.

Third, baseline assessments are a benchmark to show that learning has occurred. The baseline assessment informs both the learner and facilitator (i.e., instructor, coach) about the knowledge or skills that need to receive learner attention during training. A comparison of baseline and final test results demonstrates the amount of learning that has occurred due to the education intervention.

Fourth, a baseline assessment allows skilled individuals to "test out" of the education intervention. There is no need to complete the education intervention if they are able to meet or exceed the MPS on the baseline assessment. Participants can then advance to the next unit.

Fifth, a baseline assessment can also serve as a needs assessment for future curriculum development. For example, at Northwestern Memorial Hospital (NMH), we did not know if nurses were following best practices in CVC maintenance tasks. We created a simulated baseline assessment and tested a small cohort of nurses on these skills. The assessment results showed wide variation among nurses about adherence to best practices in CVC maintenance [18]. NMH later required all nurses who worked with CVCs to participate in training for maintenance tasks. Nurses who perform well on the baseline assessment "test out" of the intervention.

Education activities in SBML for healthcare professionals occur after the baseline assessment. These activities involve a wide spectrum of education events (Chap. 4). Approaches include lecture, small group discussion, demonstration, deliberate skills practice, and video-based demonstration. One benefit of a video-based procedure demonstration is that the facilitator need not be present when the education material is studied.

We believe the baseline assessment allows learners to have a more focused approach to education and results in less distraction during learning sessions. Standardized education activities should be used so all learners receive the same experience. Video-based or online content delivery can minimize variation. Regardless of the education strategy and method of delivery, the content must also be periodically updated to make sure it conforms with current practice standards. Content should also be peer reviewed by experts to verify accuracy and relevance of the information learned and assessed.

After viewing the video and lectures, the learners return to the simulation laboratory where they participate in deliberate practice of the learning task with the facilitator available to give guidance and feedback. Deliberate practice was first described by K. Anders Ericsson in his study of how professional musicians, chess players, and athletes reach expert levels of performance [19, 20]. Ericsson discovered that peak performers not only put in long practice hours but also that their practice was focused, systematic, and intense. Deliberate practice involves setting a well-defined task where the learner participates in focused repetitive practice. An expert coach with specific knowledge of best teaching methods for the task provides guidance and feedback. This allows the learner to practice, receive feedback, correct errors, and move toward the overall goal of continuous improvement (Chap. 4).

The learner can approach an expert level of performance with repeat cycles of deliberate practice. In medical practice, the number of procedures that doctors perform does not correlate with procedural skill if there is no mechanism for feedback and constant improvement [21]. If a surgeon performs 300 appendectomies annually, but performs each procedure incorrectly, experience is not a good teacher. Cycles of deliberate practice with feedback must be continuous to prevent skill decay (Fig. 3.3).

Figure 3.4 shows a group of learners participating in deliberate practice of resuscitation skills on a simulator. See how the simulation environment matches essential components of the clinical setting to create a learning environment that

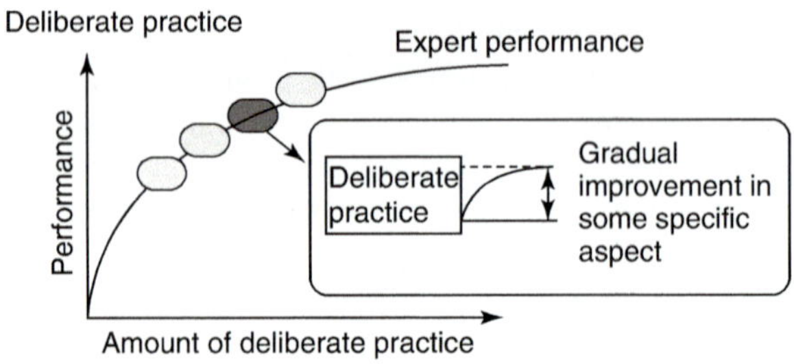

Fig. 3.3 Deliberate practice model. Without continued cycles of deliberate practice, a learner will fall back to the left of the curve. (Adapted with permission from the author as a slide in Ericsson [42])

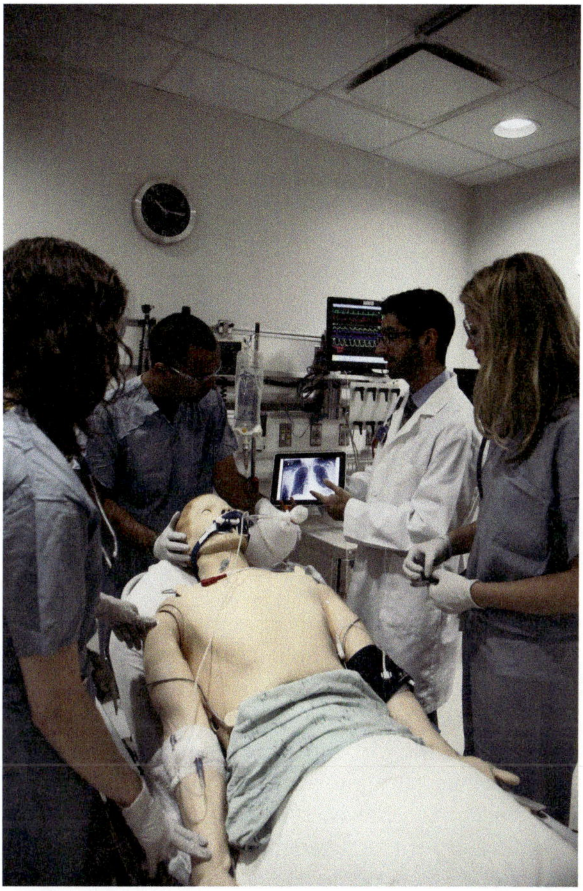

Fig. 3.4 A learner and facilitator practice deliberately to learn resuscitation skills. Notice how the learning environment resembles the clinical environment

approximates actual patient care. In this illustration, the participants are using the same equipment that is used in the hospital for an actual resuscitation. The instructor is giving the learners feedback about proper technique. The instructor may not always don personal protective equipment during practice depending on the training scenario. Deliberate practice approximates behavior performed in real clinical practice. Deliberate practice is hard work and learners are often tired at the end. Practice must be as similar as possible to how the learners perform in the real practice setting. The rule of thumb is "Practice how you play!"

Setting a MPS is the next step in designing mastery learning curricula. Decisions about whether a learner can move on to the next task (or pass the training) and care for patients has significant implications for patient safety. Decisions must be justifiable and appropriately identify healthcare providers who are ready for independent practice. This not only affects downstream patient care but also sets clear expectations for learners and training programs. The MPS can serve as a formative performance guide for learners to know expectations during training. With minimum passing standards, healthcare training programs have objective and defensible

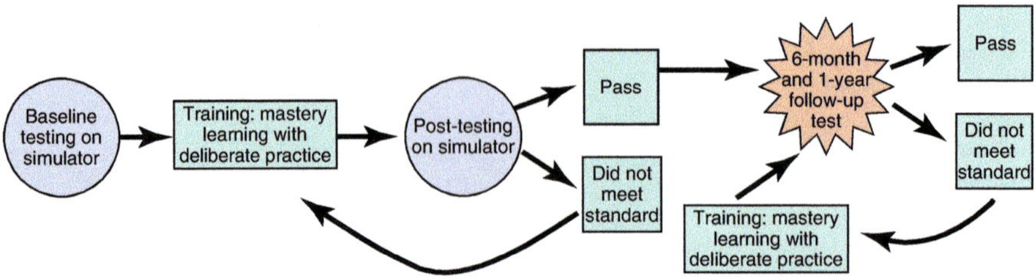

Fig. 3.5 A graphic picture of simulation-based mastery learning steps

evidence of learner summative performance and can determine readiness for practice. Four methods have been described and used to set minimum passing standards for healthcare tasks in mastery learning: Angoff, Hofstee, Mastery Angoff, and Patient-safety. A detailed discussion of these methods is found in Chap. 6. Briefly, each method convenes a sample of 8 to 12 judges who have experience and expertise in the task being assessed. Each judge independently rates the test and provides data about passing scores. Averages from the judges' decisions may be used to set the mastery standard.

Finally, as deliberate practice demonstrates that continuous cycles are needed to maintain expert performance, mastery learning also needs follow-up assessment and practice after successfully achieving the MPS and completing training. Studies demonstrate that up to 10 percent of learners do not meet the MPS in follow-up testing 6 months after the learning intervention [22, 23]. Additionally, no specific predictors of who will require follow-up training have been identified because demographic data about learners (e.g., age, gender, test performance, year of training, clinical experience, confidence) do not predict follow-up performance [22]. Patient safety is critical among healthcare providers so follow-up assessment and training is essential at least at 6 months intervals.

Figure 3.5 summarizes the steps of mastery learning curriculum from baseline assessment to long-term retention.

Curriculum Development Using Mastery Learning

The Thomas curriculum development model and the seven steps of mastery learning fit together closely (Fig. 3.6). The first steps in the Thomas model on needs assessment are the same using mastery learning principles. Mastery learning informs *goals and objectives* specifically to add that all learners are required to meet or exceed the MPS by the end of training. Session and topic difficulty progressively increase as learners reach the learning objectives. Mastery learning *education strategies* have already been defined and include a baseline test and such other entities as video demonstrations, lectures, simulation-based deliberate practice, and a posttest. Debriefing activities occur constantly both during deliberate practice and after pre- and post-assessments. *Implementation* of a mastery learning curriculum is easiest when learners are *required* to undergo training due

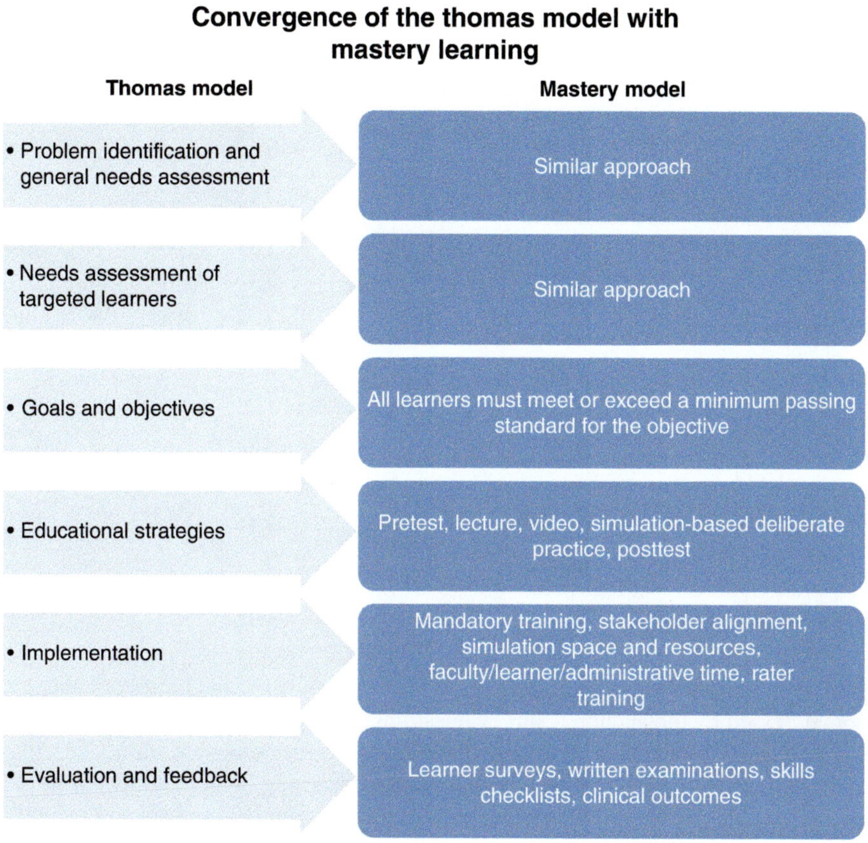

Fig. 3.6 Convergence of the Thomas model of curriculum development with mastery learning

to a patient safety warrant about meeting or exceeding a MPS set by experts. All stakeholders should be fully engaged and support training. Administrative time needs to be set to schedule the simulation laboratory, learners, and faculty for training. Raters must be calibrated and trained to assess learners identically. Time needs to be set aside for faculty not only to participate in assessments and deliberate practice sessions but also to work with the 10–20% of learners who do not meet or exceed the MPS at initial posttesting. Simulation space and resources are needed for each session including video recording and playback. More detail about implementation of mastery learning interventions is available in Chaps. 7 and 19.

Creation of course learner *assessment* and course *evaluation* tools that produce reliable data that promote valid decisions is key to mastery learning interventions. Accurate, actionable learner feedback and learner advancement decisions rely on reliable assessment data. Course evaluation is served by feedback from learner surveys that help faculty fine-tune a curriculum to better serve learner needs. An example of a learner survey administered after ACLS training is given in Table 3.3. A

Table 3.3 ACLS survey

	Strongly disagree	Disagree	Uncertain	Agree	Strongly agree
1. Practice with the medical simulator boosts my clinical skills.	1	2	3	4	5
2. It is ok to make clinical mistakes using the medical simulator.	1	2	3	4	5
3. I receive useful educational feedback from the medical simulator.	1	2	3	4	5
4. Practice with the medical simulator boosts my clinical self-confidence.	1	2	3	4	5
5. The simulator center staff is competent.	1	2	3	4	5
6. Practice sessions using the medical simulator should be a required component of residency education.	1	2	3	4	5
7. Practice with the medical simulator has helped prepare me to be a code leader better than clinical experience alone.	1	2	3	4	5
8. The medical simulator has helped prepare me to be a code leader better than the ACLS course I took.	1	2	3	4	5

comment section is included to encourage learners to write about issues or concerns not addressed by the anchored survey questions.

Written examinations or checklists have been designed to assess learner baseline and post training performance during mastery learning interventions. Multiple choice written examinations can be developed for baseline and posttesting *knowledge* training components. Detailed methods to develop written examinations are beyond the scope of this chapter. However, best practices may include creation of a test question bank based on a test blueprint that has content categories crossed by question types including knowledge, application, and interpretation (see Chap. 5). Once the test is developed, it should be pilot tested using multiple test takers. Each item should undergo analysis to determine the statistical value of the question for inclusion in the final assessment.

An added step is to derive a separate pretest and posttest that are equivalent in content, difficulty, and reliability from the test blueprint and question bank. Content categories and question difficulties are distributed evenly between the pretest and the posttest. Pilot data also permit calculation of pretest and posttest reliability coefficients. Equivalent pretests and posttests are important to have an unbiased learning assessment. This ensures learners have not simply memorized the test items and answer without thought [24]. More information on developing written tests is available from *Measurement and Assessment in Teaching* by Miller and Linn [25].

Skills are assessed using checklists for observed skill performance. Checklists can be dichotomous (done correctly vs. done incorrectly/not done) or based on a global scale. Both types of checklists can demonstrate high inter-rater reliability with appropriate anchoring and rubrics for grading. Methods for creating checklist have been described by Stufflebeam [26] and Schmutz et al. [27]. The checklist development tasks are:

1. Define task.
2. Review literature.
3. Draft checklist.
4. Review by experts.
5. Pilot test with feedback.
6. Revise checklist.
7. Calibrate checklist.
8. Revise checklist—periodically review and revise.

The first step in checklist development for a clinical procedures is defining the task that needs to be assessed. Care should be taken to ensure checklist items are not "knowledge based" but are an actual observable skill. Relevant literature should be studied to ensure the checklist produces useful data. A draft version of the procedure checklist is prepared and its items are reviewed by an expert panel. A clinical procedure checklist should have about 20–30 items. Too many items are laborious and hard to record and judge. Too few items do not allow for measurement variation or reliable assessment. The checklist should be pilot tested using learners and experts to get feedback that informs later revision. During pilot testing several raters should use the learner checklist simultaneously to refine the grading rubric and calculate inter-rater reliability. Kappa coefficients or another index should be used to measure inter-rater reliability. Items with kappa coefficients less than 0.8 should be removed or revised to improve rater agreement. Checklists should be reviewed and revised periodically to ensure accuracy and timeliness.

Chapter 5 describes the Kane and Messick models of validity and how they can be applied to show SBML interventions produce reliable data that lead to valid decisions.

Rigorous scientific methods are needed to evaluate translational science outcomes. Randomized controlled trials (RCT) are usually considered the most rigorous method to evaluate an education intervention. However, RCTs may not be ethical when evaluating SBML interventions. Research shows that powerful SBML interventions effectively improve trainee clinical skills, patient care practices, and downstream patient outcomes [28]. Therefore, withholding SBML interventions from some trainees and patients is not ethical.

Understanding how to develop SBML curricula that are rigorous and that produce reliable and valid data is paramount to a successful education and research program that is thematic, sustained, and cumulative. The rest of this chapter discusses how we converted an ACLS curriculum that was framed using the Thomas model into a successful SBML intervention. This ACLS curriculum has been sustained for over 13 years but has been consistently revised and improved.

Advanced Cardiac Life Support Mastery Learning Curriculum

Step 1: General Needs Assessment

The American Board of Internal Medicine (ABIM) requires all internal medicine (IM) residents to perform ACLS safely and effectively [29]. The American Heart Association (AHA) offers a course in ACLS in which IM residents participate to meet this goal [30]. These AHA ACLS provider courses involve a series of videos followed by skill building sessions on a simulator. Objective assessments are conducted at objective structured clinical exam-like stations where case-based scenarios are presented. The leader of the cardiac arrest is assessed in each of the various abnormal heart rhythms [30]. At the end of the course, participants take a written examination that they must pass to obtain an AHA ACLS completion card.

The quality and rigor of the AHA course varies depending on the leniency of the individual instructor and the amount of time put in by the learner. Concerns have been expressed about the adequacy of residents' ability to lead cardiac arrests in the hospital [31]. In fact, data show that the quality of cardiac resuscitation attempts by trained healthcare providers varies widely and often does not meet AHA standards [32]. The current ACLS AHA card is valid for 2 years, requiring recertification after that time. Two years may be too long for adequate retention of skill and knowledge which may lead to the wide variation in cardiac resuscitation quality. Therefore, the accepted 2-year cycle may be inadequate to ensure that healthcare providers maintain their skill and knowledge [33, 34].

Step 2: Targeted Needs Assessment

In academic medical centers, ACLS provider teams often include IM, anesthesia, and surgery residents. At NMH in Chicago, second and third year IM residents are expected to serve as code leaders once they have completed the ACLS AHA provider course. Based on nursing feedback, we discovered that cardiac arrests run by these code leaders were variable in quality and often had poor adherence to AHA ACLS guidelines. Given these observations, the IM residency program leadership was asked to work with the hospital nursing leadership and quality improvement teams to provide a solution.

Step 3: Goals and Objectives

The concerns about ACLS code leadership skills prompted the development, implementation, and evaluation of a simulation-based educational program at NMH with a goal to improve IM resident skills and management of in-hospital cardiac events. There were three basic objectives.

Objective 1 All 2nd and 3rd year IM residents will correctly follow the ACLS AHA guidelines during cardiac arrests for asystole, ventricular fibrillation, supraventricular tachycardia, ventricular tachycardia, symptomatic bradycardia, and pulseless electrical activity after simulation-based training.

Objective 2 All 2nd and 3rd year IM residents will optimally perform as an ACLS leader during cardiac arrests for asystole, ventricular fibrillation, supraventricular tachycardia, ventricular tachycardia, symptomatic bradycardia, and pulseless electrical activity after simulation-based training.

Objective 3 Evaluate simulation-trained 2nd and 3rd year IM resident code leaders' compliance with the ACLS AHA guidelines during actual hospital cardiac arrests.

Step 4: Education Strategies

The ACLS training curriculum initially implemented in 2003 was designed to train IM residents on the six most common cardiac arrest events at NMH and matched content in the 2001 AHA *ACLS Provider Manual* [30]. Simulation was the learning and teaching platform. We used realistic clinical scenarios with a high fidelity human simulator (HPS, METI LLC, Sarasota, FL). The METI simulator is a full human mannequin that is run by a computer that can mimic multiple physiologic and pharmacologic responses observed in ACLS. The mannequin has respiratory responses, heart and lung sounds, and peripheral pules. Systemic blood pressure, arterial oxygen saturation, electrocardiogram, and arterial blood pressure can be monitored. Cardiopulmonary resuscitation and defibrillation can also be performed on the mannequin.

Chief medical residents reviewed hospital cardiac arrest logs and developed scenarios based on the six most commonly occurring ACLS events at NMH. The simulation ACLS scenarios were pilot tested with attending physicians, ACLS instructors, and other content experts and revised as needed. Use of the human patient simulator in a center equipped with one-way glass and audio-visual technology allowed learners to react and care for simulated in-hospital cardiac events repeatedly while managing a team of their peers in a learning environment without posting a threat to patient safety. Participants were required to undergo a baseline assessment as a code leader, and then participated in simulation-based practice, followed by a posttest as the code leader. Feedback was provided by both an expert instructor and peers. For the initial implementation, there was no method for objectively remediating learners if they performed poorly at posttest.

Step 5: Implementation

All second and third year IM residents were required to participate in the ACLS curriculum by the residency program director. Training occurred over four, 2-hour simulation education sessions during a 2-week period. Groups of two to four residents participated in practice sessions while only two were tested together. The order of the six ACLS scenarios was randomized within each testing session. Deliberate practice and feedback sessions were run by a clinician trained in respiratory therapy who was a master ACLS teacher. The respiratory therapist ACLS teacher allowed medical faculty time to be used efficiently and enhanced the quality of the intervention.

Step 6: Evaluation and Feedback

Learner Assessment

A unique checklist was developed for each of the six ACLS conditions. Checklists were developed by a group of experts using the modified Delphi technique based on AHA ACLS guidelines. Each checklist required patient assessment, clinical examination, medication administration, adequate chest compressions, rhythm monitoring, and team work skills recommended by the AHA [30]. A dichotomous scoring scale ranging from 0 (*not done/done incorrectly*) to 1 (*done correctly*) was used for each checklist item [35]. All checklist items were given equal weight.

Faculty raters completed training and calibration during a pilot testing phase using ten volunteer learners. These sessions were video recorded and re-graded by faculty to assess inter-rater reliability using Cohen's kappa coefficients. Checklist items that did not have acceptable reliability were modified until agreement was reached. Faculty raters received feedback about their scoring and had refresher training to ensure continued high checklist scoring reliability.

Curriculum Evaluation

The first investigation of the curriculum used a randomized trial design with a wait-list control condition to evaluate if the simulation educational intervention produced significant skill acquisition results [36]. Evaluating baseline to posttest assessment differences, the education intervention produced a statistically significant 38% improvement in skill. Resident surveys showed the education intervention was well received and preferred over traditional clinical education. A follow-up study demonstrated that these IM residents' ACLS skills acquired from SBME did not decay after 6 months and 14 months [23]. Next, in an attempt to evaluate translational outcomes, a case control study of actual NMH cardiac arrests compared events that were led by a simulation-trained IM resident to those that were not. Code events led by a simulation-trained resident were 7.1 times more likely to be adherent to the AHA guidelines [37]. In an attempt to evaluate other translational outcomes, post-event survival was evaluated without significant differences between the codes led by the simulator-trained and non-simulator-trained group. However, a trend toward increased mean unadjusted survival time was seen in the simulator-trained group (195 hours vs. 107 hours; $p = 0.11$). (See Chap. 16 for a discussion of SBML with translational outcomes.)

Transformation to SBML

The ACLS intervention was converted to SBML on patient safety grounds because there were no objective means to determine if a learner needed to participate in more practice after posttesting (remediate) before safely working with patients. The seven principles of mastery learning were applied the ACLS curriculum that was revised over a 2-year period. The basic ACLS structure and instruction did not change. However, the objectives were modified to:

Objective 1 All 2nd and 3rd year residents will meet or exceed a MPS on a skills checklist based on the AHA ACLS guidelines during simulated cardiac arrests for asystole, ventricular fibrillation, supraventricular tachycardia, ventricular tachycardia, symptomatic bradycardia, and pulseless electrical activity after simulation-based training.

Objective 2 All 2nd and 3rd year IM residents will meet or exceed a MPS on a skills checklist designed to measure optimal performance as an ACLS leader during cardiac arrests for asystole, ventricular fibrillation, supraventricular tachycardia, ventricular tachycardia, symptomatic bradycardia, and pulseless electrical activity after simulation-based training.

Objective 3 Evaluate simulation-based mastery learning trained 2nd and 3rd year IM resident code leaders' compliance with the ACLS AHA guidelines during actual in-house cardiac arrests.

A MPS for the SBML curriculum needed to be established. The MPS for each ACLS skills checklist (six scenarios) was set by 12 experts using the average of Angoff and Hofstee standard setting methods (see Chap. 6) [38]. Both approaches used a panel of judges composed of individuals with expertise and experience with ACLS. The MPS was set at 74% checklist items correct for asystole, 76% for ventricular fibrillation, 72% for supraventricular tachycardia, 74% for ventricular tachycardia, 72% for symptomatic bradycardia, and 77% for pulseless electrical activity.

Deliberate practice principles were emphasized during simulation-based mastery learning training. This required more time training faculty about how to coach deliberate practice and other principles of mastery learning. Learners were also required to have the ACLS AHA algorithms memorized before coming to training sessions. This allowed more time to focus deliberate practice on team leadership skills and the cardiac arrest process. Implementation required creating more instructor and learner time to practice if the learner could not initially meet the MPS at posttesting.

Mastery learning curriculum evaluation was performed on the first 41 IM residents to participate in the SBML ACLS intervention [39]. Out of 41 residents, 33 were able to meet or exceed the MPS within the scheduled training sessions. The remaining 8 residents took additional practice time to meet mastery ranging from 15 minutes to 1 hour. These residents only needed to improve assessments for two scenarios (6 total) where they did not meet the MPS. The pretest to posttest improvement was 24% ($p \leq 0.0001$).

A second study of actual NMH cardiac arrest code leaders was performed to compare the SBML training to SBME without a mastery standard and traditional ACLS training [40]. SBML-trained resident code leaders were 88% compliant with AHA code guidelines, simulation-trained residents who were educated before the mastery learning curriculum were 68% compliant, and non-simulation trained personnel 44% compliant, $p < 0.001$. This finding confirmed that SBML is more effective than non-mastery simulation training and traditional clinical education.

Challenges to SMBL Curriculum Development

Creating SBML curriculum around clinical skills can be straightforward or challenging based on several factors. Developing curricula, assessments, and outcome measures for complex tasks such as ACLS events involving dynamic teams is difficult. Conversely, SBML programs for discrete clinical procedures and skills are relatively easy to develop when clear guidelines are available (e.g., ACLS AHA guidelines). Using SBML in scenarios that involve complex activities such as advanced clinical reasoning or decision-making is more challenging. These clinical events may not have well-articulated and easily used metrics. We do not know if clinical skills assessments in these areas can be done using SBML. However, SBML has been adapted successfully to non-procedural task such as difficult conversations (see Chap. 10) [41].

Additional challenges to developing SBML curricula include administrative support, "buy-in" from key stakeholders, and funding (addressed in more detail in Chaps. 7 and 19). Health professions educators must address each of these challenges early and often. Administrative support is required to schedule trainees and faculty for SBML. Support from stakeholders is pivotal for success to ensure backing for facilitator presence to run the education sessions and flexibility in the learner's schedule to attend all training sessions. For ACLS training, the program director for the IM residency required all residents to participate in training. Nursing and hospital leadership was in full support because the project was helping to solve a hospital safety problem (needs assessment) that was high on their agenda. Faculty are key stakeholders as well because SBML requires sufficient rater training to develop high inter-rater reliability and ensure the validity of pass/fail decisions. Faculty (and learners) may require more time to train all participants to mastery. For ACLS, the department chair supported two faculty members at 10% effort for 1 year to assist in this effort and the chief medical residents assisted in training as part of their clinical responsibilities. The costs of SBML including faculty and staff, equipment, and space must be considered. The first year of SBML ACLS training was estimated to cost approximately $45,000 and approximately $20,000 in subsequent years. The project costs were covered from an internal grant that directly resulted from stakeholder engagement.

The costs and time associated with evaluation of a program may be an additional challenge. For the ACLS curriculum, feedback from learners suggested that the curriculum could be reduced to 6 hours by removing redundant content. IM residents also requested that intensive care unit nurses participate in the simulations to improve communication. Although responding to this feedback saved some cost, it added others as the curriculum had to recently be revised and personnel added to the simulations. Because the AHA guidelines are updated every 5 years, our checklists for ACLS skills needed revision at a minimum of every 5 years, most recently in 2015. Evaluation of our ACLS curriculum helped to ensure funding for many years of training. We encourage all educators using SBML to try to extend the endpoint of their work from the simulation laboratory into the clinical realm.

Coda

Healthcare education is uneven, producing providers with wide variation in knowledge and skills. Understanding how to develop and use mastery learning curricula can help eliminate this variability. SBML ensures "excellence for all" including clinicians who become better providers and patients who receive better, safer care. Although SBML curricula are not easy to develop, they are justified by the important and sustained education and downstream clinical outcomes they yield. Health professions educators interested in creating a SBML curriculum need to consider the local environment before selecting specific targets, which highlights the importance of a needs assessment. Linkage with organizational quality initiatives is beneficial to maximize stakeholder commitment to a robust and successful SBML intervention. We challenge healthcare educators to take the extra time and effort to modify existing or create new curricula using the principles of mastery learning given the great benefit to our learners and patients.

References

1. Langdorf MI, Strom SL, Yang L, et al. High-fidelity simulation enhances ACLS training. Teach Learn Med. 2014;26(3):266–73.
2. Bell RH Jr. Why Johnny cannot operate. Surgery. 2009;146(4):533–42.
3. Barsuk JH, Cohen ER, Nguyen D, Mitra D, O'Hara K, Okuda Y, et al. Attending physician adherence to a 29-component central venous catheter bundle checklist during simulated procedures. Crit Care Med. 2016;44(10):1871–81.
4. The Core Entrustable Professional Activities for Entering Residency. Available from: https://www.aamc.org/initiatives/coreepas/.
5. Accreditation Council for Graduate Medical Education Milestones. Available from: http://www.acgme.org/acgmeweb/tabid/430/ProgramandInstitutionalAccreditation/NextAccreditationSystem.Milestones.aspx.
6. Barsuk JH, Cohen ER, Feinglass J, McGaghie WC, Wayne DB. Use of simulation-based education to reduce catheter-related bloodstream infections. Arch Intern Med. 2009;169(15):1420–3.
7. Barsuk JH, Cohen ER, Feinglass J, McGaghie WC, Wayne DB. Clinical outcomes after bedside and interventional radiology paracentesis procedures. Am J Med. 2013;126(4):349–56.

8. Barsuk JH, Cohen ER, Potts S, Demo H, Gupta S, Feinglass J, et al. Dissemination of a simulation-based mastery learning intervention reduces central line-associated bloodstream infections. BMJ Qual Saf. 2014;23(9):749–56.
9. Cook DA, Brydges R, Zendejas B, Hamstra SJ, Hatala R. Mastery learning for health professionals using technology-enhanced simulation: a systematic review and meta-analysis. Acad Med. 2013;88(8):1178–86.
10. Barsuk JH, Cohen ER, Williams MV, et al. Simulation-based mastery learning for thoracentesis skills improves patient outcomes: a randomized trial. Acad Med. 2018;93(5):729–35.
11. Thomas PA, Kern DE, Hughes MT, Chen BY. Curriculum development for medical education: a six-step approach. 3rd ed. Baltimore: Johns Hopkins University Press; 2016.
12. Stefanidis D, Colavita PD. Simulation in general surgery. In: Levine AI, DeMaria S, Schwartz AD, Sim AJ, editors. The comprehensive textbook of healthcare simulation. New York: Springer; 2013. p. 353–66.
13. Severin PN, Cortez EP, McNeal CA, Kramer JE. Considerations of pediatric simulation. In: Kyle RR, Murray WB, editors. Clinical simulation: operations, engineering and management. Burlington: Elsevier; 2008. p. 411–21.
14. Birkmeyer JD, Finks JF, O'Reilly A, et al. Surgical skill and complication rates after bariatric surgery. N Engl J Med. 2013;369(15):1434–42.
15. Bloom BS, editor. Taxonomy of educational objectives: the classification of educational goals. Handbook 1: cognitive domain. New York: David McKay; 1956.
16. McGaghie WC, Siddall VJ, Mazmanian PE, Myers J, American College of Chest Physicians Health and Science Policy Committee. Lessons for continuing medical education from simulation research in undergraduate and graduate medical education: effectiveness of continuing medical education: American College of Chest Physicians Evidence-Based Educational Guidelines. Chest. 2009;135(3 Suppl):62S–8S.
17. Davis DA, Mazmanian PE, Fordis M, et al. Accuracy of physician self-assessment compared with observed measures of competence: a systematic review. JAMA. 2006;296(9):1094–102.
18. Barsuk JH, Cohen ER, Mikolajczak A, Seburn S, et al. Simulation-based mastery learning improves central line maintenance skills of ICU nurses. J Nurs Adm. 2015;45(10):511–7.
19. Ericsson KA. Acquisition and maintenance of medical expertise: a perspective from the expert-performance approach with deliberate practice. Acad Med. 2015;90(11):1471–86.
20. Ericsson KA, Pool R. Peak: secrets from the new science of expertise. Boston: Houghton Mifflin Harcourt; 2016.
21. Barsuk JH, Cohen ER, Feinglass J, McGaghie WC, Wayne DB. Residents' procedural experience does not ensure competence: a research synthesis. J Grad Med Educ. 2017;9(2):201–8.
22. Barsuk JH, Cohen ER, McGaghie WC, Wayne DB. Long-term retention of central venous catheter insertion skills after simulation-based mastery learning. Acad Med. 2010;85(10 Suppl):S9–12.
23. Wayne DB, Siddall VJ, Butter J, et al. A longitudinal study of internal medicine residents' retention of advanced cardiac life support skills. Acad Med. 2006;81(10 Suppl):S9–S12.
24. Issenberg SB, McGaghie WC, Brown DD, et al. Development of multimedia computer-based measures of clinical skills in bedside cardiology. In: Melnick DE, editor. The eighth international Ottawa conference on medical education and assessment proceedings. Evolving assessment: protecting the human dimension. Philadelphia: National Board of Medical Examiners; 2000. p. 821–9.
25. Miller MD, Linn RL. Measurement and assessment in teaching. 11th ed. Boston: Pearson; 2013.
26. Stufflebeam DL. The checklists development checklist. Western Michigan University Evaluation Center; 2000. Available at: http://www.wmich.edu/evalctr/checklists/cdc.htm.
27. Schmutz J, Eppich WJ, Hoffmann F, et al. Five steps to develop checklists for evaluating clinical performance: an integrative approach. Acad Med. 2014;89(7):996–1005.
28. McGaghie WC, Issenberg SB, Barsuk JH, Wayne DB. A critical review of simulation-based mastery learning with translational outcomes. Med Educ. 2014;48:375–85.

29. American Board of Internal Medicine. Internal medicine policies. Available from: http://www.abim.org/certification/policies/imss/im.aspx-procedures.
30. Cummins RO, editor. ACLS provider manual. Dallas: American Heart Association; 2001.
31. Peberdy MA, Kaye W, Ornato JP, et al. Cardiopulmonary resuscitation of adults in the hospital: a report of 14720 cardiac arrests from the National Registry of Cardiopulmonary Resuscitation. Resuscitation. 2003;58(3):297–308.
32. Abella BS, Alvarado JP, Myklebust H, et al. Quality of cardiopulmonary resuscitation during in-hospital cardiac arrest. JAMA. 2005;293(3):305–10.
33. Kaye W. Research on ACLS training--which methods improve skill & knowledge retention? Respir Care. 1995;40(5):538–46; 46–9.
34. Makker R, Gray-Siracusa K, Evers M. Evaluation of advanced cardiac life support in a community teaching hospital by use of actual cardiac arrests. Heart Lung. 1995;24(2):116–20.
35. Wayne DB, Butter J, Didwania A, et al. Advanced cardiac life support checklists for simulation-based education. 2009. Available from: www.mededportal.org/publication/1773.
36. Wayne DB, Butter J, Siddall VJ, et al. Simulation-based training of internal medicine residents in advanced cardiac life support protocols: a randomized trial. Teach Learn Med. 2005;17(3):210–6.
37. Wayne DB, Didwania A, Feinglass J, et al. Simulation-based education improves quality of care during cardiac arrest team responses at an academic teaching hospital: a case-control study. Chest. 2008;133:56–61.
38. Wayne DB, Fudala MJ, Butter J, et al. Comparison of two standard setting methods for advanced cardiac life support training. Acad Med. 2005;80(10, Suppl):S63–6.
39. Wayne DB, Butter J, Fudala MJ, et al. Mastery learning of advanced cardiac life support skills by internal medicine residents using simulation technology and deliberate practice. J Gen Intern Med. 2006;21:251–6.
40. Didwania A, McGaghie WC, Cohen ER, et al. Progress toward improving the quality of cardiac arrest medical team responses at an academic teaching hospital. J Grad Med Educ. 2011;3(2):211–6.
41. Vermylen J, Wood G, Wayne DB, et al. Raising the bar: applying a mastery learning approach to communication skills training. [Abstract]. J Pain Symp Manage. 2017;53(2):388–9.
42. Ericsson KA. Why innate talent does not matter in chess, music, sports: what the study of expert performers can tell us about human modifiability. Seminar at the Center for Advanced Studies in the Behavioral Sciences, Stanford, California (February 19th); 2003.

Instructional Design and Delivery for Mastery Learning

4

William C. McGaghie, Mark Adler, and David H. Salzman

This chapter is about designing and delivering powerful instruction. The focus of instruction is health professions learners, both individually and in teams. Design and delivery of rigorous instruction is hard work and calls for thought and planning. Instructional design and delivery are deliberate decision-making processes that address all of the choices made in creating and giving birth to an educational experience. These are not a passive exercises. We start with an example from the neighbor domain of US college athletics.

The legendary University of North Carolina basketball coach Dean Smith [Michael Jordan's now deceased mentor] describes athletic skill acquisition from deliberate practice in his textbook, *Basketball: Multiple Offense and Defense* [1]. Smith writes, "The organization, the preparation, the execution, plus a coach's entire philosophy is implemented in the all-important practice session." Smith continues, "Each player's motivation should be to walk off the practice floor a better player than he was when he arrived for the session. The coach has the responsibility of helping every player meet this goal." Smith goes on to describe daily, two-hour practice sessions that are goal-directed, planned to the minute, involving praise and peer pressure, having no idle time, with only two 90-second water breaks. Coach Smith asserts, "Coaches must push players to a point beyond which the players

W. C. McGaghie (✉)
Northwestern University Feinberg School of Medicine, Departments of Medical Education and Preventive Medicine, Chicago, IL, USA
e-mail: wcmc@northwestern.edu

M. Adler
Northwestern University Feinberg School of Medicine, Departments of Pediatrics and Medical Education, Chicago, IL, USA

D. H. Salzman
Northwestern University Feinberg School of Medicine, Departments of Emergency Medicine and Medical Education, Chicago, IL, USA

W. C. McGaghie et al. (eds.), *Comprehensive Healthcare Simulation: Mastery Learning in Health Professions Education*, Comprehensive Healthcare Simulation, https://doi.org/10.1007/978-3-030-34811-3_4

would like to stop. This kind of effort builds *mental toughness* … the harder a team works to achieve its goals, the stronger will be its determination to accomplish them."

Dean Smith's teaching intensity on the basketball court is matched every day by high-performing educators in the health professions. Teachers of tomorrow's physicians, nurses, dentists, physical and occupational therapists, social workers, physician assistants, midwives, and many other health professionals engage in instructional design (planning) and delivery (execution) throughout their careers. This high-level behavioral engineering is essential, especially if the health professions educators expect individual learners and teams to achieve mastery learning goals. Learning expectations are high and education sessions are meant to be challenging. The road to mastery learning in the health professions is neither easy nor short.

Instructional design, born from health professions curriculum development (Chap. 3), is a key responsibility of education leaders. The education leaders make curriculum and instruction decisions on behalf of learners shaped by accreditation requirements, professional habits, state and local laws, and institutional customs. As pointed out in Chaps. 3 and 5, the scope of potential material to teach learners is vast. Health professions educators must decide which specific components of instruction and assessment to include and which components to leave out. Education leaders must ensure that curriculum, instruction, and assessment samples represent what competent patient care providers will do in professional practice.

Instructional design starts with a clear recognition of learner goals and expectations and proceeds to decision-making about learning activities and outcomes and how performance will be assessed (Chap. 5). Designing mastery learning curricula requires an additional step where achievement standards are set (Chap. 6). As noted elsewhere in this book, instruction and assessment are inseparable because testing and feedback are key features of the mastery learning model that leads to powerful and sustained results.

Health professions education is increasingly becoming what Anders Ericsson and Robert Pool call a "highly developed field." They write in their book, *Peak: Secrets from the New Science of Expertise*, that such fields "are blessed with highly developed, broadly accepted training methods. If one follows these methods carefully and diligently, one will almost surely become an expert" [2]. Ericsson and Pool further amplify this idea by stating "[highly developed] fields have several shared characteristics:

(a) First, there are always objective ways (win/loss of a chess competition or a head-to-head race) or semi-objective ways (such as evaluation by expert judges) to measure performance. This makes sense. If there is no agreement on what good performance is and no way to tell what changes would improve performance, then it is very difficult, often impossible, to develop effective training methods. If you do not know for sure what constitutes improvement, how can you develop methods to improve performance?

(b) Second, these fields tend to be competitive enough that performers have a strong incentive to practice and improve.
(c) Third, these fields are generally well-established, with the relevant skills having been developed over decades or even centuries.
(d) Fourth, these fields have a subset of performers who also serve as teachers and coaches and who, over time, have developed increasingly sophisticated sets of training techniques that make possible the field's steadily increasing skill level. The improvements of skills and the development of training techniques move forward hand in hand, with new training techniques leading to new levels of accomplishment and new accomplishments generating innovations in training" [2].

Ericsson and Pool provide a roadmap to develop robust mastery learning programs in health professions education. We build on these framing remarks to present chapter sections that address (a) psychological foundations, (b) instructional design, (c) instructional delivery, (d) four health professions education examples, and (e) conclusions. The intent is to describe current evidence-based instruction best practices informed by theory and experience.

Psychological Foundations

The psychological foundations of learning and instruction that underlie the mastery learning model have been addressed by several authors [3–5]. In particular, McGaghie and Harris [6] recently described the learning theory foundations of simulation-based mastery learning and focus their discussion on three individual and team outcomes: (a) behavior improvement, (b) cognitive and social construction, and (c) social cognitive self-efficacy. These foundations are discussed in Chap. 2 which describes the mastery learning model in detail.

Other foundational writings about the advancement of mastery learning in health professions education include the Arthur Chickering and Zelda Gamson "Seven principles for good practice in undergraduate education" [7] and the Issenberg et al. Best Evidence Medical Education (BEME) review on features and uses of high-fidelity medical simulations that lead to effective learning [8].

Chickering, Gamson, and colleagues point out that good instructional practice in higher and professional education uses seven principles that prompt active, not passive, *engagement* among teachers and learners [7]. Good instructional practice should:

1. Encourage contacts between students and faculty.
2. Develop reciprocity and cooperation among students.
3. Use active learning techniques.
4. Give prompt feedback.
5. Emphasize time on task.
6. Communicate high expectations.
7. Respect diverse talents and ways of thinking.

Key features and uses of high-fidelity medical simulations that lead to effective learning identified by the BEME report echo, but do not duplicate, the list above of good instruction practices [8]. In order of educational impact on learners, the BEME report argues these ten principles of simulation-based medical education (SBME) account for powerful instruction in medicine and other health professions.

1. Feedback.
2. Repetitive [deliberate] practice.
3. Curriculum integration.
4. Range of difficulty.
5. Multiple learning strategies.
6. Clinical variation.
7. Controlled environment.
8. Individualized learning.
9. Defined outcomes.
10. Simulation validity.

Active learner engagement is the key to success in health professions mastery learning settings. Strong evidence from research in science, engineering, and mathematics education supports the value of active learner engagement [9]. This contrasts with traditional Oslerian "signature pedagogies" in the health professions that rely more on passive reading and clinical observation than "hands-on" deliberate practice [10, 11] (Chap. 1).

There are at least four other lessons learned from these and other seminal writings that address mastery learning in health professions education. First, in mastery learning instruction and assessment are unitary. Rigorous assessment with actionable feedback is a key feature of education interventions [12]. Second, education with mastery learning goals needs to overcome the evaluation apprehension barrier that is so widespread in the health professions [13, 14]. Assessment data are a tool for individual and team improvement, not a weapon to expose or humiliate motivated learners. Third, health professions educators who set mastery learning goals must design and engineer rigorous learning conditions and also set high achievement standards (Chap. 6). Fourth, health professions mastery learning programs need to carefully match instruction and assessment formats with learning goals. For example, learners simply cannot master advanced cardiac life support (ACLS) skills by reading a book or watching videos. They need to receive clear learning objectives, practice ACLS skills with coaching, undergo formative assessment, receive actionable feedback about how to improve, resume practice, and get more assessment and feedback until the mastery learning standard is reached [15] (Chap. 3).

Nobel Laureate psychologist Daniel Kahneman distills these ideas and comes close to describing mastery learning in his 2011 book, *Thinking, Fast and Slow*. Kahneman writes,

> The acquisition of skills requires a regular environment, an adequate opportunity to practice, and rapid and unequivocal feedback about the correctness of thoughts and actions. When these conditions are fulfilled, skill eventually develops, and the intuitive judgments and choices that quickly come to mind will mostly be accurate [16].

Instructional Design

Health professions education instructional design is all about planning and behavioral engineering. In their book, *Instructional Design*, third edition [17], Smith and Ragan teach that the overall instructional process has three seamless steps that conform with chapters in this book: (a) perform an instruction analysis to determine "where we are going" (Chap. 3), (b) develop an instructional strategy to determine "how we will get there" (this chapter), and (c) develop and conduct an evaluation to determine "how will we know when we are there" (Chaps. 5, 15, 16, 17, 18, 19, and 20).

Such a systematic approach to health professions instruction design has at least seven benefits. Smith and Ragan assert [17] this strategy:

1. Encourages learner advocacy.
2. Supports effective, efficient, and appealing instruction.
3. Supports coordination among designers, developers, and those who will implement the instruction.
4. Facilitates diffusion and adoption.
5. Supports development for alternate embodiments or delivery systems.
6. Facilitates congruence among objectives, activities, and assessment.
7. Provides a systematic framework for dealing with learning problems.

Table 4.1 presents a scheme for instructional design and delivery for health professions mastery learning. The table has a 3 × 3 layout, structured by theory (rows) and practice (columns). The three rows address the psychological foundations of mastery learning discussed earlier: (a) behavior improvement, (b) cognitive and social construction, and (c) social and cognitive self-efficacy [6]. The three tabular columns cover instruction design practice: (a) Where are we going? (instructional objectives); (b) How will we get there? (education settings and learner experience); and (c) How will we know when we are there? The nine cells of Table 4.1 are a distillate of the instruction design conditions and decisions that health professions educators need to consider when planning powerful instruction. Theoretical rows have been mentiond earlier in this chapter and are covered in Chap. 2. Now we focus on the three columns of practice conditions.

Where Are We Going? Instructional Objectives

Instructional objectives for health professions individuals and teams and their origins are grounded in learner curriculum objectives, milestones, and entrustable professional activities (EPAs). Instructional objectives address a wide-ranging sample of possible learning outcomes including clinical skill acquisition, refinement, and maintenance; clinical reasoning, situation awareness, adaptive capacities, and other markers of cognitive and social construction; and indexes of social cognitive self-efficacy such as poise, staying cool under pressure, and professionalism. Instructional objectives express learning expectations. Instructional objectives are the mastery

Table 4.1 Instruction design and delivery for health professions mastery learning

	Where are we going? Instructional objectives	How will we get there?		How will we know when we are there?
Behavior improvement	Skill acquisition and refinement: technical and communication Skill maintenance	*Settings* Clinical education center (SPs) Simulation laboratory Clinical workplace	*Learner experience* Pretests Active engagement Observation and videos Deliberate practice Formative assessment Rigorous, actionable feedback Opportunities for practice and improvement Summative assessment	Rising formative assessment results Meeting or exceeding MPSs on measures of clinical skill acquisition Clinical skill maintenance at or above MPSs over time Faster rates of clinical skill acquisition due to mastery experiences
Cognitive and social construction	Knowledge acquisition Clinical reasoning Situation awareness Teamwork Ethics Scholarship Community engagement Advocacy Reflective practice Adaptive capacities	*Settings* Lecture hall Classroom Simulation laboratory Seminar room PBL group TBL group Library Independent study Community clinic Clinical workplace	*Learner experience* Pretests Active engagement Reading Lecture Group discussion PBL TBL Problem sets-calculations Simulation and SPs Clinical experience and community of practice Community visits and encounters Team practice exercises Case studies Formative assessment Rigorous, actionable feedback Opportunities for practice and improvement Summative assessment	Rising formative assessment results Meeting or exceeding MPSs on knowledge acquisition measures Knowledge maintenance at or above MPSs over time Improvements on quantitative and qualitative measures of professionalism, adaptive capacities, clinical reasoning and insight, teamwork, and other qualities

Table 4.1 (continued)

	Where are we going? Instructional objectives	How will we get there?		How will we know when we are there?
Social cognitive self-efficacy	Clinical self-efficacy Poise Cool under pressure Professionalism	*Settings* Clinical education center (SPs) Simulation laboratory Community clinic Clinical workplace	*Learner experience* Pretests Active engagement Practice in varied situations Formative assessments Rigorous, actionable feedback Opportunities for practice and improvement Reflection on action Summative assessment	Improved clinical self-efficacy measured quantitatively and qualitatively due to mastery experiences Improvements on quantitative and qualitative measures of professionalism, poise, responses to pressured or uncertain situations, and other qualities

SP standardized patient; *MPS* minimum passing standard; *PBL* problem based learning; *TBL* team based learning

learning targets of education interventions that are shaped by settings and learner experience.

Instructional objectives are usually more specific than curriculum goals; are expressed in behavioral, measurable language; and are subject to mastery learning standards. A variety of objective and subjective measurement tools can be used to assess achievement of different instructional goals depending on their location on a quantitative–qualitative continuum (Chap. 5). Recall the Ericsson and Pool statement about the need for "objective ways" or "at least semi-objective ways" to measure performance. In mastery learning, measured step-by-step achievement with feedback is used to prompt individual and team learner movement toward instruction objectives until a minimum passing standard (MPS) is reached. Instruction and assessment are inseparable in mastery learning.

How Will We Get There? Education Settings and Learner Experience

Instructional settings for health professions mastery learning programs vary depending on objectives, local resources, and access. Instructional settings should facilitate achievement of the specific goals and objectives of the curriculum. In many cases the settings will ideally match the ultimate setting of health professions practice. However, health professions educators must often compromise instructional perfection for "what is possible" based on local resources.

Clinical education centers using standardized patients (SPs), simulation laboratories, and clinical workplaces are common settings for performance improvement interventions. Achievement of cognitive and social construction objectives can be done in a host of settings such as classroom, seminar room, problem-based and team-based groups, library, independent study, and many others.

Planning learner experiences to promote individual and team achievement of instruction and curriculum objectives is a key responsibility of mastery learning education leaders. The education leaders must ask: How can we design or engineer a set of experiences that will increase the probability that learners will be successful? How can we help learners cross the "finish line?" (meeting the MPS threshold). What is the instruction plan that teachers or coaches intend to carry out? How can we design conditions so that all learners can practice key skills, undergo assessment, receive feedback, and improve constantly? These questions address what Ben Lovell calls coaching in medical education [18] (see also Chap. 8).

The Dean Smith intense, two-hour basketball practice sessions are a prototype, not a blueprint, for health professions educators: clear objectives; constant learner physical, intellectual, and emotional engagement; formative assessment and feedback; scheduled rest periods; and continued learner engagement, assessment, and feedback until the summative MPS is met. Individual and team learning improvement is the education focus of planned learner experiences. Learning is designed to be active [1].

The second Smith and Ragan "how will we get there?" design question has direct answers. For health professions education mastery learning programs, the primary answer for both individual and team learning experiences is embodied in two entities: (a) the mastery learning bundle [19, 20] and deliberate practice [21–24]. Both entities are covered in Chap. 2 yet warrant repetition here.

The *mastery learning bundle* has seven essential features.

1. Baseline, i.e., diagnostic testing.
2. Clear learning objectives, units ordered by difficulty.
3. Education activities (e.g., deliberate skills practice) focused on the objectives.
4. Minimum passing *mastery* standard for each unit.
5. Formative testing + feedback → *mastery* of each unit.
6. Advancement if performance ≥ MPS.
7. Continued practice or study until the MPS is reached.

Deliberate practice (DP) is the highway toward acquisition and maintenance of knowledge, self-efficacy, and professionalism attributes in the health professions. Ericsson points out that

> … expert performance … acquisition requires a systematic and deliberate approach. Deliberate practice is therefore designed to improve specific aspects of performance in a

> manner that assures that attained changes can be successfully measured and integrated into representative performance. Research on deliberate practice in music and sports shows that continued attempts for mastery require that the performer always try, by stretching performance beyond its current capabilities, to correct some specific weakness, while preserving other successful aspects of function. This type of deliberate practice requires full attention and concentration, but even with that extreme effort, some kind of failure is likely to arise, and gradual improvements with corrections and repetitions are necessary [23].

Deliberate practice complements the mastery learning bundle with its ten integrated components.

1. Highly motivated learners with good concentration;
2. Engagement with a well-defined learning objective or task at an;
3. Appropriate level of difficulty with;
4. Focused, *repetitive practice* that leads to;
5. Rigorous, precise measurements that yield;
6. Actionable feedback from education sources (e.g., simulators, teachers) and where;
7. Trainees also monitor their learning experiences and correct strategies, errors, and levels of understanding, engage in more DP, and continue with;
8. Assessment to reach a *mastery* standard and then;
9. Advance to another task or unit;
10. Goal: constant improvement.

Together, these instruction design features of the mastery learning experience are a powerful education intervention that leads to skill acquisition. Citations to health professions mastery learning education and evaluation research programs described in Chap. 2 underscore the utility of the model. Another example of a mastery learning education program [actually an approximation to mastery learning] from the music profession reinforces the model's utility.

Dorothy DeLay was a virtuoso violin teacher at the Juilliard School of Music in New York City who enjoyed a career that spanned over 50 years. Her long list of proteges includes such celebrated artists as Nora Chastain, Misha Keylin, Itzhak Perlman, Joel Smirnoff, and Won Bin Yim. Biographer Barbara Lourie Sand provides a detailed account of DeLay's educational skills in the book *Teaching Genius: Dorothy DeLay and the Making of a Musician* [25]. DeLay asked herself in a reflective moment, "What do I want my students to be able to do? I want them to work independently and know what they are doing." DeLay thought about experts' (Toscanini, Heifetz, Casals) reactions to concert performances and decided "… this is what my kids have to know when they play, and the practice sheets I made up are a condensation of those ideas." Barbara Lourie Sand proceeds to report about the rigorous practice sessions DeLay's violin students endured.

> DeLay's practice sheets include a schedule: the first hour is spent on basics—articulation, shifting, and vibrato exercises for the left hand, and various bow strokes for the right; the second hour is for passages from repertoire, arpeggios, and scales; the third for etudes or

Paganini; the fourth on concerto; and the fifth for practicing Bach or the student's recital repertoire. Students are instructed to limit themselves to the first, third, and fourth hours on orchestra rehearsal days, and to rest at least ten minutes between hours

Virtuoso cellist Pablo Casals was a student of Dorothy DeLay. During his 81st year of life with a professional career that spanned over 60 years, Casals was asked by a syndicated newspaper columnist, "Why do you continue to practice four and five hours a day?" Casals replied, *"Because I think I am making progress"* [26].

A similar story is told about the motivation, dedication, ceaseless deliberate practice, and grueling physical, intellectual, and tough team work needed to reach very high-performance standards to become a US Navy SEAL [27]. SEALs excel at their professional craft. They are the most elite warriors in the US military.

The role of mastery learning educators—curriculum development, instruction design, instruction delivery in many settings—is very active, not passive. Mastery learning educators plan curricula and instruction sessions; set learning conditions in specific settings; organize people, education apparatus such as simulators and materials; schedule personnel and facilities; plan assessments; deliver actionable feedback; and expect constant improvement among health professions individuals and teams (Chap. 7). This is hard and indispensable work. Anders Ericsson notes that "… more accomplished individuals in the domain, such as professional coaches and teachers, will always play an essential role in guiding the sequence of practice activities for future experts in a safe and effective manner" [23]. Much of this behavior is no different from the work done by excellent health professions educators in traditional programs.

Health professions educators who instruct individuals and teams to mastery learning standards need not be from the same profession as the learners. Medical instruction can be presented by psychologists, respiratory therapists, physical therapists, physician assistants, nurses, and technicians. Nurse education can be done by many other health professionals and clinical specialists. For example, a respiratory therapist was the lead educator in a rigorous ACLS instructional program for internal medicine residents to mastery standards [15]. Physical therapists have effectively educated medical students on the musculoskeletal examination with instructional ratings equal to physician instructors [28]. Surgical technicians have been used effectively to teach fourth year medical students subcuticular suturing. Authors of the surgery education evaluation research report state, "Training by either a non-surgeon skills coach or a faculty surgeon resulted in no difference in performance on a basic surgical skill" [29].

How Will We Know When We Are There?

We have asserted regularly that instruction and assessment coalesce in mastery learning contexts—they are inseparable. Mastery learning assessments are best considered as assessment programs rather than singular measures or methods [12] (Chap. 5). We have also stated that assessment in mastery learning must be psychologically safe to reduce or eliminate evaluation apprehension which is widespread among health professions learners at all levels. A briefing before training can help with this goal. Mastery learning assessments must also be linked tightly to instructional objectives, educational settings, and learner experiences.

Instructional objectives that address behavior improvement focus on boosting clinical skill acquisition and maintenance. The two principal achievement aims are to increase learner skill sets via formative assessment, feedback, and practice. The final mastery learning goal for each instructional unit is to have all learners meet or exceed the MPS, which is a summative unit decision. Assessment methods and measures commonly used for behavior improvement include checklists and rating scales, clinical simulations and SPs, haptic sensors, observations by faculty and peers, and many other technologies. Mastery learning in service of behavior improvement goals frequently relies on a variety of assessment technologies that together produce data to inform mastery decisions.

Mastery decisions about learner achievement in cognitive and social construction can also be formative and summative. In the health professions, these decisions are usually about the acquisition and maintenance of knowledge using objective tests and examinations. However, there is also great concern across the health professions about learner development regarding professionalism, adaptive capacities, clinical reasoning and insight, teamwork, and many other attributes. Such learning outcomes are now assessed using observational ratings, peer judgments, longitudinal portfolios, and other subjective methods.

Mastery decisions about social cognitive self-efficacy are rarely done in health professions education. This is because social cognitive self-efficacy is usually considered a collateral consequence of mastery learning rather than an intentional instructional objective. Advice about how to construct objective measures of clinical self-efficacy is available from Albert Bandura for health professions educators who may choose to assess such learning outcomes in the short-run and longitudinally [30].

Instructional Delivery

An organized course design plan is essential to achieve the three instructional design questions: Where are we going? How will we get there? How will we know when we are there? A course designer can develop a plan for instructional delivery after addressing the three questions.

Consider the following example. Medical students are expected to demonstrate mastery of a core set of clinical competencies, including communicating with nurses on the telephone regarding patient care issues before graduation. In their future roles as residents, telephone communication will be a daily activity that impacts patient care. To ensure the students are able to effectively perform this skill at the end of their medical school training, a mastery learning course was developed and implemented in a fourth year transition to residency course. All students must demonstrate mastery at responding to pages as a course requirement.

Exhibit 4.1 presents a practical instructional delivery plan for a mastery learning simulation session for communication skills. This example demonstrates the instructional design decisions made during the development of this course to ensure soon-to-graduate medical students are prepared to perform an important clinical skill.

Exhibit 4.1 Instructional Design Plan for Mastery Learning Simulation Session
Basic Information

- Course Title: Interprofessional Communication
- Course Director: *Linda Todd, RN*
- Primary Learners: 4th year medical students

Where Are We Going?

- Overall goals of the course: To improve learners' ability to communicate with healthcare providers (RNs, typically) about urgent care concerns.
- Specific objectives – All participants will achieve mimimum passing standards (MPSs) at postest as measured by checklists evaluating the learners' abililty to:
  - *Demonstrate* professional behavior in conversations with others.
  - *Identify* clinical concerns using clarifying questions and read back.
  - *Develop and communicate* next steps for care.
  - *Confirm* plan for when they will follow up with the other clinician.
- Needs assessment:
  - *Learning environment:* Conducted in simulation lab or any clinical space with patient care equipment (computer, phone)
  - *Learners:* Clinicians who are responsible for the management of patients who would be asked about a clinical concern (e.g., call or question from a bedside nurse or junior trainee)
  - *What are our instructional needs/targets?*

    Respectful and professional communication
    Sharing one's mental model
    Using closed-loop communication
    Articulating a clear and actionable plan based on input from others
  - *What is currently being done to address this problem?*

    Physicians-in-training are immediately responsible for patient care questions from a variety of sources; they do not routinely receive training.

    Without a formal curriculum incorporating best practices including an opportunity to receive feedback and improve, learners will not consistently communicate well.

How Will We Get There?

- *Primary goal:* Improve the quality and professionalism of 4th year medical student communication with care team members.

- *Implementation:*
  - *Pretest*: Each participant will undergo a 20 min pretest individually. The pretest will include a pre-brief regarding expectations and an introduction to the standardized clinicians they will be speaking with. The learners will receive a simulated handoff on a panel of patients about whom they will answer clinical questions from a page. The simulation will begin when the participant is either called or asked a clinical question directly. There are six distinct cases used as clinical prompts.
  - *Pre-learning:* Each learner is given a communication skills expectations primer prior to the intervention.
  - *Intervention:* Learners will engage in practice using communication skills (introducing yourself, addressing other persons by name, listening to issue and clarifying and reading back issues, identifying and communicating a plan, and seeking other's understanding of plan. We provide 90 min for practice in small groups to allow students to work in pairs.
  - *Posttest:* A 20-min individual session, with the same format as the pretest, will be conducted 1 week after the intervention. Participants must meet the MPS. Those that do not will complete more training with deliberate practice and re-take the posttest until the MPS is achieved.
  - *Faculty:* Experienced healthcare providers with experience in conducting a mastery learning intervention will be instructors for the intervention. *(Names and specific experience are included here.)* Each rater will receive training on the instrument using example videos.
- *Funding: (Example)* Faculty will be provided by the medical school. Trained nurse raters are a budgeted cost.

How Will We Know We Have Arrived?

- How will learner achievement be assessed? Learners will meet or exceed the MPS. After the first year, we will assess posttest achievement and adjust the practice time and modify the curriculum based on the number of participants who do not meet the MPS at the first posttest. The MPS setting exercise was led by Dr. Harriett Matthews who has experience at managing such events. Two standard setting sessions were conducted with content and education experts.
- What types of assessments will be used? Our novel checklist tool was designed, following the Schmutz et al. protocol [31], before curriculum implementation. Instrument validation data were collected to support the use of the checklist in this setting.
- Content mapping: Our checklist items map to specific medical school milestones and our Professional Communication Entrustable Professional Activity with conviction to not over-represent any specific domain.

Health Professions Examples

This detailed account of mastery learning instruction delivery in a medical school fourth year curriculum is informative and useful. Communication between learners and other healthcare team members is a necessary skill for the soon-to-be residents with clear connection to patient care quality. In this curriculum, learners practice, undergo assessment, receive feedback, and work to improve; and learners continue to work hard on these skills until the MPS is reached. Teachers toil to help residents meet or exceed the mastery learning MPSs. We conclude this chapter section on instruction delivery by highlighting four other examples—the last an approximation—of mastery learning programs in health professions education. The four examples are about rigorous education in (a) nursing, (b) surgery, (c) dermatology, and (d) psychotherapy.

Nursing

Brittany Dahlen and her colleagues at Children's Hospital in Minneapolis, Minnesota, developed and tested a mastery learning curriculum for experienced cardiovascular intensive care unit (CVICU) hospital nurses on central line dressing changes [32]. The curriculum includes a rigorous skills pretest, feedback, instruction based on pretest results, and a posttest. Assessment and instruction for each of the 20 CVICU nurses was continued until each mastered the curriculum at a 100% MPS. Dahlen and colleagues report, "None of the participants achieved the MPS in the pretest. Common missteps include maintaining sterile protocol and masking the patient. MPS was achieved by 55% in the second attempt and 89% in the third attempt." All of the 20 CIVCU nurses eventually met the flawless MPS on the checklist measure of central line dressing changes. The authors conclude, "Despite self-reporting of high confidence in the pretest questionnaire, there was no correlation … between achieving mastery and pretest self-reported confidence in the ability to execute a dressing change…" [32].

Surgery

Northwestern University surgeon Ben Schwab and his colleagues created a simulation-based mastery learning (SBML) curriculum for surgical residents on laparoscopic common bile duct exploration (LCBDE) [33]. They performed a study to compare clinical outcomes among patients treated with LCBDE versus endoscopic retrograde cholangiopancreatography, the usual standard of care. The SBML training involved a baseline skills assessment (pretest) and then deliberate practice sessions using a LCBDE simulation with immediate feedback given by an expert instructor.

To answer the "how will we get there" component of the instructional design process, the authors used a previously developed LCBDE simulator [34]. The curriculum and deliberate practice were embedded as a mandatory component on a minimally invasive surgery service and learners continued to practice until the MPS was achieved. Learner instruction occurred over the course of 3 years with senior residents initially trained by a single expert instructor, and then trained as a team in the second year, and finally in the third year, senior residents who had achieved mastery served as trainers. This process allowed for a design which developed a "self-sustaining 'train the trainer' model" [33]. The multiple components of SBML require a considerable amount of coaching, assessments, and designing a structure that facilitates a sustainable long-term approach to teaching and giving feedback. However, the SBML model may yield a much higher likelihood of programmatic continuation (see also Chap. 12).

The authors report the results of the program:

> Of the 22 residents, 21 (95%) failed the pretest and all 22 passed the posttest. The average total curriculum time was 4 hours, which was divided into weekly 1-hour practice sessions. During the same period, 2 surgical faculty members voluntarily underwent the same SBML curriculum. Both failed the pretest and passed the posttest [33].

Downstream, comparative clinical results are also informative. Patients treated with LCBDE had a reduced length of stay compared to the usual standard of care. In addition, "Cost savings … resulted in a 3.8 to 1 return on investment from curriculum implementation" [33] (see also Chap. 19).

Dermatology

June Robinson and a team of dermatologists, primary care providers (PCPs), and medical educators at Northwestern University created a mastery learning curriculum on melanoma opportunistic screening skills and practice intended for instruction to PCPs [35]. The PCPs were community-based physicians and physician assistants who routinely screen ambulatory patients for skin diseases. The mastery learning curriculum contained 450 clinical and dermoscopic real patient images verified with pathological diagnoses. Robinson and colleagues state, "PCPs underwent training on the identification of at-risk patients and lesions suspicious for melanoma, consisting of three units: (a) visual and dermoscopic assessment, (b) diagnosis and management, and (c) deliberate practice."

To design the course and answer the "how will we get there" component of instructional design, the authors had to determine which content to include and a method and structure for deliberate practice. Highlighting the concept from earlier in the chapter about the hard work required to design a mastery learning curriculum, the authors indicate that the course was "developed over 11 months by a team of dermatologists, PCPs, and medical educators." To deliver the content, an online program was developed, algorithmic aids created, and the program divided into phases. To answer the final component of instructional design, "how will we know when we are there?" the authors elected to use the patient safety approach to standard setting (see Chap. 6) given the critically important nature and impact on patient safety of correct and early melanoma diagnosis. The Robinson team also points out that all seven features of the mastery learning bundle (e.g., pretest, MPS, posttest) were included in the melanoma screening mastery learning curriculum.

The investigators conducted a randomized trial to compare the melanoma opportunistic screening skills of PCPs who completed the mastery learning curriculum versus PCPs who had not received the education intervention. Results show that "PCPs in the intervention group answered more melanoma detection questions correctly on the post-test compared to control group PCPs." PCPs who underwent mastery training "… had fewer false-positive and no false-negative melanoma diagnoses and referred fewer benign lesions including nevi, seborrheic keratosis, and dermatofibromas than control PCPs." Finally, "Those receiving training referred significantly more melanomas than controls, mostly located on the head and neck" [35]. Robinson and colleagues conclude, "Mastery learning improved PCPs ability to detect melanoma on a standardized post-test and may improve referral of patients with suspected melanoma" [35].

Psychotherapy

Education and training of psychotherapists has traditionally relied on many hours of supervised clinical experience and qualitative judgments about whether an individual is competent for independent practice. Psychotherapy learning goals and objectives are frequently opaque. Supervised practice of psychotherapy skills varies widely in quality and intensity, and objective measures of skill acquisition and maintenance, except for standardized knowledge tests, are absent. Rigorous MPSs for psychotherapy skill acquisition are not imposed. Traditional psychotherapy education resembles Winston Churchill's Cold War description of the Soviet Union, "… a riddle, wrapped in a mystery, inside an enigma."

However, the psychotherapy education paradigm is beginning to show signs of change. Psychotherapy clinician-educators including Daryl Chow and colleagues [36] and Tony Rousmaniere [37] have successfully introduced the idea of deliberate practice into clinical education. These steps are a far cry from a fully engaged mastery learning approach to the education of psychotherapists yet represent a solid point-of-departure for future curriculum and measurement development.

These examples of mastery learning programs indicate the many decisions that health professions educators must make throughout the process of instructional design and delivery. The decisions are not simple and rarely "one off" events because instructional design and delivery for mastery learning in the health professions undergoes frequent refinement due to evaluation data and educational experience. Continuous quality improvement (CQI) is one of the pillars of mastery learning. Our learners and the patients they serve deserve no less.

Coda

Instructional design and delivery to achieve mastery learning goals in the health professions requires clear purpose, thoughtful planning, and hard work. Educators need to set clear objectives for learners at all levels; organize settings and educational experiences that challenge learners to engage in deliberate practice, receive feedback, and regularly improve; and develop assessment programs that permit formative and summative judgments about learners using quantitative and qualitative data. Instructional design and delivery in the health professions should undergo frequent upgrades to fulfill CQI goals.

References

1. Smith D. Basketball: multiple offense and defense. Boston: Allyn and Bacon; 1999.
2. Ericsson A, Pool R. Peak: secrets from the new science of expertise. Boston: Houghton Mifflin Harcourt; 2016.
3. Mayer RE. Applying the science of learning: evidence-based principles for the design of multimedia instruction. Am Psychol. 2008;63(8):760–9.
4. Mayer RE. Applying the science of learning to medical education. Med Educ. 2010;44:543–9.
5. McGaghie WC, Fisichella PM. The science of learning and medical education. Med Educ. 2014;48:106–8.
6. McGaghie WC, Harris IB. Learning theory foundations of simulation-based mastery learning. Simul Healthc. 2018;13(3S Suppl 1):S15–20.
7. Chickering AW, Gamson ZF, Associates. Seven principles for good practice in undergraduate education. AAHE Bull. 1987;39(7):2–6.
8. Issenberg SB, McGaghie WC, Petrusa ER, et al. Features and uses of high-fidelity medical simulations that lead to effective learning: a BEME systematic review. Med Teach. 2005;27(1):10–28.
9. Freeman S, Eddy SI, McDonough M, et al. Active learning increases student performance in science, engineering, and mathematics. PNAS. 2014;111(23):8410–5.
10. Harris I. Conceptions and theories of learning for workplace education. In: Hafler CJ, editor. Extraordinary learning in the workplace. New York: Springer; 2011.
11. Karani R, Fromme HB, Cayea D, Muller D, Schwartz A, Harris IB. How medical students learn from residents in the workplace: a qualitative study. Acad Med. 2014;89:490–6.
12. van der Vleuten CPM, Schuwirth LWT. Assessing professional competence: from methods to programmes. Med Educ. 2005;39:309–17.
13. McGaghie WC. Evaluation apprehension and impression management in clinical medical education. Acad Med. 2018;93(5):685–6.
14. Rosenblum L. Cursed by knowledge—building a culture of psychological safety. N Engl J Med. 2019;380(8):786–90.
15. Wayne DB, Butter J, Siddall VJ, et al. Mastery learning of advanced cardiac life support skills by internal medicine residents using simulation technology and deliberate practice. J Gen Intern Med. 2006;21:251–6.
16. Kahneman D. Thinking, fast and slow. New York: Farrar, Straus and Giroux; 2011.
17. Smith PL, Ragan TJ. Instructional design. 3rd ed. Hoboken, NJ: Wiley; 2005.
18. Lovell B. What do we know about coaching in medical education? A literature review. Med Educ. 2018;52:376–90.
19. WC MG, Siddall VJ, Mazmanian PE, Meyers J. Lessons for continuing medical education from simulation research in undergraduate and graduate medical education. Effectiveness of

continuing medical education: American College of Chest Physicians evidence-based educational guidelines. Chest. 2009;135(Suppl):62S–8S.
20. McGaghie WC. Mastery learning: it is time for medical education to join the 21st century. Acad Med. 2015;90(11):1438–41.
21. Ericsson KA, Krampe RT, Tesch-Römer C. The role of deliberate practice in the acquisition of expert performance. Psychol Rev. 1993;100(3):363–406.
22. Ericsson KA. Deliberate practice and the acquisition and maintenance of expert performance in medicine and related domains. Acad Med. 2004;79(10, Suppl):S70–81.
23. Ericsson KA. The influence of experience and deliberate practice on the development of superior expert performance. In: Ericsson KA, Charness N, Feltovich PJ, Hoffman RR, editors. The Cambridge Handbook of expertise and expert performance. New York: Cambridge University Press; 2006.
24. Ericsson KA. Acquisition and maintenance of medical expertise: a perspective from the expert-performance approach with deliberate practice. Acad Med. 2015;90(11):1471–86.
25. Sand BL. Teaching genius: Dorothy DeLay and the making of a musician. Montclair, NJ: Amadeus Press; 2000.
26. Casals P. Quote. Available at: https://quoteinvestigator.com/2014/02/12/casals-progress/.
27. Wasdin HE, Templin S. Seal team six: memoirs of an elite navy seal sniper. New York: St. Martin's Press; 2011.
28. McGaghie WC, Kowlowitz V, Renner BR, et al. A randomized trial of physicians and physical therapists as instructors of the musculoskeletal examination. J Rheumatol. 1993;20:1027–32.
29. Kim MJ, Boehler ML, Ketchum JK, Bueno R, Williams RG, Dunnington GL. Skills coaches as part of the educational team: a randomized controlled trial of teaching of a basic surgical skill in the laboratory setting. Am J Surg. 2010;199(1):94–8.
30. Bandura A. Guide for constructing self-efficacy scales. In: Pajares F, Urdan T, editors. Self-efficacy beliefs in adolescents. Greenwich, CT: Information Age Publishing; 2006.
31. Schmutz J, Eppich WJ, Hoffmann F, et al. Five steps to develop checklists for evaluating clinical performance: an integrative approach. Acad Med. 2014;89(7):996–1005.
32. Dahlen B, Finch M, Lambton J. Simulation-based mastery learning for central venous line dressing changes. Clin Simul Nurs. 2019;27:35–8.
33. Schwab B, Teitelbaum EN, Barsuk JH, et al. Single-stage laparoscopic management of choledocholithiasis: an analysis after implementation of a mastery learning resident curriculum. Surgery. 2018;163:503–8.
34. Santos BF, Reif TJ, Soper NJ, et al. Development and evaluation of a laparoscopic common bile duct exploration simulator and procedural rating scale. Surg Endosc. 2012;26:2403–15.
35. Robinson JK, Jain N, Marghoob AA, et al. A randomized trial on the efficacy of mastery learning for primary care provider melanoma opportunistic screening skills and practice. J Gen Intern Med. 2018;33(6):855–62.
36. Chow DL, Miller SD, Seidel JA, et al. The role of deliberate practice in the development of highly effective psychotherapists. Psychotherapy. 2015;52(3):337–45.
37. Rousmaniere T. Deliberate practice for psychotherapists: a guide to improving clinical effectiveness. New York: Routledge; 2017.

Assessment in Mastery Learning

5

Celia Laird O'Brien, Mark Adler, and William C. McGaghie

The purpose of assessment in mastery learning is to promote learner improvement. In mastery learning, assessment and instruction in all forms are inseparable. Assessment and instruction are complementary features of the 7-part mastery learning bundle described in Chap. 2. The mastery learning bundle features and the assessment focus of each are presented in Table 5.1.

Assessment in mastery learning is *criterion-referenced,* designed to measure progressive within-person gains. This contrasts with *norm-referenced* assessment which focuses on highlighting traditional learning outcomes as individual differences between learners [1]. The criterion-referenced approach does not gauge the achievement of individuals or teams compared to a reference group or a normal curve. Instead, achievement is compared to a minimum passing standard (MPS) that is uniform for all learners as seen in Fig. 5.1. "Excellence for all" is the expectation in mastery learning. Mastery learning assessment is used to gauge, reinforce, and boost learner progress and also to confirm achievement of learning outcomes [2].

The idea of criterion-referenced learner assessment is not new [1] and has close synonyms in such testing concepts as dynamic testing [3] and assessment embedded as a vital feature in learning programs rather than in measurement instruments [4].

C. L. O'Brien (✉)
Northwestern University Feinberg School of Medicine, Department of Medical Education, Chicago, IL, USA
e-mail: celia.obrien@northwestern.edu

M. Adler
Northwestern University Feinberg School of Medicine, Departments of Pediatrics and Medical Education, Chicago, IL, USA

W. C. McGaghie
Northwestern University Feinberg School of Medicine, Departments of Medical Education and Preventive Medicine, Chicago, IL, USA

W. C. McGaghie et al. (eds.), *Comprehensive Healthcare Simulation: Mastery Learning in Health Professions Education*, Comprehensive Healthcare Simulation, https://doi.org/10.1007/978-3-030-34811-3_5

Table 5.1 Assessment focus for each mastery learning bundle feature

Mastery learning bundle feature	Assessment focus
1. Baseline or diagnostic testing	Set individual or team performance baseline, provide actionable feedback about performance improvement, motivate study and deliberate practice
2. Clear learning objectives sequenced as units usually in increasing difficulty	Learning objectives derived from needs assessments and expert performance analysis (Chap. 3)
3. Engagement in educational activities (e.g., deliberate practice, calculations, data interpretation, reading) focused on reaching the objectives	Indexes of learner engagement, curriculum implementation, fulfill education requirements and expectations (Chap. 4)
4. A set minimum passing standard (MPS) for each educational unit. MPSs can be set for written tests, checklists, haptic devices, and many other measures of clinical performance	Standard setting using state-of-the-art methods (Chap. 6) or professional consensus
5. Formative testing to gauge unit completion at a preset mastery MPS	Criterion-referenced assessment to measure progressive within-person gains to approximate, meet, or exceed the MPS
6. Advancement to the next education unit given measured achievement at or above the MPS	Progressive curriculum achievements documented by performance data
7. Continued practice or study on an education unit until the MPS is reached	Deliberate practice and repeat performance measurement until the MPS is reached (Chap. 4)

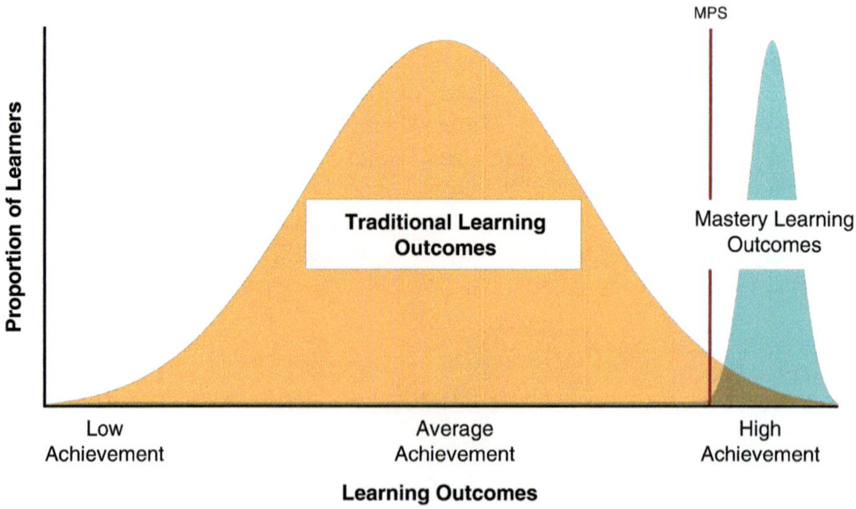

Fig. 5.1 Comparison of traditional learning outcomes with mastery learning outcomes

However, criterion-based learner assessment runs counter to current psychometric culture because it minimizes the importance of variation in education data (except for mastery learning pretests) and has greater interest in high and uniform learner achievement [5]. This is a radical shift from the psychometric foundations in individual differences that have governed educational measurement and data interpretation for the past century.

The key idea for mastery learning in the health professions is that assessment chiefly serves formative learning goals—*assessment for learning*. By contrast, psychometric assessment usually addresses summative learning goals—*assessment of learning* [4, 5]. In mastery learning settings instruction and assessment coalesce and their separation is opaque.

Health professions educators are fortunate to work on behalf of learners who have weathered very selective and competitive school admission screening; have high academic aptitude; are motivated and hard working; and aspire to become great nurses, physicians, physical therapists, pharmacists, physician assistants, and other health professionals. Academic failure rates in most health professions education programs and settings are very low. There is no reason to believe that, with a few exceptions, the persons who are recruited and selected for careers in the health professions should be anything less than topnotch performers. The only way to gauge the acquisition and maintenance of topnotch performance is via rigorous learner assessment, feedback, and constant improvement—all cornerstones of mastery learning.

Mastery learning grounded in rigorous and frequent learner assessment depends on a new teacher-learner relationship. Mastery learning is done under conditions of psychological safety, without learner evaluation apprehension or fear of failure, where education assessment data are used as a tool for improvement not as a weapon for humiliation or punishment [6, 7]. Mastery learning depends on a teacher-learner partnership that sets high education expectations; engages all parties in active, strenuous, deliberate practice; measures the growth of competence and provides frequent, actionable feedback; and boosts individual and team morale. Mastery learning is not at all passive for learners or teachers.

The criterion-referenced focus of mastery learning depends on a health professions culture of improvement and accountability. Values of excellence, service, and patient care trump the importance of competition with one's peers that is the tacit foundation of psychometric assessment.

The rest of this chapter is organized as six consecutive sections that address the formation, context, measures, data, and consequences of assessment in mastery learning. The six sections are (a) curriculum and objectives, (b) validity argument, (c) assessment context, (d) assessment measures, (e) data, and (f) decisions. This chapter is not meant to be a comprehensive report on the numerous assessment methods available to measure learner progress. Instead we intend to provide an overview of mastery learning assessment that can be applied to many curricula and workplaces. Most important, we aim to show that assessment in mastery learning is not a "one off," stand-alone procedure. Assessment in mastery learning is the backbone that unites the six following sections (Fig. 5.2). Paraphrasing social scientist Laurel Richardson, "… like a true spine, it [assessment] bears weight, permits movement, [and] links parts together in a functional, coherent whole" [8].

Curriculum and Objectives

Curriculum and Assessment Integration

Mastery learning curriculum design and development using the Thomas et al. approach [9] is discussed in detail in Chap. 3. There is a reciprocal relationship

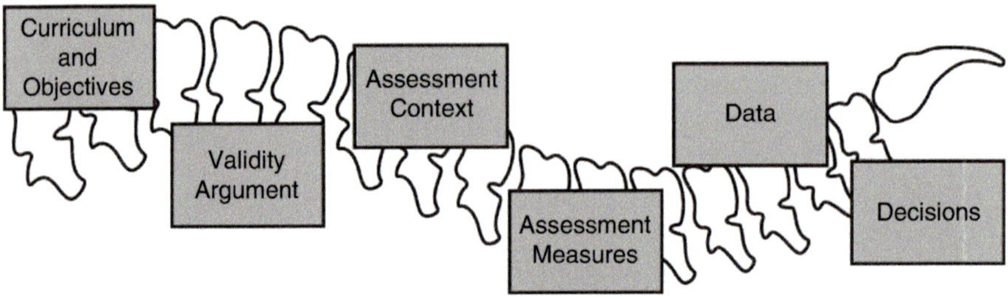

Fig. 5.2 Six features of assessment in mastery learning

between writing curriculum and learning objectives and preparing an assessment plan to make sure each learner achieves the objectives. Mechanisms of curriculum design, expression of learning objectives, and learner assessment inform each other dynamically and constantly. This reasoning underlies the argument of van der Vleuten and Schuwirth that "… assessment is not merely a measurement problem, as the vast literature on reliability and validity seems to suggest, but that it is also very much an instructional design problem and includes educational, implementation and resources aspects" [4].

This interdependence applies to curriculum and learning objectives and learner assessment with each process informing the others. Learner assessments originate from curriculum and learning objectives. Assessments and the data they yield contribute to accurate decisions about learner advancement and promotion. Assessment data also show if the curriculum objectives are "on target" and contribute to a validity argument about the education and measurement plan. Table 5.2 points out these relationships for a core clinical skill in medicine and nursing, the clinical breast examination (CBE). Health professions educators who endorse mastery learning need to pay careful attention to the linkages among curriculum and objectives, validity argument, assessment context, assessment measures, data, and decisions at all times.

What Do We Aim to Produce?

Recall from Chap. 2 and as seen in Table 5.2 that the learning theory foundations of mastery learning address (a) *behavior improvement* (clinical performance), (b) *cognition and social construction* (knowledge creation and interpretation of clinical representations, situation awareness and clinical decision-making, communication with patients, families, and the healthcare team, clinical data recording and updating), and formation of (c) *social cognitive self-efficacy* [see also ref. 10]. In clinical education and professional settings, these three categories operate simultaneously and often seamlessly. Learner assessment tactics need to address these three curriculum categories both individually and as a unified construct.

Behavior improvement comes from deliberate practice of key clinical skills in a simulation laboratory or in patient care settings [11–13]. Deliberate practice, of

Table 5.2 Clinical breast examination curriculum and objectives, assessment context, assessment measures, data, decisions, and validity argument

Clinical skill	Curriculum and objectives	Validity argument	Assessment context	Assessment measures	Data	Decisions
Clinical breast examination (CBE)	*Behavior improvement* Clinical performance	Content Response process Relationships to other variables	Clinical education center Simulation laboratory Clinic or bedside	Checklist detailing key CBE actions, haptic sensors, observational ratings	Checklist items and haptic records that show the power of mastery learning education interventions	Learner acquisition of clinical skill ≥ MPS Learner maintenance of clinical skill
	Cognitive and social construction Knowledge of indications, contraindications, and complications; create and interpret clinical representations	Content Internal structure Relationships to other variables	Classroom Clinical education center Simulation laboratory Clinic or bedside	Multiple-choice examination, mini-CEX Clinical records Standardized patients (SPs) Faculty and peer judgments	Pre- and posttest scores of acquired knowledge Clinical experience logs Ratings that show improved clinical representations	Learner acquisition of knowledge and clinical representations ≥ MPS Learner maintenance of knowledge and clinical representations
	Situation awareness (SA) and clinical decision-making (CDM) about when to perform CBE	Content Response process Consequences of assessment use Relationships to other variables	Clinical education center Simulation laboratory Clinic or bedside	Problem sets, computer simulation Clinical records/EHR audits? Faculty and peer judgments	Learner responses, ratings, faculty and peer records on improved SA and CDM	Learner demonstration of SA and CDM ≥ MPS Learner maintenance of SA and CDM
	Communication skill (CS) with patients, families, and the healthcare team	Content Response process Consequences of assessment use Relationships to other variables	Clinical education center Simulation laboratory Clinic or bedside	Checklist, global rating scale Faculty and peer judgments?	Items that show mastery learning improves discourse skills	Learner demonstration of CS ≥ MPS Learner maintenance of CS
	Clinical data recording and updating	Content Response process Relationships to other variables	Clinical education center Simulation laboratory Clinic or bedside	Simulated and real electronic health record (EHR) audit	Archival data from EHR records	Learner records of EHR skills ≥ MPS Learner maintenance of EHR skills
	Social cognitive self-efficacy Confidence in one's clinical skills and reliability	Content Internal structure Consequences of assessment use Relationships to other variables	Clinical education center Simulation laboratory Clinic or bedside	Self-reports of clinical self-efficacy (S-E)	Item and scale responses on CBE self-efficacy	Increased S-E due to clinical learning and practice Learner maintenance and enhancement of S-E

course, must be accompanied by rigorous measurement, actionable feedback, high standards, and opportunities for improvement. Assessment of clinical behavior improvement is usually accomplished using checklists, haptic sensors, and observational ratings. Chapter 4 covers such mastery learning instruction design and delivery in greater detail.

Constructivist knowledge, creation and interpretation of clinical representations, situation awareness, communication skills, and data recording are very difficult to assess in the health professions. Assessment of learner cognitive and social construction of clinical events calls for different evaluation approaches including multiple-choice tests, mini clinical evaluation exercises (mini-CEXs), faculty and peer judgments, problem sets, simulations, checklists, specific and global rating scales, and simulated and real electronic health record audits. Longitudinal measures that span an extended timeframe and multiple clinical problems and settings are needed to obtain a reliable sample of learner competence.

Formation of social cognitive self-efficacy is a product of planned simulated and real clinical encounters with follow-up and feedback, mentoring, reading and reflection, and observing experts. Unguided, random clinical experience is not a good teacher [6] and human beings are notoriously bad at self-assessment [14, 15]. However, reliable external data and guidance from a trusted mentor has been shown to improve accuracy of self-assessment [16]. Assessment of social cognitive self-efficacy formation is typically done using quantitative self-reports [17] and more qualitative global ratings.

Integrated learner assessment that captures behavior improvement, growing constructivist sophistication, and better social cognitive self-efficacy cannot be done using single measurements or simple thinking. Mastery learning assessment *programs* are needed to evaluate complex competencies among individuals and teams in the health professions. van der Vleuten and Schuwirth assert this "requires quantitative and qualitative information from different sources as well as professional judgment. Adequate sampling across judgments, instruments, and contexts can ensure both validity and reliability" [4]. Other scholarly writings in health professions education assessment reinforce this argument [18–21]. Learner assessment programs in the health professions that rely on longitudinal electronic portfolios illustrate such an integrative approach [22].

The growing movement in health professions education to develop curricula and assessment plans that focus on developmental milestones and entrustable professional activities is compatible with the mastery learning model. Chapter 17 addresses such ideas in great detail.

Validity Argument

"Validity is an overall evaluative judgment of the degree to which empirical evidence and theoretical rationales support the *adequacy and appropriateness of interpretations and actions* based on test scores or other modes of assessment" [23].

Current validity frameworks are those proposed by Samuel Messick [23] and Michael Kane [24]. These frameworks have been summarized by Cook and colleagues [25, 26] and Boulet and colleagues [27]. Lineberry and colleagues have located these ideas squarely within the mastery learning context [5]. The concept was described in older models using such terms as face, concurrent, and predictive validity. These models have been modernized to form a view that validity is now a unitary construct.

Different streams of evidence support a validity argument that is ongoing, never finished. Key features of current ideas about validity include:

- Validity is a property of data and decisions rather than a feature of an instrument or a measurement procedure.
- Validity is specific to a purpose such as a mastery decision and for a specific population, e.g., student nurses in a foundations course. Validity is not transferable.
- Validity is neither dichotomous nor ever fully settled.
- Validity is a hypothesis-driven inquiry to support an argument about the measured performance of specific persons or healthcare teams under specific conditions.
- Health professions educators draw conclusions about assessment data and the ability to make accurate decisions from available evidence and the persuasiveness of a validity argument.

A validity argument is a continuous discussion about how to collect, interpret, and use assessment data in many forms to reach valid decisions about the advancement and entrustment of individual health professionals and health professions teams. Questions and answers in the give-and-take discussion enrich an ongoing dialogue about how and when learners and teams should move forward in education settings and later be judged fit to care for patients.

Current thinking holds that valid decisions are grounded in six sources of assessment evidence [23–27].

1. *Interpretations and uses for mastery learning assessments*—what does mastery mean and what is the best evidence for mastery assessment?
2. *Content*—coverage of skills, information, and attributes of professionalism that represent professional practice.
3. *Response process*—the degree to which learner responses captured by assessments simulate responses in professional practice.
4. *Internal structure and reliability*—the degree to which individual assessment items or methods converge on a common construct or competency.
5. *Relationships to other variables*—how mastery assessment data correlate with conceptually similar measures.
6. *Consequences of assessment use*—the impact of mastery assessment data and decisions on health professions individuals and teams and the patients they serve.

Lineberry and colleagues state that "Sound assessment is the cornerstone of mastery learning systems" [5]. They continue to "outline key issues in the validation and justification of mastery learning assessments … [organized] by the key tenets of modern assessment validity theory" [5]. The work of this group is summarized in List 5.1, which lists six key considerations for the validation and justification of mastery learning assessments, drawn chiefly from Michael Kane's scholarship [24]. List 5.1 is reproduced from *Academic Medicine* [5] with permission from Wolters Kluwer.

List 5.1 Key considerations for the validation and justification of mastery learning assessments

Interpretations of and Uses for Mastery Learning Assessments

- Specify what degree of achievement or readiness to progress is meant by mastery
- Specify how long learners are meant to retain mastery
- Specify how complete mastery within a particular content area must be (compensatory versus non-compensatory scoring)
- Specify how scores will be used to make decisions and actions about learners

Sources of Validity Evidence: Content

- Develop sufficient assessment content to allow for high-volume retesting as needed
- Use best practices for generating multiple equivalent retests
- When appropriate, assess aspects of performance beyond achievement of content (e.g., automaticity of performance)

Sources of Validity Evidence: Response Process

- Examine whether learners' response processes on retests are consistent with true mastery, rather than with memorization of the particulars of the assessment content

Sources of Validity Evidence: Internal Structure and Reliability

- Use adjusted reliability estimates for the mastery versus non-mastery distinction
- Carefully consider how to derive estimates of reliability and internal structure for mastery posttests, when learner performance is likely to be restricted in range
- If non-compensatory scoring is used, adjust reliability estimates accordingly

Sources of Validity Evidence: Relationships to Other Variables

- Carefully consider how to derive estimates of relationships to other variables for mastery posttests, when learner performance is likely to be restricted in range

- Collect evidence as to whether a given mastery assessment relates to satisfactory versus unsatisfactory progress in later educational units and/or subsequent patient care

Sources of Validity and Justification Evidence: Consequences of Assessment Use

- Examine potential positive and negative effects of mastery assessment for curriculum and instruction, individual learners, patient outcomes, and society

  Lineberry et al. [5]. Reprinted with permission from Wolters Kluwer.

Regular attention to these validity argument issues among health professions educators will enrich our ideas about what clinical mastery learning really means and how to improve our future thinking and practice.

Assessment Context

Learner assessment in health professions education is always situated in context. The contexts are cast in two general categories: (a) controlled education settings like classrooms and clinical education centers including simulation laboratories and (b) workplace education settings including in- and out-patient clinics, community health centers, first-responder emergency situations, and military trauma scenes where little or no education control can be exercised. Controlled and workplace contexts shape and drive the assessment experiences that learners receive. The assessment context is a key part of the health professions education experience [18–20].

Controlled Education Settings

Controlled health professions education settings include classrooms, seminars, problem-based learning (PBL) groups, and clinical education centers such as simulation laboratories and standardized patient (SP) programs. Controlled education settings allow health science learners and their teachers to engage in knowledge and skill acquisition exercises without distraction. The emphasis in controlled settings is on reading, discussion, problem-solving, and deliberate practice with actionable feedback toward mastery learning goals.

Assessment conditions in controlled education settings are standardized, uniform for everyone, and best suited to address acquisition and measurement of basic clinical skills. Checklists, haptic sensors, standardized patients (SPs), and observational ratings are used to assess CBE skills (Table 5.2) and many other clinical education outcomes such as advanced cardiac life support (ACLS), intubation, central venous catheter (CVC) insertion, and communication with patients and their families. These are T1 outcomes [28] assessed in a controlled education setting, chiefly *assessments for learning* [4, 5]. Chapter 16 describes assessment in controlled settings and their translational results in detail.

Workplace Education Settings

Learner assessment in workplace education settings like outpatient primary care clinics, physical therapy practices, pediatric emergency departments, and surgical intensive care units is a very different project than assessment in controlled settings. Workplace-based learner assessments are frequently rendered under disorderly conditions where patient care goals replace education objectives [29]. There is a presumed trade-off in workplace-based assessment between the reliability of evidence from controlled settings and the validity of "real world" assessments in frequently chaotic clinical environments.

Singh and Norcini point out that workplace-based assessment in the health professions has great value for at least five reasons. First, it allows for assessment of knowledge, skill, and attributes of professionalism that are directly aligned with workplace expectations. Second, observation and assessment of single clinical encounters can be done using the mini-CEX. Third, procedural skills can be observed directly in the real clinical context. Fourth, learners' clinical work samples can be assessed for breadth and saturation of coverage. Fifth, individual clinical cases can be discussed in detail with formative feedback given to learners [29]. Workplace-based assessments may also stretch the measurement endpoint to capture translational education outcomes such as improved patient care practices (T2) and patient outcomes (T3) [28]. Translational education outcomes are the subject of Chap. 16.

Despite the lack of control, workplace-based assessment addresses clinical learning goals that complement learning goals that are taught, learned, and evaluated in more controlled education environments. Learner assessment situated in the clinical workplace extends assessment performed in a controlled clinical education center or health professions simulation education laboratory.

Assessment Measures

Assessment measures in health professions education mastery learning programs originate from four key sources: (a) sampling, (b) blueprinting, (c) granularity, and (d) instrumentation. These four sources cascade to allow health professions educators to make data-based, accurate decisions about learner advancement and competence.

Sampling

Clinical practice in the health professions is a very complex enterprise. Competent clinical practice involves a broad and deep portfolio of professional attributes: basic

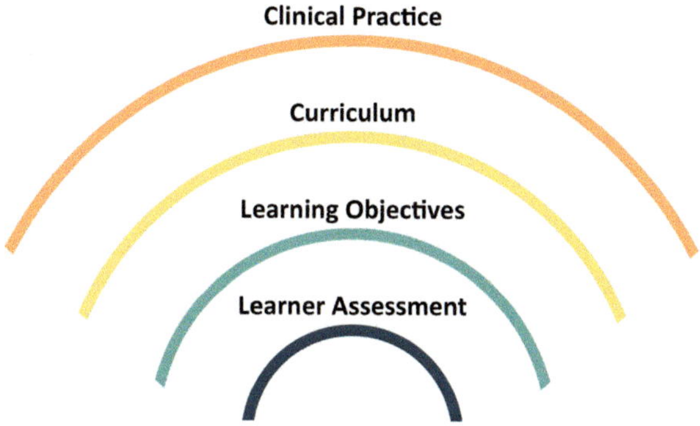

Fig. 5.3 Learner assessment as a sample of learning objectives, curriculum, and clinical practice

science and clinical knowledge; procedural skills; teamwork; diagnostic and treatment acumen; setting clinical priorities, communication with patients, families, and healthcare team members; awareness of healthcare economics; attention to ethical issues; and many other matters. Thus the universe of healthcare clinical practice is nearly endless, spanning a wide array of cognitive foundations, skills and abilities, character traits, and features of professionalism. As health professions educators, we can neither teach nor assess this entire universe.

Figure 5.3 is a graphic that portrays this situation as a sampling plan that depends on professional judgment by health professions educators. The curricula we create and present are a small sample of the clinical practice universe. Learning objectives are a curriculum sample. Learner assessments are an even smaller sample of the learning objectives we set for students, residents, and fellows and for continuing education programs. Data derived from learner assessments need to be accurate and useful to make decisions about individual and healthcare team competence. The accuracy and utility of assessment data stem from the degree that the content sampling plan that "trickles down" from clinical practice to curriculum, learning objectives, and learner assessment is sensible and representative.

Educational measurement scholar Samuel Messick has addressed content and learning performance sampling under the heading of *content relevance and representativeness*. Messick writes,

> A key issue for [measurement] content … is the specification of the boundaries of the content domain to be assessed—that is, determining the knowledge, skills, and other attributes to be revealed by the assessment tasks. The boundaries and structure of the construct domain can be assessed by means of job analysis, task analysis, curriculum analysis, and especially domain theory—that is, scientific inquiry into the nature of the domain processes and the ways in which they combine to produce effects on the outcome [23].

Messick continues, "The intent is to ensure that all important parts of the construct domain are covered, which is usually described as selecting tasks that sample domain processes in terms of their functional importance" [23].

Mastery learning assessment programs in health professions education must therefore have focus on a select sample of knowledge, clinical skills, and attributes of professionalism derived from research, tradition, and expert judgment. Such an assessment sampling plan is first captured as an assessment blueprint which in turn leads to decisions about adoption or creation of assessment instruments and tools.

Blueprinting

A test blueprint is an operational definition of the purpose and scope of an assessment. An assessment blueprint identifies the cases, tasks, or other content to be included (and, by inference, excluded) in an assessment and how they will challenge the trainee. The next two paragraphs and Table 5.3 are taken from a 2009 chapter publication about assessment blueprinting [30]. The text and table are reprinted with permission from Taylor & Francis.

Table 5.3 Test blueprint for clinical cardiology using the "Harvey" CPS

Evaluation goals	Identify finding	Identity finding and correlate it with underlying pathophysiology	Identify finding and correlate it with underlying disease process and differential diagnosis	Identify finding and correlate it with the severity of the underlying disease process and clinical management	
Cardinal auscultatory findings					Total
1. Second sound splitting	10%		5%		15%
2. Third sound		5%	5%		10%
3. Fourth sound				10%	10%
4. Systolic clicks		5%	5%		10%
5. Innocent murmur	5%			10%	15%
6. Mitral regurgitation		5%		5%	10%
7. Aortic stenosis					0%
8. Aortic regurgitation	5%		10%		15%
9. Mitral stenosis		10%			10%
10. Continuous murmur					0%
11. Tricuspid regurgitation	5%				5%
12. Pericardial rub					0%
Total	25%	25%	25%	25%	100%

Reproduced with permission of "Assessment in Health Profession Education" [30] April 2009, Taylor & Francis Group LLC Books

"Table 5.3 presents an *example* blueprint of a simulation-based assessment in clinical cardiology using the 'Harvey' cardiology patient simulator (CPS) [30, 31]. The example is for a test of second year internal medicine residents who are completing a four-week cardiology rotation. This illustrative blueprint shows that recognition of the 12 cardinal auscultatory findings can be assessed against four separate and increasingly complex evaluation goals. They range from (a) identify finding to (b) identify finding and correlate it with underlying pathophysiology, (c) correlate the finding with underlying disease process and differential diagnosis, and (d) correlate the finding with the severity of the underlying disease process and clinical management. Tabular cell entries show the distribution of test content for this example. The cell entries and marginal totals indicate that assessment of second sound splitting, innocent murmur, and aortic regurgitation are emphasized over other options. Cells and marginals also show that identify finding is weighted equally with the other three more complex evaluation goals. Other health professions education programs (e.g., nursing, pharmacy, physical therapy) and levels of testing (i.e., beginner to advanced) may have very different evaluation weighting schemes.

The point of Table 5.3 is that health science educators who use simulation and other technologies for learner assessment must make conscious decisions about what the tests will cover (and not cover) and with what emphasis. This involves professional judgment and choice shaped by reason, experience, and anticipation about future professional practice needs of today's learners. Test blueprint development and use, combined with clinical educators' judgment and choice, contributes content-related validity evidence to learner assessment practices. This is a basic building block of an assessment program that makes valid decisions about learner competence" [30].

The blueprinting process should not be done in isolation. Educators should rely on peer-reviewed publications and experts in the field as well as their own professional experience when considering which contexts, cases, and items will compose the assessment. Practical advice about how to frame and create blueprints for a variety of assessment formats is available from a textbook on educational measurement and evaluation [32]. Examples of blueprints that have been used as foundations for educational assessments in the health professions are available from the National Council of State Boards of Nursing [33] regarding the licensure examination for registered nurses, for a nephrology in-training examination [34], about a certification examination in child and adolescent psychiatry [35], and for a medical licensing examination in Korea [36].

Granularity

The idea of granularity in health professions education assessment refers to the detail of measurement. Granularity is not equivalent to reliability, which is a property of data. Highly granular assessments focus on discrete elements of, say, a clinical skill like the surgical procedures presented in Chap. 12. Checklists can be used for granular assessment of surgical skills where attention to specific surgical steps, often in an ordered sequence, is the key to a successful operation [37]. Many invasive and noninvasive clinical skills in nursing, dentistry, medicine, and other health professions require granular assessment to gauge achievement toward a mastery standard.

By contrast, the opposite pole of the granularity continuum in health professions education assessment evaluates clinical skills and behavior that defy reduction to a checklist or rating scale. Here educators acknowledge the importance of assessing such clinical learning outcomes as teamwork, professionalism, and managing complex clinical problems that have more than one correct answer and where experts disagree about the best course of action. Such assessments rely on global ratings, expert judgment, and peer group evaluations to reach assessment decisions, including mastery verdicts [4].

Health professions educators must use informed judgment about the best location on the granularity continuum to situate each assessment. Just like assessment sampling and blueprinting, informed judgment by individuals and faculty groups is needed to settle granularity questions.

Instrumentation

Instrumentation focuses on the "hows" of mastery learning measurement and assessment. What is the best way to assess a student nurse's skill at urinary catheter insertion? How can physician assistant teachers judge young clinicians' acumen about medication reconciliation? What's the best approach for faculty assessors to gauge the operative skill of novice orthopedic surgeons?

The key to making good decisions about assessment instruments in health professions education is to focus on the match of assessment goals and measurement tools. Returning to Table 5.2 we present examples of the goals-tools match regarding assessment of learner skill at performing the clinical breast examination (CBE). If the intent is to assess CBE clinical performance, reliance on simulated breast models with embedded haptic sensors that address normal tissue and pathological lesions is a sensible approach. Several measurement tactics including a checklist to assess CBE technique with live and video-recorded observations together with embedded haptic sensors to assess the location and depth of palpation pressure provide a partial sample of CBE competence [38, 39]. The CBE competence sample is amplified from multiple-choice measures of acquired knowledge; SPs; problem sets and computer simulations on situation awareness and clinical decision-making; faculty and peer judgments; checklists and rating scales to measure various communication skills; probes of real and simulated electronic health records to assess data recording and updating [40]; and self-reports about the growth of self-efficacy as a result of mastery education experience.

A variety of assessment instruments are needed to acquire a confluence of data so education leaders can make formative decisions about learner progress and summative decisions about professional certification and licensure.

Data

Data are information derived from assessment instruments and procedures. Data come in two generic forms: (a) quantitative numbers from a variety of sources and (b) qualitative words, symbols, pictures, and fabricated products. Different but sometimes overlapping methods are used to collect, interpret, and use quantitative and qualitative assessment data together. These are called mixed-method approaches—simultaneous use of numbers and words [41].

Data Use

In mastery learning settings, data are collected and used to serve at least four purposes, to (a) provide actionable feedback to learners about how to improve, (b) inform faculty decisions about learner advancement and entrustment (Chap. 17), (c) judge education program efficiency and effectiveness, and (d) contribute to health professions education science and scholarship.

Actionable feedback for learner performance improvement is a core concept in mastery learning (Chap. 8). The aim of performance improvement depends on an understanding that assessment data are used to gauge and improve professional progress, not as a weapon to humiliate or belittle learners. Use of assessment data for actionable feedback requires the educator to do the hard work of creating a safe space for learning that can mitigate evaluation apprehension [6, 7]. Feedback based on reliable assessments must be sought, not avoided, to boost constant improvement from deliberate practice and reach mastery learning goals. Basketball superstar Michael Jordan wrote about his legendary coach Dean Smith, "I love the competition of practice [with feedback]. I got that from Coach Smith who would make every drill competitive. I took pride in the way I practiced" [42].

Accurate faculty decisions about learner advancement in a health professions curriculum rely on trustworthy data. Multiple-choice test scores, checklist summaries, clinical ratings, haptic recordings, EHR trails, and many other metrics can be used to inform faculty decisions about learner advancement and entrustment, maybe the need for more study and deliberate practice, and mastery of curriculum components. A variety of quantitative and qualitative data are needed to make accurate decisions about learner progress.

The efficiency and effectiveness of health professions education programs are gauged in large part by learner achievement measures. What is the number and percentage of student nurses who have mastered protocols for the care and treatment of pressure sores among bedridden nursing home patients? How many graduating medical students can counsel primary care patients about smoking cessation, prudent diet, exercise, alcohol consumption, and safe sex? How effective are surgical technicians at preparing sterile trays for tomorrow's operations? These are questions that are addressed by education program outcome data. Curriculum efficiency and effectiveness is chiefly judged from learner results.

Health professions teachers and scientist-scholars use data derived from assessment instruments to document learner achievement; evaluate the impact of novel education interventions; study correlates of classroom, clinical, and simulation learning experiences; and calculate "downstream," translational outcomes of education interventions on patient care practices and patient outcomes [28] (see also Chap. 16). Given thoughtful planning and approval from a local Institutional Review Board (IRB), nearly all data collected and used for learner assessment and feedback can also be used for research and academic writing. Scholarship and publications drawn from these data-based activities enrich the knowledge base about mastery learning in health professions education and spawn new and better education approaches.

Data Quality and Utility

The quality and utility of data derived from instruments and procedures used for assessments in mastery learning settings is gauged using methods and standards that resemble those used for psychometric data. However, the methods and standards are not identical because criterion-based assessment focuses on within-person (or within-group) improvement rather than variation between persons and groups. Reliability in quantitative mastery learning clinical skill acquisition projects is best estimated by indexes of inter-rater agreement or generalizability theory for observational data [43, 44]. The Cohen's kappa coefficient is used for nominal data, Kendall's coefficient of concordance is used for ordinal data, and the intra-class correlation coefficient is used to estimate the reliability of interval observational data. Generalizability theory, described by Robert Brennan, offers another comprehensive method that provides information about sources of score variance including information about rater agreement [44]. Routine calibration of haptic sensors ensures the reliability of the data they produce just like any other piece of laboratory measurement apparatus. Reliability in qualitative mastery learning projects is determined by accumulation of subjective data, repetition, saturation, agreement, and member checking [4, 18, 19]. Qualitative data reliability estimation is no less rigorous than quantitative data reliability estimation, just different.

Data reliability indexes that rely on individual differences variation are used sometimes in mastery learning projects for measures of attitude and self-efficacy (Cronbach's alpha) and acquired knowledge (KR-20 and 21). These data reliability estimates are most useful to gauge the quality of mastery learning pretest data, but not posttest data, where variation due to individual differences is irrelevant.

Decisions

The ability to make accurate decisions about the educational advancement of individuals and teams in a mastery learning setting depends on two variables: (a) a carefully defined minimum passing standard (MPS) and (b) trustworthy, reliable data.

Small and large units of a mastery learning curriculum need to have MPSs to assess and judge learner readiness for advancement. Examples include a clinical skill acquisition exercise like ACLS; a basic science course unit such as renal physiology; or a larger curriculum component like a 6-week rotation in outpatient psychiatry. What is the "bottom line" MPS for each of these three curriculum components? How is "good enough" performance defined and expressed? Who has responsibility and authority to set and enforce the MPS? What are the consequences for learners and health professions education programs when mastery and not-yet-mastery advancement decisions are reached? These and other MPS issues are covered in Chap. 6, "Standard Setting for Mastery Learning," and in recent scholarly writing [45].

The value and utility of reliable quantitative and qualitative assessment data has been discussed in the previous section. Accurate, reliable decisions about individual learners and learner teams simply cannot be made without trustworthy data. Returning to Table 5.2, however, we note that not all education decisions need to employ a mastery learning MPS. To illustrate, in the curriculum category of social cognitive self-efficacy (S-E)—confidence in one's clinical skills and personal reliability—measured S-E growth due to the curriculum and clinical experience without imposing a MPS can contribute evidence that the curriculum is working, provided that learners are informed by accurate feedback on their performance.

Coda

Assessment in mastery learning curricula in the health professions is an essential feature of the education intervention. Instruction and learner assessment are inseparable. Health professions mastery learning assessment acknowledges the complex social context of learning and professional practice, relies on multiple quantitative and qualitative measurement methods, insists on the production and use of reliable data, and advocates for assessment programs instead of individual measures to render mastery (entrustment) decisions about learners [46]. Such assessment programs blend the best of psychometric traditions with new ideas about gauging the learning achievements of individuals and teams [47]. Overall, assessment in mastery learning endorses the view of Watling and Ginsburg, "… regular injections of test-based assessment into a curriculum can enhance both learning and retention" [48].

Reliable decisions about the advancement and entrustment of individuals and teams is a cornerstone of mastery learning programs [5]. Such decisions contribute to a validity argument about the utility of mastery learning as an education intervention and the assessment programs embedded in mastery learning curricula.

References

1. Popham WJ. Criterion-referenced measurement. Englewood Cliffs, NJ: Prentice-Hall; 1978.
2. McGaghie WC. Mastery learning: it is time for medical education to join the 21st century. Acad Med. 2015;90(11):1438–41.
3. Grigorenko EL, Sternberg RJ. Dynamic testing. Psychol Bull. 1998;124(1):75–111.

4. van der Vleuten CPM, Schuwirth LWT. Assessing professional competence: from methods to programmes. Med Educ. 2005;39(3):309–17.
5. Lineberry M, Park YS, Cook DA, Yudkowsky R. Making the case for mastery learning assessments: key issues in validation and justification. Acad Med. 2015;90(11):1445–50.
6. McGaghie WC. Evaluation apprehension and impression management in clinical medical education. Acad Med. 2018;93(5):685–6.
7. Rosenbaum L. Cursed by knowledge—building a culture of psychological safety. N Engl J Med. 2019;380(8):786–90.
8. Richardson L. Writing strategies: reaching diverse audiences, Qualitative research methods series, vol. 21. Newbury Park, CA: Sage Publications; 1990.
9. Thomas PA, Kern DE, Hughes MT, Chen BY. Curriculum development for medical education: a six-step approach. 3rd ed. Baltimore: Johns Hopkins University Press; 2016.
10. McGaghie WC, Harris IB. Learning theory foundations of simulation-based mastery learning. Simul Healthc. 2018;13:S15.
11. Ericsson KA. Deliberate practice and the acquisition and maintenance of expert performance in medicine and related domains. Acad Med. 2004;79(10, Suppl):S70–81.
12. Ericsson KA, Whyte J, Ward P. Expert performance in nursing: reviewing research on expertise in nursing within the framework of the expert-performance approach. Adv Nurs Sci. 2007;30(1):E58–71.
13. Ericsson KA. Acquisition and maintenance of medical expertise: a perspective from the expert-performance approach with deliberate practice. Acad Med. 2015;90(11):1471–86.
14. Davis DA, Mazmanian PE, Fordis M, et al. Accuracy of physician self-assessment compared with observed measures of competence: a systematic review. JAMA. 2006;296:1094–102.
15. Eva KW, Cunnington JPW, Reiter HI, et al. How can I know what I don't know? Poor self-assessment in a well-defined domain. Adv Health Sci Educ Theory Pract. 2004;9(3):211–24.
16. Sargeant J, Mann K, van der Vleuten C, Metsemakers J. "Directed" self-assessment: practice and feedback within a social context. J Contin Educ Health Prof. 2008;28:47–54.
17. Bandura A. Guide for constructing self-efficacy scales. In: Pajores P, Urdan T, editors. Self-efficacy beliefs of adolescents. Greenwich, CT: Information Age Publishing; 2006. p. 307–37.
18. Schuwirth L, Ash J. Assessing tomorrow's learners: in competency-based education only a radically different holistic method of assessment will work. Six things we could forget. Med Teach. 2013;35:555–9.
19. Hodges B. Assessment in the post-psychometric era: learning to love the subjective and collective. Med Teach. 2013;35:564–8.
20. Lockyer J, Carraccio C, Chan M-K, et al. Core principles of assessment in competency-based medical education. Med Teach. 2017;39960:609–16.
21. Gruppen LD, ten Cate O, Lingard LA, et al. Enhanced requirements for assessment in a competency-based, time variable medical education system. Acad Med. 2018;93:S17–21.
22. O'Brien CL, Sanguino SM, Thomas JX, Green MM. Feasibility and outcomes of implementing a portfolio assessment system alongside a traditional grading system. Acad Med. 2016;91(11):1554–60.
23. Messick S. Standards of validity and the validity of standards in performance assessment. Educ Meas Issues Pract. 1995;14(4):5–8.
24. Kane MT. Validating the interpretations and uses of test scores. J Educ Meas. 2013;50(1):1–73.
25. Cook DA, Brydges R, Ginsburg S, Hatala RA. A contemporary approach to validity arguments: a practical guide to Kane's framework. Med Educ. 2015;49(6):560–75.
26. Cook DA, Hatala RA. Validation of educational assessments: a primer for simulation and beyond. Adv Simul. 2016;1(1):31.
27. Boulet JR, Jeffries PR, Hatala RA, et al. Research regarding methods of assessing learning outcomes. Simul Healthc. 2011;6(Suppl):S48–51.
28. McGaghie WC. Medical education research as translational science. Sci Trans Med. 2010;2:19cm8.
29. Singh T, Norcini JJ. Workplace-based assessment. In: McGaghie WC, editor. International best practices for evaluation in the health professions. London: Radcliffe Publishing Ltd; 2013.

30. McGaghie WC, Issenberg SB. Simulations in assessment. In: Downing SM, Yudkowsky R, editors. Assessment in health professions education. New York: Routledge; 2009. p. 245–68.
31. Gordon MS, Issenberg SB. Instructor guide for Harvey the cardiovascular patient simulator. University of Miami Miller School of Medicine, Gordon Center for Research in Medical Education; 2006.
32. Miller MD, Linn RL, Gronlund NE. Measurement and assessment in teaching. 11th ed. New York: Pearson; 2013.
33. National Council of State Boards of Nursing. NCLEX – RN Examination: detailed test plan for the National Council licensure examination for registered nurses. Chicago: NCSBN; 2015.
34. Jurich D, Duhigs LM, Plumb TJ, et al. Performance on the nephrology in-training examination and ABIM nephrology certification examination outcomes. Clin J Am Soc Nephrol. 2018;13(5):710–7.
35. American Board of Psychiatry and Neurology. Certification examination in child and adolescent psychiatry: 2017 content blueprint and 2017 content outline. Available at: https://www.abpn.com/wp-content/uploads/2016/11/2017_Child_and_Adolescent_Psychiatry_CERT_Conteny_specifications.pdf.
36. Korea Health Personnel Licensing Examination Institute. Health professional examination guides. Available at: http://www.kuksiwon.or.kr/EngHome?context.aspx?page=sub_2_1&sub=1#.
37. Gallagher AG, O'Sullivan GC. Fundamentals of surgical simulation. New York: Springer; 2012.
38. Laufer S, D'Angelo A-LD, Kwan C, et al. Rescuing the clinical breast examination: advances in classifying technique and assessing physician competency. Ann Surg. 2017;266(6):1069–74.
39. Laufer S, Cohen ER, Kwan C, et al. Sensor technology in assessments of clinical skill (research letter). N Engl J Med. 2015;372(8):784–6.
40. Heiman HL, Rasminsky S, Bierman JA, et al. Medical students' observations, practices, and attitudes regarding electronic health record documentation. Teach Learn Med. 2014;26(1):49–55.
41. Cresswell JW, Plano Clark VL. Designing and conducting mixed methods research. 3rd ed. Thousand Oaks, CA: Sage Publications; 2018.
42. Jordan M. For the love of the game. New York: Crown Publishers; 1998.
43. Downing SM. Reliability: on the reproducibility of assessment data. Med Educ. 2004;38:1006–12.
44. Brennan RL. Generalizability theory. Educ Meas Issues Prac. 1992;11(4):27–34.
45. Barsuk JH, Cohen ER, Wayne DB, et al. A comparison of approaches to mastery learning standard setting. Acad Med. 2018;93(7):1079–84.
46. Govaerts MJB, van der Vleuten CPM, Holmboe ES. Managing tensions in assessment: moving beyond either-or thinking. Med Educ. 2019;53:64–75.
47. Schoenherr JR, Hamstra SJ. Psychometrics and its discontents: an historical perspective on the discourse of the measurement tradition. Adv Health Sci Educ. 2016;21:719–29.
48. Watling CJ, Ginsburg S. Assessment, feedback and the alchemy of learning. Med Educ. 2019;53:76–85.

Standard Setting for Mastery Learning

6

Diane B. Wayne, Elaine R. Cohen, and Jeffrey H. Barsuk

Mastery learning is an educational approach in which *time* varies and *outcomes* are uniform [1, 2]. In mastery learning, pass-fail decisions are made depending on individual achievement of predetermined objective standards. These individualized decisions are not affected by overall group performance. Assessments used in mastery learning have a minimum passing standard (MPS) that all learners must meet or exceed to advance in a curriculum or complete training. Defensible standard setting in health professions education is critical for two reasons. First, a fair MPS informs learners about their performance compared to objective standards rather than subjective caprice. Second, use of a defensible MPS holds training programs accountable to graduate clinicians with the clinical skills needed to care for patients safely [3].

Educators using the mastery model in health professions education must know about standard setting techniques to set fair and defensible passing standards. Many educators believe mistakenly that standard setting is complex and labor intensive. This misconception results in "seat of the pants" standard setting practices like using arbitrary normative approaches (e.g., 1.5 standard deviations below a group mean) that can change due to group performance. This method does not represent education best practices or fit into contemporary models of competency-based education. Use of normative standards does not answer such important questions as "How much knowledge does each learner need to advance in the curriculum?" or "How much knowledge is needed to perform a clinical skill safely on real patients?" Instead, when normative standard setting methods are used, learners with low achievement levels routinely advance to the next unit of study [3].

D. B. Wayne (✉) · J. H. Barsuk
Northwestern University Feinberg School of Medicine, Departments of Medicine and Medical Education, Chicago, IL, USA
e-mail: dwayne@northwestern.edu

E. R. Cohen
Northwestern University Feinberg School of Medicine, Department of Medicine, Chicago, IL, USA

W. C. McGaghie et al. (eds.), *Comprehensive Healthcare Simulation: Mastery Learning in Health Professions Education*, Comprehensive Healthcare Simulation, https://doi.org/10.1007/978-3-030-34811-3_6

By contrast, in a mastery learning environment, rigorous standard setting promotes "excellence for all" by requiring that each learner demonstrate knowledge and skills to a predetermined level. The standard is set by content experts and is considered appropriate for advancement to the next unit of study. Each learner is "well prepared" rather than being judged "minimally competent." Time is flexible to allow each learner to achieve the MPS and downstream patient safety is an important and routine concern [3].

Foundation Principles

Normative Versus Criterion-Based Standards

Normative education achievement standards depend on group performance that may change over time. These standards are expressed relative to a group, for example, students who score two standard deviations below the mean fail the examination (Fig. 6.1). Normative standards are not appropriate for the individualized assessments needed for competency-based education.

Criterion-based or absolute standards reflect an individual's performance and are not affected by group performance. An example is a passing standard set as achieving a score of at least 75% correct on an examination. We recommend that educators assemble a panel of expert judges and use an accepted standard setting approach to set criterion-based standards. Standard setting is best accomplished after a mastery learning curriculum (including assessment tools) has been developed and pilot tested (Chap. 3).

Judge Selection

Selection of judges for standard setting exercises is a critical component toward setting a fair MPS. Based on prior scholarship [4, 5], and our own experiences [6–11], we recommend the following:

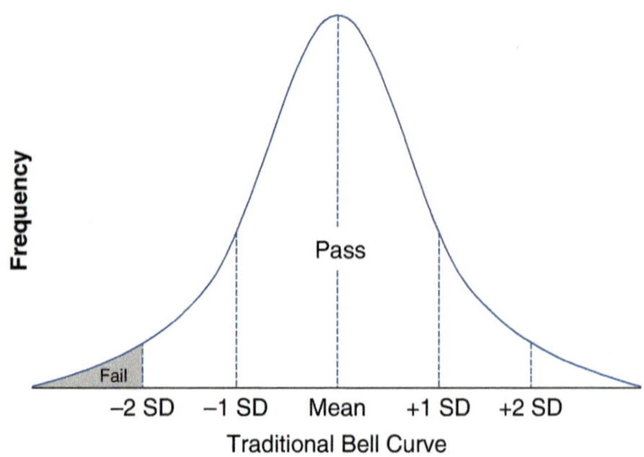

Fig. 6.1 A traditional bell curve with a normal distribution of scores. Trainees who score two standard deviations below the mean fail the examination

1. A minimum of 8 and preferably 10–12 judges should participate in a standard setting exercise.
2. Curriculum developers and instructors should in general not serve as judges to allow a broad a perspective into standard setting.
3. We prefer a multidisciplinary group of standard setting experts representing professions and specialties. For example, in setting a standard for advanced cardiac life support (ACLS)-simulated clinical scenarios, we might consider board certified physicians representing anesthesiology, critical care medicine, internal medicine, cardiology, and advanced practice nurses from similar disciplines. When approaching standard setting for end-of-life discussions, we would recruit experienced chaplains and social workers as expert judges in addition to physicians, physician assistants, and nurses.
4. Judges should be actively performing and supervising the skills and procedures they are asked to assess.
5. We recommend repeating the standard setting exercise after at least 6 weeks to ensure stability of judgments over time (test-retest reliability).

Recruitment of clinicians and other subject experts to participate in standard setting is rarely a barrier. In fact, most are enthusiastic participants in standard setting because they are passionate about their professional work and want to ensure high-quality performance among learners. Over the past decade we have never lacked willing judges with requisite expertise across various stakeholder groups including physicians, nurses, program directors, peer evaluators, and patients [6–11].

Standard Setting Exercise

When scheduling a standard setting exercise, we recommend the following:

1. Schedule the session over the lunch hour and provide a modest meal.
2. Reserve a quiet room; ask participants to sign over pagers and turn off cell phones.
3. Prepare standard setting packets in advance that contain step-by-step instructions for completing the exercise including:
   (a) Description of the education intervention.
   (b) Consequences of a pass or not pass decision for learners from the assessment.
   (c) Baseline performance data from a pilot study group (see below).
   (d) Copies of checklists and other assessment tools used by trained raters.
   (e) Forms for each judge to provide ratings.

Use of the standardized packet helps the session facilitator keep an orderly flow and enable the group to finish all content within the scheduled timeframe. A sample standard setting packet is in the chapter appendix (Appendix 6.1).

We use the first part of the session to orient judges to the assessment under review and how it fits into the overall training program assessment system. We discuss the stakes of the examination and not reaching mastery such as not performing the procedure on actual patients or returning to the simulation lab for additional practice. Because the judges are subject matter experts, we typically review the curriculum and assessment protocol in approximately 10–15 minutes. For complex interventions such as ACLS scenarios, it is useful to have judges observe teaching and assessment sessions before engaging in standard setting.

During the standard setting exercise, we recommend that the session leader focus the expert judges on performance expectations. Comments and feedback about nonessential items related to the curriculum and assessment tools are deferred until the standard setting exercise is finished. This recommendation is based on the need to complete standard setting "on time" due to the busy schedules of expert panelists. Mastery learning curricula benefit from refinement and updating, and it is possible to receive helpful suggestions and feedback from judges during standard setting. However, standard setting is different from curriculum development and should not occur until after the curriculum and assessment tools are developed and pilot tested (see Chaps. 3 and 5).

Mastery learning curricula require individualized assessments and the use of criterion-based standards. There are several established methods that may be used to set a defensible minimum passing standard (MPS) including the traditional Angoff and Hofstee approaches and the newer Mastery Angoff and patient-safety methods.

Standard Setting Methods

Angoff

The traditional Angoff standard setting method is an item-based approach [12]. Judges evaluate each question or checklist item individually. Judges are asked to consider the performance of a "borderline" trainee, one who has a 50–50% chance of passing the examination. Judges are asked "What percentage of borderline trainees would perform each specific item correctly?" If the assessment tool uses a rating scale, judges are asked what rating a "borderline" trainee would obtain on each item. Ratings are then averaged across items and judges to determine the final MPS. The traditional Angoff approach is used by licensing and certification agencies such as the National Board of Medical Examiners [13].

Hofstee

The traditional Hofstee standard setting approach considers the entire examination [14]. Judges are asked four questions: (a) What is the minimum acceptable passing score? (b) What is the maximum acceptable passing score? (c) What is the minimum acceptable failure rate? (d) What is the maximum acceptable failure rate? Questions about minimum and maximum passing rates ask judges to provide a range for the acceptable passing score. The minimum acceptable failure rate asks judges to assess if any examinees must fail the examination regardless of performance. The maximum acceptable failure rate asks judges to assess if any examinees must pass the examination regardless of performance.

The most frequent result in simulation-based mastery learning (SBML) standard setting is a determination of 0% for the minimum acceptable failure rate and 100% for the maximum acceptable failure rate. This is because judges know that learners in SBML curricula can retake the examination as many times as necessary without penalty because the ultimate goal is clinical skill acquisition and downstream patient safety.

Once these four questions are answered, actual performance data are used to plot a Hofstee graph. These performance data are used to plot the cumulative percentage of test scores on the Y axis, with percent of test items correct on the X axis. Vertical lines are plotted for the minimum and maximum acceptable passing scores, while horizontal lines are plotted for the minimum and maximal acceptable failure rates. Finally, a diagonal line is drawn from the intersection of the minimum acceptable passing score and minimum acceptable fail rate lines to the intersection of the maximum acceptable passing score and maximum acceptable failure rate lines. The point on the X axis where the diagonal line intersects the actual cumulative percent curve of trainees is the Hofstee MPS.

The Hofstee approach has a long history of use in clinical skills assessment. Some authors prefer the Hofstee to the Angoff approach due to perceived ease of use [15].

Pros and Cons of Angoff and Hofstee

The Angoff and Hofstee are well-studied approaches that produce stable data after weeks or even years [6, 7, 16]. Both have been used successfully in a multi-year research program linking rigorous SBML to downstream improvements in patient care quality and reduced health care costs [17–22]. However, the Angoff method frequently results in MPSs that are too lax while the Hofstee MPSs are too stringent. Therefore, the recommended approach for SBML has traditionally been to use the mean of the Angoff and Hofstee passing scores.

An additional challenge with the Angoff method is that assessing the performance of a "borderline" trainee is often difficult for even expert judges to conceptualize. Providing performance data to judges is helpful when using the Angoff method. Performance data demonstrate which steps or questions are the most challenging and grounds overall judgments in reality, avoiding setting a MPS that is too lenient or impossibly stringent.

Earlier work from our research group showed that providing performance data increased the Angoff and Hofstee MPSs for simulated central venous catheter (CVC) insertion skills [7]. In a subsequent study, the CVC insertion MPSs increased significantly when judges reviewed data showing that performance had improved over time and many trainees were exceeding the previously established MPS even without training [10]. Similar findings were shown regarding judges' use of performance data in an Angoff standard setting exercise for a medical licensing examination [13]. Judges significantly modified their assessments based on performance data, suggesting that reliance on data may supersede content expertise of how a "borderline" trainee would perform. Based on these factors, our long-standing preference has been to provide performance data to judges when using the Angoff and Hofstee methods.

A reasonable question is whether traditional Angoff and Hofstee standard setting methods are the best approach in mastery learning settings. SBML imposes different conditions than traditional learning environments. In SBML, the normal distribution of test scores is bent into a J curve (Fig. 6.2) because all learners acquire high skill levels, frequently expressed as academic grades, before completing training.

A foundation principle of mastery learning is that all learners achieve maximum skill acquisition with little outcome variation. Allowing "borderline" trainees to complete a curriculum and advance to clinical care is not consistent with mastery learning principles. Use of the traditional Hofstee method in mastery settings is also problematic. The Hofstee method considers minimum and maximum acceptable failure rates, yet in mastery learning, additional practice and retesting is offered to trainees until the MPS is reached. To address these issues, two new standard setting methods were created for mastery learning environments: the Mastery Angoff and the patient-safety methods [3, 23].

Mastery Angoff

The Mastery Angoff method is an item-based approach [3]. Judges evaluate each question or checklist item individually. Judges are asked to consider the performance of a "well prepared" trainee who would perform each step on an actual patient with minimum or no supervision, safely and effectively. Judges are asked, "What percentage of well-prepared trainees would perform each specific item correctly?" Ratings are then averaged across items and judges to determine the final MPS.

When comparing traditional Angoff and Mastery Angoff approaches for CVC insertion, we found that the Mastery Angoff led to more stringent passing standards [16]. Using the MPS derived from traditional Angoff and Hofstee approaches,

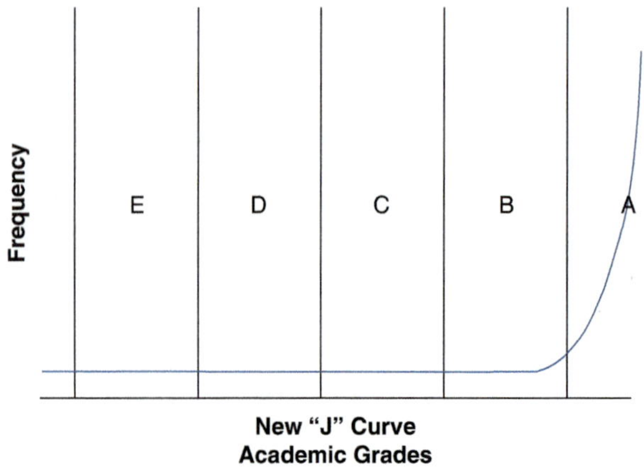

Fig. 6.2 Traditional education yields a normal score distribution. In mastery learning, the outcome distribution is a "J" curve where all learners achieve high performance with minimum variation

learners could miss up to 3 items on the CVC insertion checklist. However, judges using the Mastery Angoff approach determined that learners could only miss 1 item without returning to the simulation laboratory for additional practice before engaging in patient care [16]. Based on the historical performance of internal medicine and emergency medicine residents in CVC insertion SBML, applying the newer MPS would result in additional practice and retesting of 55/123 residents (45%) who had previously passed the internal jugular vein clinical skills examination and 36/130 residents (28%) who had previously passed the subclavian vein clinical skills examination [16]. More research is needed to determine if the stringency of the Mastery Angoff MPS provides additional downstream clinical benefit to patients.

In addition to being more stringent, judgments made using the Mastery Angoff method are less impacted by performance data than traditional standard setting approaches. Prenner and colleagues used the Mastery Angoff method to set standards for a written examination of cardiac telemetry monitoring [24]. They found that in contrast to the traditional Angoff method, baseline data had no impact on the final Mastery Angoff MPS. The authors conclude this occurred because judges have a better idea of what constitutes a "well prepared" trainee than a "borderline" trainee.

Patient-Safety

The patient-safety method is both item-based and test-based. In the patient-safety method, judges are asked to review each checklist item and determine whether it has implications for patient safety, comfort, or clinical outcomes [23]. If the item has implications for patient safety, comfort, or clinical outcomes, it is considered a critical item. If the item does not have these implications, it is considered a non-critical item. Judges set separate MPSs for critical and non-critical items. After review of the entire examination, the judges might determine that the MPS for critical items is 96% items correct while the MPS for non-critical items is 75% correct.

Several studies compared MPSs derived from the patient-safety approach to those derived from traditional approaches. Yudkowsky and colleagues compared the patient-safety and traditional Angoff approaches in a study of a five-station objective structured clinical examination for medical students [23]. The authors found that the patient-safety method was more stringent than the Angoff method—allowing 0 missed checklist items compared to 3. The patient-safety derived MPS was identical to that achieved using the Mastery Angoff method when applied to CVC insertion checklists [16].

Additional Considerations

Two issues frequently arise during standard setting exercises. The first is whether to provide judges with baseline performance data. As described earlier, we have provided these data historically to judges using the traditional Angoff and Hofstee approaches to prevent setting a MPS that is either too lenient or too stringent. Our research suggests that baseline data influence judges and can impact the stringency of the MPS using the Angoff and Hofstee methods [7], yet more recent work shows little impact of baseline data on Mastery Angoff results [16]. Thus we present baseline data when using the traditional Angoff and Hofstee methods. However, it is optional to present performance data to judges when using the Mastery Angoff or patient-safety approaches.

An additional question that frequently comes up during standard setting is how to address "compulsory" items. For example, an individual judge may feel that a checklist item such as "maintain sterile technique" cannot be missed in addition to achieving the MPS on the overall assessment. In general, we have addressed this at the end of the standard setting session where we ask the group to reach consensus on mandatory items. If consensus is reached, the final MPS might read as follows:

An overall score of 92% on the examination must be achieved and checklist items 1, 3, and 5 must be completed correctly.

In this scenario, not achieving an overall score of 92% or missing items 1, 3, or 5 would result in the learner returning to the education setting for additional skills practice and retesting.

A third question that may arise is how to determine a MPS if an assessment contains both a checklist and a global rating scale (GRS). Checklists ask judges to determine the performance of specific actions often using a dichotomous done correctly vs. not done or done incorrectly rating. In contrast, GRSs ask judges to rate overall performance. While both have advantages, we have historically used checklists in our SBML interventions because they provide step-by-step performance feedback to trainees. GRSs have several advantages as shown on a recent systematic review [25]. Specifically, GRSs may have higher average inter-item and inter-station reliability, capture some elements of performance not shown on checklist items, and can be used across multiple assessments. In cases where both a checklist and GRS are used, we recommend addressing the checklist first and then determining the MPS for the GRS. In this case of a checklist used with a GRS with four possible scores of novice, beginner, competent, and expert, the final MPS might read as follows:

An overall score of 92% on the checklist examination must be achieved and the examinee must receive an overall global rating of "competent" or higher.

In this scenario, not achieving an overall score of 92% or receiving a global rating of "novice" or "beginner" would result in the learner returning to the education setting for additional skills practice and retesting.

Recommendations

Standard setting is an essential part of mastery learning curriculum development and implementation. Several evidence-based standard setting approaches are available including the traditional and well-studied Angoff and Hofstee methods. Use of these methods in SMBL curricula has been linked to downstream improved patient care practices, patient outcomes, and impressive return on investment results. In recent years, the Mastery Angoff approach, focused on the "well-prepared" rather than the "borderline" trainee, has gained popularity due to ease of use and fit with mastery learning curriculum goals. This approach, while not as well studied as traditional methods, also does not require baseline performance data and is much easier for judges to understand and use than the traditional Angoff method. For these reasons, we recommend the Mastery Angoff approach as the best current standard setting option for health professions educators. We acknowledge that additional research is needed to compare the Mastery Angoff to traditional approaches and to specifically evaluate its impact on downstream patient care outcomes. Finally, all parts of a mastery learning curriculum require regular review and updating. MPSs should be reevaluated periodically to ensure that they represent current best practices and are embedded in curricula achieving relevant education and patient care goals.

Appendix 6.1: Standard Setting Packets for Traditional Angoff and Hofstee and Mastery Angoff and Patient-Safety Methods for Simulated Lumbar Puncture

Performance data (reviewing these data may be useful for traditional Angoff and Hofstee approaches)

This table shows sample pretest and posttest data from a pilot group of 57 internal medicine residents performing a simulated lumbar puncture procedure. Overall pretest and posttest means/standard deviations are displayed as well as the frequency of each overall score at pre- and posttest

% Correct	Pretest frequency	Posttest frequency
10%	1	0
19%	1	0
24%	6	0
29%	4	0
33%	5	0
38%	7	0
43%	6	0
48%	6	0
52%	3	1
57%	3	0
62%	4	0
67%	5	1
71%	1	0
76%	3	0
81%	1	1
86%	1	5
90%	0	8
95%	0	15
100%	0	26
	Mean = 46.3%	Mean = 94.4%
	SD = 17.6%	SD = 8.5%

A. *Traditional Angoff Method*

1. Select the judges.
2. Discuss the purpose of the test, the curriculum and assessment, the nature of the examinees, and what constitutes adequate and inadequate skills/knowledge. Review baseline performance data.
3. Define the "borderline" group, a group that has a 50–50 chance of passing.
4. Read the first item.
5. Each judge estimates the proportion of the borderline group that would perform it correctly.
6. The ratings are recorded for all to see, discuss, and change as appropriate.
7. Repeat steps 4–6 for each item.
8. Calculate the passing score by averaging the estimates of all judges for each item and summing the items.
9. Use the checklist below[a] to do this exercise.

Checklist item	Pilot pretest data (%)	% of borderline residents who perform each step correctly
Clean the skin with betadine (may not use chlorhexidine) × 3	30	
Drape the patient	91	
Use 1% lidocaine to form a wheal at intended site	54	
Numb deeper structure (larger needle)	54	
Insert spinal needle advancing toward umbilicus (may be more cephalad depending on how flexed the spine)	65	
Bevel must be in correct direction	46	
Slowly advance the needle with periodic checking for CSF (removal of stylet) until enter space	23	
Measure opening pressure	14	

[a]This is a partial checklist adapted from Barsuk et al. [26]. *In an actual standard setting exercise, insert complete assessment tool with performance data*

B. *Traditional Hofstee Method*

1. Select the judges.
2. Discuss the purpose of the test, the curriculum and assessment, the nature of the examinees, and what constitutes adequate and inadequate skills/knowledge. Review baseline performance data.
3. Review the test in detail.
4. Ask the judges to answer four questions:
   (a) What is the minimum acceptable required passing score?
   (b) What is the maximum acceptable required passing score?
   (c) What is the minimum acceptable fail rate?
   (d) What is the maximum acceptable fail rate?
5. After the test is given, graph the distribution of scores and select the cut score as described by De Gruiter[a]

Clinical skill standard setting Hofstee method				
	Minimum acceptable required passing score	Maximum acceptable required passing score	Minimum acceptable fail rate	Maximum acceptable fail rate
Clinical skill				

[a]De Gruiter [27]

C. *Mastery Angoff Method*

1. Select the judges.
2. Discuss the purpose of the test, the curriculum and assessment, the nature of the examinees, and what constitutes adequate and inadequate skills/knowledge.
   (a) Mastery learning: residents can continue to practice and retest until they achieve the passing standard (no penalty for taking a longer time or multiple retests).
   (b) Past performance data is not relevant, since residents can keep practicing until they can accomplish even difficult items.
3. Define the "well prepared to succeed" group: the standard reflects the expected performance *in the sim lab* of residents who are:
   (a) Well prepared to perform the procedure
   (b) Safely and successfully
   (c) On live patients
   (d) With minimal supervision
4. Read the first item.
5. Each judge estimates the proportion of the "well prepared" group that would get it right (or the probability that any individual "well prepared" resident would get it right).
6. The ratings are recorded for all to see, discuss, and change as appropriate.
7. Repeat steps 4–6 for each item.
8. Calculate the passing score by averaging the estimates of all judges for each item and summing the items.
9. Use the checklist below[a] to do this exercise.

Checklist item	% of *well-prepared* residents who accomplish this item correctly *in the sim lab*
Clean the skin with betadine (may not use chlorhexidine) × 3	
Drape the patient	
Use 1% lidocaine to form a wheal at intended site	
Numb deeper structure (larger needle)	
Insert spinal needle advancing toward umbilicus (may be more cephalad depending on how flexed the spine)	
Bevel must be in correct direction	

Checklist item	% of *well-prepared* residents who accomplish this item correctly *in the sim lab*
Slowly advance the needle with periodic checking for CSF (removal of stylet) until enter space	
Measure opening pressure	

[a]This is a partial checklist adapted from Barsuk et al. [26]. *In an actual standard setting exercise, insert complete assessment tool*

D. *Patient-Safety Method*
1. Select the judges.
2. Discuss the purpose of the test, the curriculum, assessment, and the nature of the examinees.
   (a) Mastery learning: *residents can continue to practice and retest until they achieve the passing standard (no penalty for taking a longer time or multiple retests).*
3. Determine dimensions relevant to patient safety.
   In this case we will *consider relevant dimensions to be*
   (a) *Patient or provider safety*
   (b) *Patient comfort*
   (c) *The outcome of the procedure*
4. For each item, each judge indicates whether performance or non-performance of this item would impact each of these dimensions.
5. Do this for the skills checklist below[a]
6. Set standards separately for *critical* and *non-critical* items.
   (a) An item that impacts any one of the three dimensions is considered a critical item.
   (b) An item that does not impact any one of these dimensions is considered a non-critical item.
7. Average across judges to determine:
   (a) Which items are critical or non-critical
   (b) Passing scores for critical and non-critical items
8. Standards are *not connected.* Accomplishing non-critical items does not compensate for non-performance of critical items.

Checklist item[a]	Impacts safety?		Impacts comfort?		Impacts outcome?	
Clean the skin with betadine (may not use chlorhexidine) × 3	Yes	No	Yes	No	Yes	No
Drape the patient	Yes	No	Yes	No	Yes	No
Use 1% lidocaine to form a wheal at intended site	Yes	No	Yes	No	Yes	No
Numb deeper structure (larger needle)	Yes	No	Yes	No	Yes	No
Insert spinal needle advancing toward umbilicus (may be more cephalad depending on how flexed the spine)	Yes	No	Yes	No	Yes	No
Bevel must be in correct direction	Yes	No	Yes	No	Yes	No
Slowly advance the needle with periodic checking for CSF (removal of stylet) until enter space	Yes	No	Yes	No	Yes	No
Measure opening pressure	Yes	No	Yes	No	Yes	No

[a]This is a partial checklist adapted from Barsuk et al. [26]. *In an actual standard setting exercise, insert complete assessment tool*

Setting the Standard

The passing standard represents performance *in the simulation lab,* before performing the procedure on live patients. Residents can continue to practice and retest until they achieve the passing standard; there is no penalty for taking a longer time or multiple retests.

1. What should be the passing standard for *critical* items, i.e., items that impact patient or provider safety, patient comfort, or procedure outcome? What proportion of critical items should residents perform correctly in the sim lab before performing the procedure on live patients with minimal supervision?
   ______%
2. What should be the passing standard for *non-critical items*, i.e., items that do *not* impact patient or provider safety, patient comfort, or procedure outcome? What proportion of non-critical items should residents perform correctly in the sim lab before performing the procedure on live patients with minimal supervision?
   ______%

Please add any comments you may have about these standard setting procedures:

References

1. McGaghie WC, Miller GE, Sajid A, Telder TV. Competency-based curriculum development in medical education. Public Health Paper No. 68. Geneva: World Health Organization; 1978.
2. McGaghie WC. Mastery learning: it is time for medical education to join the 21st century. Acad Med. 2015;90(11):1438–41.
3. Yudkowsky R, Park YS, Lineberry M, Knox A, Ritter EM. Setting mastery learning standards. Acad Med. 2015;90(11):1495–500.
4. Norcini J, Guille R. Combining tests and setting standards. In: Norman GR, Van der Vleuten CPM, Newble DI, editors. International handbook of research in medical education. Dordrecht: Kluwer Academic Publishers; 2002. p. 811–34.
5. Downing SM, Tekian A, Yudkowsky R. Procedures for establishing defensible absolute passing scores on performance examinations in health professions education. Teach Learn Med. 2006;18:50–7.
6. Wayne DB, Fudala MJ, Butter J, Siddall VJ, Feinglass J, Wade LD, McGaghie WC. Comparison of two standard-setting methods for advanced cardiac life support training. Acad Med. 2005;80(10 Suppl):S63–6.
7. Wayne DB, Barsuk JH, Cohen E, McGaghie WC. Do baseline data influence standard setting for a clinical skills examination? Acad Med. 2007;82(10 Suppl):S105–8.
8. Wayne DB, Cohen E, Makoul G, McGaghie WC. The impact of judge selection on standard setting for a patient survey of physician communication skills. Acad Med. 2008;83(10 Suppl):S17–20.
9. Wayne DB, Butter J, Cohen ER, McGaghie WC. Setting defensible standards for cardiac auscultation skills in medical students. Acad Med. 2009;84(10 Suppl):S94–6.
10. Cohen ER, Barsuk JH, McGaghie WC, Wayne DB. Raising the bar: reassessing standards for procedural competence. Teach Learn Med. 2013;25(1):6–9.
11. Sharma R, Szmuilowicz E, Ogunseitan A, Montalvo J, O'Leary K, Wayne DB. Evaluation of a mastery learning intervention on hospitalists' code status discussion skills. J Pain Symptom Manag. 2017;53(6):1066–70.
12. Angoff WH. Scales, norms, and equivalent scores. In: Thorndike RL, editor. Educational measurement. 2nd ed. Washington, DC: American Council on Education; 1971. p. 508–600.

13. Clauser BE, Mee J, Baldwin SG, Margolis MJ, Dillon GF. Judges' use of examinee performance data in an Angoff standard-setting exercise for a medical licensing examination: an experimental study. J Educ Meas. 2009;46:390–407.
14. Hofstee WKB. The case for compromise in educational selection and grading. In: Anderson SB, editor. On educational testing. San Francisco: Jossey-Bass; 1983. p. 107–27.
15. Schindler N, Corcoran J, DaRosa D. Description and impact of using a standard-setting method for determining pass/fail scores in a surgery clerkship. Am J Surg. 2007;193(2):252–7.
16. Barsuk JH, Cohen ER, Wayne DB, McGaghie WC, Yudkowsky R. A comparison of approaches for mastery learning standard setting. Acad Med. 2018;93:1079.
17. McGaghie WC, Issenberg SB, Barsuk JH, Cohen ER, Wayne DB. Translational educational research: a necessity for effective health-care improvement. Chest. 2012;142(5):1097–103.
18. Wayne DB, Didwania A, Fudals M, Barsuk JH, Feinglass J, McGaghie WC. Simulation-based education improves quality of care during cardiac arrest team responses at an academic teaching hospital: a case-control study. Chest. 2008;133:56–61.
19. Barsuk JH, Cohen ER, Feinglass J, McGaghie WC, Wayne DB. Use of simulation-based education to reduce catheter-related bloodstream infections. Arch Intern Med. 2009;169(15):1420–3.
20. Gossett DR, Gilchrist-Scott D, Wayne DB, Gerber SE. Simulation training for forceps assisted vaginal delivery and rates of maternal perineal trauma. Obstet Gynecol. 2016;128(3):429–35.
21. Cohen ER, Feinglass J, Barsuk JH, Barnard C, O'Donnell A, McGaghie WC, Wayne DB. Cost Savings from reduced catheter-related bloodstream infection after simulation-based education for residents in a medical intensive care unit. Simul Healthc. 2010;5:98–102.
22. Barsuk JH, Cohen ER, Feinglass J, Kozmic SE, McGaghie WC, Wayne DB. Cost savings of performing paracentesis procedures at the bedside. Simul Healthc. 2014;9(5):312–8.
23. Yudkowsky R, Tumuluru S, Casey P, Herlich N, Ledonne C. A patient safety approach to setting pass/fail standards for basic procedural skills checklists. Simul Healthc. 2014;9(5):277–82.
24. Prenner SB, McGaghie WC, Chuzi S, Cantey E, Didwania A, Barsuk JH. Effect of trainee performance data on standard setting judgments using the mastery Angoff method. J Grad Med Educ. 2018;10:301.
25. Ilgen JS, Ma IW, Hatala R, Cook DA. A systematic review of validity evidence for checklists versus global rating scales in simulation-based assessment. Med Educ. 2015;49(2):161–73.
26. Barsuk JH, Cohen ER, Caprio T, McGaghie WC, Simuni T, Wayne DB. Simulation-based education with mastery learning improves lumbar puncture skills. Neurology. 2012;79(2):132–7.
27. De Gruijter DNM. Compromise models for establishing examination standards. J Educ Meas. 1985;22(4):263–9.

Implementing and Managing a Mastery Learning Program

7

Elaine R. Cohen, Kenzie A. Cameron, Jeffrey H. Barsuk, and Diane B. Wayne

Planning for Mastery Learning

Health professions educators must have adequate resources and support to plan and implement a mastery learning curriculum. Identification of necessary resources is the first step in the planning process and must include personnel, time, equipment, supplies, facilities, and funding. Successful mastery learning programs are often linked to institutional quality goals [1]. Securing internal resources for mastery learning programs is easier when this alignment occurs.

Table 7.1 presents a mastery learning implementation checklist. The text that follows amplifies the tabular items and provides details about planning, pilot testing, implementing, and continuously managing a mastery learning education program.

The Mastery Learning Team

> Good teams are not a matter of luck; they result from hard work, careful planning, and commitment from the sponsoring organization [2]. – Leigh Thompson PhD Kellogg School of Management, Northwestern University

E. R. Cohen (✉)
Northwestern University Feinberg School of Medicine, Department of Medicine, Chicago, IL, USA
e-mail: elaine.cohen@northwestern.edu

K. A. Cameron
Northwestern University Feinberg School of Medicine, Departments of Medicine, Medical Education, Medical Social Sciences, and Preventive Medicine, Chicago, IL, USA

J. H. Barsuk · D. B. Wayne
Northwestern University Feinberg School of Medicine, Departments of Medicine and Medical Education, Chicago, IL, USA
e-mail: dwayne@northwestern.edu

W. C. McGaghie et al. (eds.), *Comprehensive Healthcare Simulation: Mastery Learning in Health Professions Education*, Comprehensive Healthcare Simulation, https://doi.org/10.1007/978-3-030-34811-3_7

Table 7.1 Mastery learning implementation checklist

Planning

- ☐ Form team – including lead faculty member(s) and administrative coordinator
- ☐ Plan curriculum and assessment
- ☐ Develop evaluation measures including course evaluation questionnaires
- ☐ Ensure support from relevant stakeholders (e.g., department chair, GME program coordinator, curriculum dean)
- ☐ Obtain funding for approved budget
- ☐ Secure protected time for faculty and learners
- ☐ Develop slide sets and videos
- ☐ Select practical location for training
- ☐ Obtain materials and equipment including any medical supplies, simulators, and AV needs
- ☐ Submit IRB application

Pilot testing

- ☐ Select non-study subjects to pilot test the intervention
- ☐ Note and address issues related to space, simulators, AV equipment, etc
- ☐ Faculty rater training
- ☐ Standardize instructions, teaching content, and debriefing methods
- ☐ Use pilot data to calculate inter-rater reliability (IRR) with additional training and pilot testing as needed
- ☐ Debrief with course faculty; make adjustments as needed
- ☐ Prepare data management files to track education outcomes (pre- and posttest results, written examinations, course evaluation questionnaire responses, etc.)

Implementation

- ☐ Engage learners and set expectations regarding attendance, clinical coverage, and other logistics before the training session
- ☐ Prepare the following items for each training session:
  - ☐ Consent forms with current IRB approval stamp
  - ☐ Standardized material for faculty use (instructions before the simulation, simulation content, debriefing)
  - ☐ Written reading materials and/or examination questions
  - ☐ Assessment checklists
  - ☐ Course evaluation questionnaires
- ☐ Enter and track results in spreadsheet or other electronic format using IRB-approved methods
- ☐ Record any encountered issues about participants, faculty, staff, or setting to discuss at team meeting
- ☐ Evaluate curriculum effectiveness through analysis of educational outcomes

Continuous management

- ☐ Continue periodic team meetings
- ☐ Plan for manuscript preparation
- ☐ Review training sessions and assessments for consistency and re-calibrate if needed
- ☐ Continue to collect and enter data
- ☐ Submit IRB renewals, report enrollment numbers, and prepare progress reports for funding sources

Creating a supportive learning environment is necessary for a mastery learning program to thrive. Identifying key personnel to form a group committed to program success is an important first step. Mastery learning team members should include education leaders such as program or clerkship directors, faculty instructors, administrative staff, and researchers. Team members with diverse strengths create the supportive environment and set the stage for a successful mastery learning curriculum [3]. Program and clerkship directors support trainees, advocate for the education program, and ensure the curriculum is relevant for board certification or graduation requirements. Faculty instructors, often including the main curriculum developer (Chaps. 3 and 4), should include educators and content experts. For the mastery learning program to be successful, faculty instructors must fully commit to the project and have adequate protected teaching time.

Administrative staff provide critical support by performing all the day-to-day activities for the mastery learning program. They prepare institutional review board (IRB) submissions for research projects, maintain and distribute course materials, track course logistics, coordinate schedules for instructors and learners, collect and maintain data, and manage expenses. Finally, researchers serve an important role to oversee outcome measurement and evaluation. Education research should not be an extraordinary event. Rather, rigorous outcome measurement should be embedded in everyday activities so results may be tracked and shared [4].

Once the team is identified, an initial team meeting is essential to set expectations, review individual responsibilities, and discuss plans for research reporting (including authorship criteria and order). Although all team members will contribute individually, we recommend identification of a single team leader with responsibility for the overall program. Regular meetings should take place so team members can share updates and ask questions related to the program. Highly successful teams do the following [5]:

- Establish a compelling mission, goals, and shared commitment;
- Mutually define how the team will make and process decisions;
- Define and structure team members' roles;
- Maintain a stable team membership;
- Provide a safe place to innovate and challenge the status quo;
- Coach by delivering specific and ongoing feedback;
- Emphasize a combination of individual and team-based rewards; and
- Enable a culture of continuous improvement.

Time and Logistics

The time needed to develop, teach, and assess a mastery learning program should be taken into account during curriculum development. The team leader must have enough time to oversee implementation and management. Faculty instructors need time to prepare, pilot test, and deliver the curriculum. Time estimates must include sessions for learners who do not initially meet the mastery standard. These are people who need more education and evaluation time after standard training and assessment.

Securing protected time for faculty can be challenging, especially for educators with significant clinical responsibilities. One way to reduce this burden is to have more than one faculty instructor trained to teach the curriculum. Physician faculty are often not required to educate medical or other health professionals. Standardized patients, research assistants, and other clinicians can be trained to score skills checklists provided they are properly calibrated with the primary instructor(s). Successful examples using highly trained non-physician raters include mastery learning of advanced cardiac life support (ACLS), paracentesis training for residents, and common clinical conditions by graduating medical students [6–8].

Administrative staff support the program by preparing course materials (videos, lectures, written materials, data collection forms, surveys) and managing logistics (AV, classroom space, faculty and learner scheduling) so that faculty instructors can focus on teaching. Administrative support is critical for successful implementation and should be considered during early planning and budgeting.

Mastery learning programs are often added to clinical education requirements. This means learners also require protected time to fully engage the curriculum. Learner time includes preparation, training, assessment, and feedback so program and clerkship director support is imperative. We also acknowledge the benefit of engaging residency and clerkship program coordinators who have deep knowledge of resident and student schedules and duty hour requirements. For example, internal medicine residents at the McGaw Medical Center of Northwestern University are required to master a set of clinical skills before starting the intensive care unit (ICU) rotation. To achieve ICU readiness, residents train to mastery standards in patient ventilator management [9] and central venous catheter (CVC) insertion [10, 11], at various times during blocks when they do not have on-call responsibilities. A long-standing partnership between Department of Medicine staff (residency program director, program coordinator, chief residents) and mastery learning faculty has been essential for the success of this program.

Requiring mastery training immediately before or after education transitions is a proven option to ensure that trainees are prepared to provide clinical care. At Northwestern, all medical students complete a mastery learning capstone course linked to the entrustable professional activities endorsed by the Association of American Medical Colleges before graduation [8]. Similarly, a Northwestern "intern boot camp" uses simulation-based mastery learning (SBML) for individualized training, assessment, and documentation of competence *before* interns provide medical care [12]. Interns are trained in skills such as cardiac auscultation [13], procedures such as paracentesis [7] and lumbar puncture [14], management of critically ill patients [9], and communication with patients [15] all over a 3-day period. In addition to trainee and faculty participation, success of the boot camp program requires institutional support – in this case 3 days of salary for new interns to complete SBML before beginning clinical rotations.

Facilities and Equipment

Many mastery learning curricula are taught in classrooms using low fidelity mobile equipment and standardized patients [7, 14–16]. Institutions may charge to use a simulation or clinical education center, but use of specialized space is not always necessary. Considering other options may also be more convenient for learners. For example, if a resident physician is primarily working in the hospital, mastery learning would ideally occur in a hospital location rather than in a simulation center located in another building.

We acknowledge that some curricula require advanced equipment and supplies such as high fidelity patient simulators, computers, or cadavers that require using a specialized space. For example, resident training in ACLS uses a sophisticated simulator that displays multiple physiologic and pharmacologic responses observed in ACLS situations. Additionally, the simulator is located in a center equipped with one-way glass and AV technology that allows residents to react and care for simulated in-hospital cardiac events while managing a team of their peers and receiving feedback in a "mistake forgiving" environment [17, 18] (Fig. 7.1).

In SBML, learners are asked to do everything they would perform during an actual patient encounter. This includes using medical supplies and equipment needed to perform a procedure or clinical skill. Creativity often reduces supply costs. For example, many procedure kits can be reused and companies may be willing to donate outdated supplies. Borrowing more expensive equipment (e.g., ultrasound machines) is also an option. Extensive evidence shows that creating a realistic learning environment is worthwhile as several mastery learning programs have demonstrated a significant return on investment [1, 19, 20] (Chap. 19).

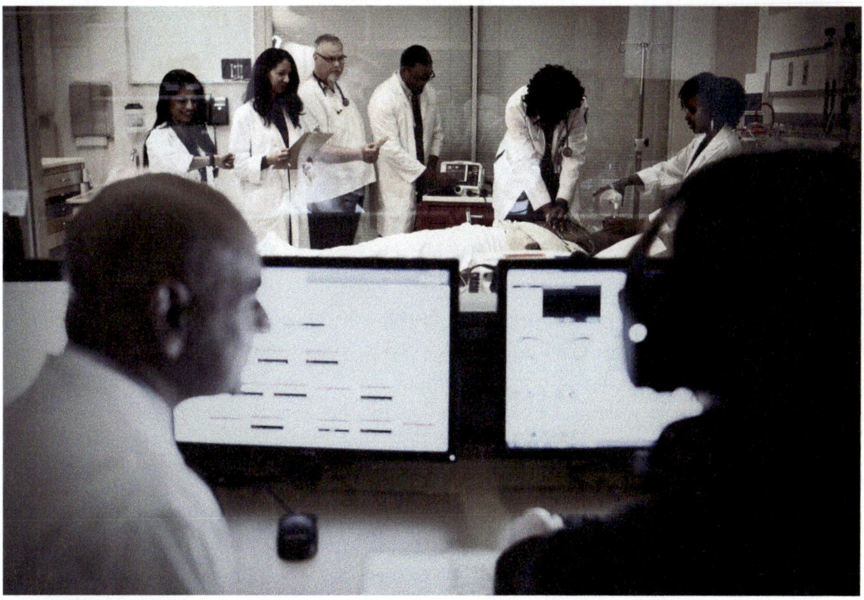

Fig. 7.1 SBML training for internal medicine residents on ACLS events in a medical simulation laboratory

Pilot Testing

Pilot testing is a mandatory component of mastery learning programs. Pilot testing ensures that the curriculum is feasible in the allotted time, clinical scenarios are clear, realistic, and run smoothly, equipment is adequate, and the program achieves its education goals. Adjustments can be made in time, supplies, and equipment based on the results of pilot testing. During the pilot test, educators can also change curriculum delivery. Pilot testing should include the following components of a mastery learning curriculum: (a) standardized instructions; (b) pretest; (c) lecture or other didactic content; (d) hands-on deliberate practice; (e) individualized feedback; (f) posttest; and (g) debriefing.

We have successfully used faculty members and trainees such as chief residents to pilot test new curricula. We endorse use of a variety of subjects for pilot testing of clinical scenarios used for teaching and assessment. For example, the goal of Northwestern's ACLS mastery learning course is to prepare residents to lead actual ACLS patient care events. A review of actual ACLS events produced a list of common clinical scenarios faced by resuscitation teams at our major clinical affiliate. Clinical scenarios based on these cases were developed, embedded in the high fidelity simulator, and pilot tested with attending physicians, ACLS instructors, and other content experts. After feedback, the scenarios were revised as needed before resident training began [18].

Pilot testing also includes rater training and calibration and assessment of inter-rater agreement. Documentation of data reliability is critical to draw any conclusions from study results. For this reason, all assessment tools must be pilot tested to ensure they generate reliable data that can be used to support valid pass/fail judgments about learner competence [21]. Use of more than one assessor is required to obtain estimates of inter-rater reliability [22]. All raters should be trained and calibrated to use assessment tools consistently. If low levels of inter-rater reliability are found, additional training and calibration is needed. Assessment tools can also be edited or recalibrated as needed.

We used these recommended steps in a pilot study of medical students participating in a SBML breaking bad news (BBN) curriculum. First, all pre- and posttest conversations were scored by one examiner. Next, a second examiner reviewed a 50% random sample of video recorded conversations using the same assessment tool to evaluate inter-rater reliability. As BBN conversations can be difficult to assess, some inconsistencies between raters were found. The course developers revisited the scoring rubric. After this revision, the examiners rescored the set of videos and high inter-rater reliability was achieved [23].

Data collected during pilot testing may be helpful for standard setting exercises. Providing pilot performance data to standard setting judges can help inform the minimum passing standard (MPS), although this may not be required [24]. Performance data demonstrates which steps or questions on the assessment tools are most challenging. This gives the judges some context in order to set a MPS that is neither too lenient nor stringent (Chap. 6).

Implementation

After time and hard work is spent developing, planning, and pilot testing, the time is ready to put the mastery learning program into action. Before implementation begins, faculty instructors should be comfortable teaching the curriculum and using the assessment tools. All simulation scenarios must be finalized and raters calibrated.

Program Management

Administrative staff should schedule the first group of learners and instructors. Detailed and clear communication should be sent to all participants (learners and instructors) including a brief curriculum overview; date, time, and duration of training; location; readings or other materials to review; and any other important information (e.g., bring stethoscope and white coat). Clear expectations should be set in advance about cell phone use and forwarding pages to a colleague who can provide clinical coverage during the mastery learning activity. An additional note from a clinical operations leader or the program or clerkship director offering support for the program often creates buy-in for learners.

Instructors should be prepared with all data collection tools before the training session. Predetermined study outcome measures (Chap. 5) should be used to evaluate program success. Data collection can be done using paper or electronic forms. If training sessions or assessments require video recording, cameras should be set up beforehand and consent obtained from trainees and instructors. After introductions, expectations for the learners and instructors should be stated clearly. If trainees are being asked to participate in a research study, informed consent must be documented before any training begins.

Baseline data collection forms including participant demographics, clinical experience, and self-confidence surveys should be completed before training begins. Next, instructors read a standardized clinical scenario and trainees perform a pretest of a specific clinical skill. Completing the pretest allows learners to focus on key areas during training and provides information for faculty to use to give actionable feedback. After the pretest, learners participate in didactic training including demonstration of the procedure or clinical skill. Next they participate in deliberate practice with individualized feedback. Debriefing and evaluation often conclude the first session of a mastery learning curriculum. In a separately scheduled session (ideally on a different day), learners return and complete a posttest. If a trainee meets or exceeds the MPS, she can move on to the next task or skill. If a trainee does not meet or exceed the MPS, she participates in more deliberate practice and retesting until the MPS is met. After the posttest, learners complete a post-course satisfaction survey. These data support the program and allow faculty to improve the curriculum based on learner feedback.

A good example of successful pilot testing and implementation is a cardiac auscultation SBML curriculum for third-year medical students [13, 25]. Local clerkship directors saw a need for improved assessment and training in core skills such as cardiac auscultation. A curriculum was developed and pilot tested [25] with 100 medical students from three Chicago medical schools using the UMedic tutorial and Harvey® cardiac patient simulator [26]. Expert judges used the pilot test data to set a defensible MPS for the previously validated computer-based assessment.

For the SBML study, 77 third- and 31 fourth-year students were assessed in cardiac auscultation proficiency using the computerized case-based examination and auscultation of actual patients. Third-year students participated in the entire SBML curriculum, while fourth-year medical students (traditionally trained) did not receive the intervention and served as controls.

All students provided informed consent and completed baseline demographic surveys. Third-year students completed the computerized assessment before the intervention (pretest). Next they participated in the curriculum, which featured approximately 1 hour of deliberate practice on 12 major cardiac findings. The SBML intervention included a computer-based, interactive self-study tutorial (UMedic) [26], didactic instruction, deliberate practice, and self-assessment. After the self-directed portion of the curriculum, third-year students received 30–40 minutes of focused review using a cardiac simulator (Harvey®) led by an experienced clinician educator. Third-year students then completed a posttest where they were expected to meet or exceed the MPS of 75% items correct on the computerized assessment as set by the expert panel. Fourth-year students completed the assessment but did not receive the SBML intervention.

At baseline, third-year students $M = 67.3\%$, SD = 18.85, scored similar to fourth-year students $M = 73.9\%$, SD = 14.1% (p = NS). However, after SBML training, third-year students improved their scores significantly to $M = 93.8\%$, SD = 11.6% ($p < 0.001$), compared to their baseline score and performed better than traditionally trained fourth-year students ($p < 0.001$).

To assess the impact of SBML on actual patient care, all students evaluated four to five patients recruited from internal medicine or cardiology practices based on the presence of at least one important cardiac finding. Third-year students who completed SBML more accurately assessed patients with cardiac findings ($M = 81.8\%$, SD = 8.8%) compared to fourth-year students ($M = 75.1\%$, SD = 13.4%) ($p = 0.003$) who did not complete SBML but had more clinical experience.

In addition to the impact on education and clinical care, results from the course evaluation revealed that the students reported the curriculum improved their cardiac auscultation skills, was a useful adjunct to clinical experience, and was enjoyable.

Outcome Assessment

Collecting outcome data during implementation allows health professions educators to determine the effectiveness and impact of a curriculum (Chap. 5). Educators must be able to describe the properties of all of the measurements or assessments they have adopted or developed for use as outcome measures. The primary outcome measure answers the main research question of the study. All other outcomes are secondary. Details including how (which assessment tools) and when (at what time point) each outcome is measured should be determined. Various types of data may be collected to evaluate a mastery learning program including written examinations [27], and checklists [28] or global rating scales [29]. Self-assessments are not recommended as a stand-alone outcome measure given their generally poor relationship to objective outcome measures [30, 31]. Data collection is performed using a unique identifier and either paper forms or an electronic format. Data collected using paper forms should be returned to administrative staff and entered into a secure database as soon as possible.

Data can undergo analysis after data collection is complete. Data tables can be generated and shared with the rest of the mastery learning team. This information is helpful to revise the curriculum and assess it over time – even if an active research study is not underway.

A study of CVC insertion SBML illustrates the importance of continuous data collection and review. Once the intervention was in place for several years, faculty instructors noted that second-year residents seemed to be performing better during pretest assessments of internal jugular and subclavian CVC insertion skills over time. Because meticulous records had been kept, an evaluation of pretest scores across 3 years including 102 residents was possible. Analysis of pretest data revealed that a statistically significant increase in pretest scores had in fact occurred leading to almost 40% of second-year residents meeting or exceeding the MPS even before training began. We found that this unexpected impact of SBML was due to teaching and role modeling by more senior residents who trained the junior residents during their first-year rotations leading to improved results as second-year trainees. As a result of these findings [32], standard setting exercises were redone and a more stringent MPS imposed on subsequent resident cohorts [33].

Continuous Management

Ongoing management of a mastery learning program is necessary for it to continue to thrive. This includes regular team meetings, reviewing teaching sessions, continuous data collection, maintaining paperwork and approvals, and periodic curriculum revision.

The mastery learning team should continue to meet periodically to review data, address implementation issues, and update the curriculum as needed. Time should also be set aside for manuscript writing and revision. It is important to offer continuous feedback to instructors who are teaching curriculum repetitions. Options include observing a training session live or video recording it for group review. If more than one team member is completing assessments, rater calibration should take place periodically to ensure they stay consistent. Additional training and calibration should occur if low levels of inter-rater reliability are found.

Data collection continues while the mastery learning program is being implemented. Data should be entered on a regular basis to avoid a backlog. The database should be maintained by administrative staff and backed up on a server. If competency is being documented as part of residency or clerkship, mastery learning completion certificates should be filed in trainee records.

Various administrative tasks must also be addressed on a regular basis. These include submitting IRB renewals and updates, reporting consent and enrollment numbers to the institution, and preparing progress reports for funding agencies.

Mastery learning curricula are complex and face several threats to ongoing success. First, personnel changes may pose challenges. For example, keeping a mastery learning curriculum alive without a primary faculty sponsor is difficult. Close alignment with programmatic goals and backing from trainees who have completed the intervention are key to maintaining support and navigating personnel changes. A thriving research environment and strong team culture may also help attract other faculty who wish to participate. Second, funding sources may change longitudinally. The close alignment to institutional priorities (especially those regarding patient safety and clinical outcomes) described earlier may help programs raise additional funds to support mastery learning programs over time. Third, competing priorities will arise and need to be addressed. Keeping a current SBML program while developing new ones may raise issues about learner and faculty bandwidth. These issues are real and need to be carefully addressed with the team and clinical/departmental sponsors. Finally, a successful mastery learning program should always be evolving. This requires continuous maintenance and curriculum enhancement. It is critical to keep up with the mastery learning literature as well as relevant clinical guidelines related to specific topic areas. For example, ACLS guidelines are updated every 5 years. Previous revisions have changed the focus of ACLS training from airway-breathing-circulation (ABC) to circulation-airway-breathing (CAB) [34, 35] requiring updates to our ACLS skills checklists to reflect current clinical practice guidelines [36].

Other Considerations

Change Management and Implementation Science

Even a well-planned and perfectly implemented SBML intervention will have limited impact over the long-term if an organization is not ready to change, or if careful review of the impact of the project is not performed. Furthermore, understanding culture, setting, and the downstream collateral impact of SBML is critical when planning dissemination of SBML to additional locations and settings.

There are several theories, models, and frameworks regarding how to effectively implement change, many of which have some overlap [37]. Kotter's change management model is one we use frequently and find very effective [38]. This model has eight major steps including (a) establishing a sense of urgency, (b) forming a coalition of stakeholders with institutional power to lead change, (c) creating a vision, (d) communicating the vision, (e) empowering others to act on the vision, (f) planning for and creating short-term wins, (g) consolidating improvements and producing more change, and (h) institutionalizing new approaches. Although a detailed review of change management is beyond the scope of this text, we urge readers interested in SBML project leadership to thoughtfully consider the buy-in that is needed for projects to succeed and how to thoughtfully manage the changes brought about by new training models such as SBML.

Once a project begins, the field of implementation science provides more background about why some projects succeed and others fail. Understanding implementation science can help ensure project success. Several implementation science theories and frameworks exist [39–43]. Diffusion of Innovations [39] and the Consolidated Framework for Implementation Research (CFIR) [40] are theories and frameworks that are often used in healthcare and have been used to evaluate SBML implementations [44–46]. Diffusion of Innovations identifies five components that influence the adoption and sustainability of an innovative intervention/idea. These include (a) the innovation itself, (b) the adopter, (c) the social system, (d) the individual adoption process, and (e) the diffusion system [47]. Thinking about the characteristics of individuals and teams involved and impacted by SBML, as well as the larger organizational culture, helps project leaders understand and identify potential barriers and facilitators to project success. CFIR identifies critical constructs between and among existing implementation science theories and presents a consolidated framework for implementation research. CFIR also describes four activities that are present in the implementation process: planning, engaging, executing, and reflecting/evaluating. Although a detailed review of implementation science is beyond the scope of this chapter, we urge readers leading SBML projects to thoughtfully consider the environmental changes brought about by SMBL and how these changes impact long-term project success.

An example of using implementation science principles to disseminate a SBML program from one site to another is given in Table 7.2. In this instance, a local community hospital adopted a previously developed SBML curriculum in CVC insertion that significantly reduced infection rates at Northwestern [46].

Table 7.2 Use of implementation science to disseminate SBML to a second site

Setting	Implementation science theory used	Example of how implementation was performed	Outcome
Local academic community hospital wanted to use the Northwestern University protocol for central venous catheter SBML to address a high rate of central line-associated bloodstream infections	Consolidated Framework for Implementation Research (CFIR)	*Planning*: Site visits, weekly phone calls, audits of training, pilot testing *Engagement*: Early involvement of and buy-in from hospital administration, medical education, nursing and infection control leaders *Execution*: Replication of training materials including videos/ lectures, data collection forms *Evaluation*: Multi-year follow-up	74% reduction in central line-associated bloodstream infections

Adapted from [46] with permission from BMJ Publishing Group Ltd

Dissemination of SBML to New Settings and Locations

The critical steps for success in SBML planning and implementation have been covered above. Success of SBML in its initial location depends upon these steps in addition to thoughtful attention to the principles of change management and implementation science. After a SBML project is successfully launched and maintained, project and administrative leaders may consider dissemination to other clinical areas or locations. Dissemination beyond a single institution is also possible with careful attention to culture, planning, and implementation [44–46]. Dissemination of a SBML intervention can impact greater numbers of patients, yielding even more downstream clinical benefit.

Coda

Implementation and continuous management of a SBML curriculum is a complex but worthwhile endeavor. Each step must be carefully managed to ensure achievement of educational and translational science outcomes. A successful theatrical production similarly requires much more than just a script. It involves multiple components including an excellent cast and musicians, sufficient funding, experienced production staff, and the proper location, set, and costumes. Rehearsals and previews help prepare for a successful opening night and feedback from critics may lead to modifications or adjustments. Launching a national production tour requires each of these steps to be replicated once again with identical attention to detail. Implementation and ongoing management of a successful SBML curriculum requires each of these steps: rigorous curriculum (script), expert faculty (actors), sufficient funding, appropriate location, realistic pilot testing (dress rehearsals), and meticulous evaluation (reviews). Dissemination (national production tour) is also possible with the proper time and attention.

Mastery learning curricula must be implemented and managed carefully and may seem laborious. However, educators need not be intimidated. Maintaining a well-oiled mastery learning program is really no different from managing any other program of clinical skill acquisition if it is done right. With the proper guidance, including the steps outlined in this chapter (Table 7.1), anyone can make a mastery learning curriculum a reality.

References

1. Cohen ER, Feinglass J, Barsuk JH, et al. Cost savings from reduced catheter-related bloodstream infection after simulation-based education for residents in a medical intensive care unit. Simul Healthc. 2010;5(2):98–102.
2. Thompson LL. Making the team: a guide for managers. 6th ed. New York: Pearson Education; 2016.

3. Salas E, Rosen MA, Burke CS, et al. The making of a dream team: when expert teams do best. In: Ericsson KA, Charness N, Feltovich PJ, Hoffman RR, editors. The Cambridge handbook of expertise and expert performance. New York: Cambridge University Press; 2006.
4. McGaghie WC, Pugh CM, Wayne DB. Fundamentals of educational research using clinical simulation. In: Kyle RR, Murray WB, editors. Clinical simulation: operations, engineering, and management. Burlington: Academic Press; 2008.
5. Stagl KC, Salas E, Burke CS. Best practices in team leadership: what team leaders do to facilitate team effectiveness. In: Conger J, Riggio R, editors. The practice of leadership: developing the next generation of leaders. San Francisco: Jossey-Bass; 2007.
6. Wayne DB, Didwania A, Feinglass J, Fudala MJ, Barsuk JH, McGaghie WC. Simulation-based education improves quality of care during cardiac arrest team responses at an academic teaching hospital: a case-control study. Chest. 2008;133(1):56–61.
7. Barsuk JH, Cohen ER, Vozenilek JA, O'Connor L, McGaghie WC, Wayne DB. Simulation-based education with mastery learning improves paracentesis skills. J Grad Med Educ. 2012;4(1):23–7.
8. Salzman DH, McGaghie WC, Caprio TW, et al. A mastery learning capstone course to teach and assess components of three entrustable professional activities to graduating medical students. Teach Learn Med. 2019;31(2):186–94.
9. Schroedl CJ, Corbridge TC, Cohen ER, Fakhran SS, Schimmel D, McGaghie WC, Wayne DB. Use of simulation-based education to improve resident learning and patient care in the medical intensive care unit: a randomized trial. J Crit Care. 2012;27(2):219.e7–219.e13.
10. Barsuk JH, McGaghie WC, Cohen ER, Balachandran JS, Wayne DB. Use of simulation-based mastery learning to improve the quality of central venous catheter placement in a medical intensive care unit. J Hosp Med. 2009;4(7):397–403.
11. Barsuk JH, McGaghie WC, Cohen ER, O'Leary KJ, Wayne DB. Simulation-based mastery learning reduces complications during central venous catheter insertion in a medical intensive care unit. Crit Care Med. 2009;37(10):2697–701.
12. Cohen ER, Barsuk JH, Moazed F, Caprio C, Didwania A, McGaghie WC, Wayne DB. Making July safer: simulation-based mastery learning during intern bootcamp. Acad Med. 2013;88(2):233–9.
13. Butter J, McGaghie WC, Cohen ER, Kaye M, Wayne DB. Simulation-based mastery learning improves cardiac auscultation skills in medical students. J Gen Intern Med. 2010;25(8):780–5.
14. Barsuk JH, Cohen ER, Simuni T, Caprio T, McGaghie WC, Wayne DB. Simulation-based education with mastery learning improves residents' lumbar puncture skills. Neurology. 2012;79(2):132–7.
15. Szmuilowicz E, Neeley KJ, Sharma RK, Cohen ER, McGaghie WC, Wayne DB. Improving residents' code status discussion skills: a randomized trial. J Palliat Med. 2012;15(7):768–74.
16. Gossett DR, Gilchrist-Scott D, Wayne DB, Gerber SE. Simulation training for forceps-assisted vaginal delivery and rates of maternal perineal trauma. Obstet Gynecol. 2016;128(3):429–35.
17. Wayne DB, Butter J, Siddall VJ, et al. Mastery learning of advanced cardiac life support skills by internal medicine residents using simulation technology and deliberate practice. J Gen Intern Med. 2006;21(3):251–6.
18. Barsuk JH, Cohen ER, Wayne DB, Siddall VJ, McGaghie WC. Developing a simulation-based mastery learning curriculum: lessons learned from 11 years of advanced cardiac life support. Simul Healthc. 2016;11(1):52–9.
19. Schwab B, Teitelbaum EN, Barsuk JH, Soper NJ, Hungness ES. Single-stage laparoscopic management of choledocholithiasis: an analysis after implementation of a mastery learning resident curriculum. Surgery. 2018;163(3):503–8.
20. Barsuk JH, Cohen ER, Feinglass J, et al. Cost savings of performing paracentesis procedures at the bedside after simulation-based education. Simul Healthc. 2014;9(5):312–8.
21. Downing SM, Tekian A, Yudkowsky R. Procedures for establishing defensible absolute passing scores on performance examinations in health professions education. Teach Learn Med. 2006;18(1):50–7.

22. Downs SH, Black N. The feasibility of creating a checklist for the assessment of the methodological quality both of randomised and non-randomised studies of health care interventions. J Epidemiol Community Health. 1998;52(6):377–84.
23. Vermylen JH, Wood GJ, Cohen ER, Barsuk JH, McGaghie WC, Wayne DB. Development of a simulation-based mastery learning curriculum for breaking bad news. J Pain Symptom Manag. 2019;57(3):682–7.
24. Barsuk JH, Cohen ER, Wayne DB, McGaghie WC, Yudkowsky R. A comparison of approaches for mastery learning standard setting. Acad Med. 2018;93(7):1079–84.
25. Wayne DB, Butter J, Cohen ER, McGaghie WC. Setting defensible standards for cardiac auscultation skills in medical students. Acad Med. 2009;84(10 Suppl):S94–6.
26. Miami Group. UMedic user manual. Miami: Gordon Center for Research in Medical Education, University of Miami Miller School of Medicine; 2008.
27. Downing SM, Haladyna TM. Handbook of test development. Mahwah: L. Erlbaum; 2006.
28. Stufflebeam DL. The checklists development checklist. 2000. Available at: https://wmich.edu/sites/default/files/attachments/u350/2014/guidelines_cdc.pdf. Accessed 10 Dec 2018.
29. Adler MD, Vozenilek JA, Trainor JK, et al. Comparison of checklist and anchored global rating instruments for performance rating of simulated pediatric emergencies. Simul Healthc. 2011;6(1):18–24.
30. Dunning D, Heath C, Suls JM. Flawed self-assessment: implications for health, education, and the workplace. Psychol Sci Public Interest. 2004;5(3):69–106.
31. Davis DA, Mazmanian PE, Fordis M, Van Harrison R, Thorpe KE, Perrier L. Accuracy of physician self-assessment compared with observed measures of competence: a systematic review. JAMA. 2006;296(9):1094–102.
32. Barsuk JH, Cohen ER, Feinglass J, McGaghie WC, Wayne DB. Unexpected collateral effects of simulation-based medical education. Acad Med. 2011;86(12):1513–7.
33. Cohen ER, Barsuk JH, McGaghie WC, Wayne DB. Raising the bar: reassessing standards for procedural competence. Teach Learn Med. 2013;25(1):6–9.
34. International Liaison Committee on Resuscitation and Emergency Cardiovascular Care Science with Treatment Recommendations. Circulation. 2005;112(Suppl III):III-1-136. [Context Link].
35. Proceedings of the 2005 international consensus on cardiopulmonary resuscitation and emergency cardiovascular care science with treatment recommendations. Resuscitation. 2005;67:157–341.
36. Wayne DB, Nitzberg M, Reddy S, et al. Advanced cardiac life support checklists for simulation-based education. MedEdPORTAL. 2014. Available at: https://www.mededportal.org/publication/9697/. Accessed 10 Dec 2018.
37. Robbins S. Organizational behavior. 10th ed. Upper Saddle River: Prentice Hall; 2003.
38. Kotter JP. Leading change. Boston: Harvard Business Review Press; 2012.
39. Rogers EM. Diffusion of innovations. New York: Free Press of Glencoe; 1962.
40. Damschroder LJ, Aron DC, Keith RE, Kirsh SR, Alexander JA, Lowery JC. Fostering implementation of health services research findings into practice: a consolidated framework for advancing implementation science. Implement Sci. 2009;4:50.
41. Feldstein AC, Glasgow RE. A practical, robust implementation and sustainability model (PRISM) for integrating research findings into practice. Jt Comm J Qual Patient Saf. 2008;34(4):228–43.
42. Glasgow RE. The REAIM model. In: Glanz K, Lewis FM, Rimer BK, editors. Health behavior and health education. San Francisco: John Wiley & Sons; 2002.
43. Kitson A, Harvey G, McCormack B. Enabling the implementation of evidence based practice: a conceptual framework. Qual Health Care. 1998;7:149–58.
44. Cameron KA, Cohen ER, Hertz JR, Wayne DB, Mitra D, Barsuk JH. Barriers and facilitators to central venous catheter insertion: a qualitative study. J Patient Saf. 2018. [Epub ahead of print].

45. Cohen ER, Barsuk JH, Hertz JR, et al. Healthcare providers' awareness and understanding of competency requirements for central venous catheter insertion. AMEE MedEDPublish. 2018. Available at: https://doi.org/10.15694/mep.2018.0000012.1.
46. Barsuk JH, Cohen ER, Potts S, et al. Dissemination of a simulation-based mastery learning intervention reduces central line-associated bloodstream infections. BMJ Qual Saf. 2014;23(9):749–56.
47. Dearing JW. Applying diffusion of innovation theory to intervention development. Res Soc Work Pract. 2009;19(5):503–18.

8 Feedback and Debriefing in Mastery Learning

Nahzinine Shakeri, David H. Salzman, Mark Adler, and Walter J. Eppich

Feedback and Debriefing

The terms feedback and debriefing are often used interchangeably, but feedback and debriefing are different. *Feedback* is objective, observable performance data compared to a standard or a goal that is communicated from a provider to a learner. Feedback is one-way communication with the intent of improving learner performance [1]. Feedback characteristics include the content, aim, feedback recipient and provider, feedback format, provider preparation, information source, context, and communication conditions (Table 8.1) [1]. Sources of feedback may include experts, peers, self-reflection, sensorized devices, video recordings, or other media [1, 2].

Feedback has several key features. Feedback should be specific, actionable, tailored to the learner, and timely. Feedback should acknowledge and reinforce performance that meets or exceeds expectations and identify areas for improvement [3]. Effective feedback is based on observable aspects of performance, is usually

N. Shakeri (✉)
Northwestern University Feinberg School of Medicine, Department of Emergency Medicine, Chicago, IL, USA
e-mail: nahzinine.shakeri@northwestern.edu

D. H. Salzman
Northwestern University Feinberg School of Medicine, Departments of Emergency Medicine and Medical Education, Chicago, IL, USA

M. Adler · W. J. Eppich
Northwestern University Feinberg School of Medicine, Departments of Pediatrics and Medical Education, Chicago, IL, USA

W. C. McGaghie et al. (eds.), *Comprehensive Healthcare Simulation: Mastery Learning in Health Professions Education*, Comprehensive Healthcare Simulation, https://doi.org/10.1007/978-3-030-34811-3_8

Table 8.1 Characteristics of feedback

Characteristic	Description
Content	Specific information about performance, difference between performance and standard
Aim	Motivation for improvement, to promote reflection
Feedback recipient	Individual receiving the feedback
Feedback provider	Individual or device providing the feedback
Format	Oral, written, from a device
Provider preparation	Collecting results or observing the feedback recipient beforehand
Information source	Information from a person (internal feedback) or from another source (external feedback)
Context	Timing and location of communication
Communication conditions	Timeliness, directness, clarity of communication

Adapted from van de Ridder et al. [1]. Reprinted with permission from Wiley Blackwell.

delivered by an expert provider, contains specific information, compares learner performance to a clear standard, is given with the aim of skill improvement, prompts action, and is part of a plan to observe learner performance regularly [1].

Feedback from multiple sources increases learning [4]. Feedback devices, instruments that provide quantitative information about performance metrics, are another source of information. Several studies demonstrate improvement in performance due to feedback devices. The research reports describe improved adherence to resuscitation algorithms [5, 6] and better CPR skill acquisition and retention [7, 8]. Research does not yet show that learner feedback alone improves translational patient outcomes (Chap. 16). However, feedback devices are considered a helpful adjunct to high-quality training [5–7, 9].

Debriefing in health professions education, in contrast with one way feedback, is defined as an interactive conversation to facilitate learner reflection about performance with the goal of improving future clinical care [10, 11]. The flow of communication in debriefing is interactive between the facilitator and participant(s) rather than one-way. Tannenbaum and Cerasoli define four critical features of debriefing [12]:

1. Debriefing involves active self-learning by the participant.
2. The intent of debriefing is education rather than judgment or punishment.
3. Debriefing involves reflection about specific events rather than on global performance.
4. Debriefing should include information obtained from several sources.

Characteristics of debriefing to consider are summarized in Table 8.2.

Numerous studies have demonstrated that feedback and debriefing are effective education interventions that can improve the performance of both individuals and teams [4, 12–17]. Both feedback and debriefing should integrate objective performance observations. Past research demonstrates no correlation between self-assessment by clinicians and their actual performance measured objectively [18]. In

Table 8.2 Characteristics of debriefing

Characteristic	Description
Who – Who is debriefing?	Number of individuals debriefing Facilitator training Role of debriefing individuals: peers, supervisors, confederates, standardized patients Same discipline vs. multidisciplinary
What – What is the purpose, content, and method of debriefing?	Purpose: formative vs. summative Content: communication, algorithm-based performance and/or procedural skills Method: advocacy-inquiry, plus/delta, nonjudgmental, scripted, self-assessment, etc.
When – When is the debriefing occurring?	Pre-briefing Within event debriefing (micro-debriefing) Immediate post-simulation debriefing Delayed post-simulation debriefing
Where – In what environment is the debriefing occurring?	In situ, in debriefing room, in simulation room
Why – What theoretical framework supports the debriefing?	Experiential learning, mastery learning, reflective practice, corrective feedback, mental frameworks

Adapted from Raemer et al. [11]. Simulation in Healthcare is a publication of the Society for Simulation in Healthcare. Reprinted with permission from Wolters Kluwer Health.

fact, several studies report that the least skilled clinicians tend to be very confident about their competence but are the least able to self-assess with accuracy [18]. This is consistent with findings from other professions [18, 19]. Because self-assessment correlates poorly with actual skill, clinicians require external, objective measurements to boost skill improvement. These objective performance measurements address two categories: (a) task work and (b) teamwork. *Task work* describes specific technical skills clinicians must employ to advance patient care such as communication strategies, delivering bad news, procedural skills, and using algorithm-based practice. By contrast, modern healthcare requires *teamwork*, which emphasizes how team members work together and communicate to fulfill task work [20] (Chap. 11).

Feedback and Debriefing in Simulation

Multiple factors influence the effectiveness of feedback and debriefing. Sawyer and colleagues summarize debriefing best practices and outline seven essential elements of debriefing: (a) ensuring psychological safety, (b) establishing ground rules for debriefing, (c) setting a debriefing stance or "basic assumption," (d) establishing a shared mental model, (e) addressing key learning objectives, (f) asking open-ended questions, and (g) using silence [21].

Psychological safety is the ability to "behave or perform without fear of negative consequences to self-image, social standing or career trajectory" [22]. Psychological safety promotes learner engagement which increases individual reflection, receptivity to feedback, and willingness to practice at the edge of one's ability level [23, 24]. Similarly, team psychological safety encourages learning behaviors which, in turn, improve team performance, such as asking for help, admitting errors, and seeking feedback [25].

The facilitator should actively work to create a safe and supportive learning environment to establish psychological safety and foster learner engagement with educational activities. This critical step begins in the pre-simulation briefing. During this introduction, the facilitator should clarify learning objectives, describe roles of the learner and facilitator, and state learner expectations [23]. Participants and facilitators should agree on basic *ground rules for debriefing*. These rules should include confidentiality, the need for universal participation, and the importance of focusing on performance improvement rather than criticism [21–27]. Establishing rules ahead of time can boost psychological safety and increase learner engagement [28].

The facilitator should discuss the role of error and normalize mistakes, framing them as an engine for learning and improvement. Similarly, facilitators should clarify whether learners will be evaluated formally, and if so, whether this assessment is formative (for learning) or summative (of learning) (Chap. 5). Summative assessment, which is used to make decisions about advancement in training, often triggers evaluation apprehension [24, 29]. Finally, the facilitator should emphasize a commitment to respecting learners and valuing their perspectives [23–26]. Simply labeling the learning environment as "safe" is not enough. Facilitators should work to cultivate psychological safety by delivering feedback and debriefing in a candid but nonthreatening manner.

To help establish psychological safety, facilitators should communicate a *debriefing stance or "basic assumption"* [21]. The basic assumption is an overarching statement that unites the learner and facilitator behind a shared perspective about the abilities and motivations of the individual learner or learner team. For example, "We believe that everyone participating in this simulation is intelligent, capable, cares about doing their best, and wants to improve" [23]. The basic assumption establishes positive regard for others and fosters genuine curiosity among the learners and facilitator when an error is made or if the learner or team performs differently than expected [21, 23, 27]. In addition to contributing to psychological safety, research shows that evoking positive emotion during debriefing can increase learning [21, 23].

After agreeing about basic rules of engagement, experts recommend beginning a debriefing with a short description of the scenario to *establish a shared mental model*. This can be accomplished by asking the learners to review and summarize simulation events using an introductory question such as, "In one to two sentences, can someone please summarize the key scenario components?" Learners must have a shared understanding of the events that transpired during the simulation to discuss them together. Asking learners to summarize a case prompts a common comprehension and helps participants build a shared mental model [21, 27, 28].

As with any education intervention, and as discussed in Chaps. 3 and 4, a simulation scenario should be grounded in *key learning objectives* [21, 27–35]. The debriefing facilitator should know the learning objectives and expectations about learner performance. Addressing concepts relevant to the learning objectives during the debriefing focuses simulation-based education [21, 28].

The types of questions asked during a debriefing will affect discussion quality. The facilitator should use *open-ended questions* which allow for an in-depth exploration of the reasons why an action was or was not performed. The conversation should avoid close-ended or "yes or no" questions. Open-ended questions are a good way to stimulate reflection, promote discussion, and encourage learners to share their perspectives [21, 27–33]. By probing learner perspectives, the facilitator can better tailor the discussion to highlight specific learning gaps where expectations have not been met and reinforce aspects of successful performance.

Following an open-ended question, the facilitator should refrain from immediately answering his or her own question. Instead, there should be *time for silence*. Silence allows learners to reflect and make connections. Periods of silence following open-ended questions can be used as an effective debriefing tool to help learners perform critical analysis and gel what they have learned [21, 35].

Debriefing Models

Many specific debriefing methods have been described. There is little evidence comparing the effectiveness of different debriefing approaches to support one technique versus another [21]. Instead, educators must choose from a variety of frameworks and tools. Some blended models, such as PEARLS and Team GAINS, combine several different conversational approaches [31, 32]. Educators should keep the goals of the SBML curriculum in mind when structuring feedback and debriefing because these are a key component of the education program. Certain debriefing techniques may be better suited to specific performance domains. Educators can select focused strategies for debriefing different skills. Debriefing models are summarized in Table 8.3.

Debriefing Timing

The timing of feedback debriefing during a SBML session should be considered carefully. Debriefing may occur during ("within-event debriefing" or "micro-debriefing") or after the simulation ("post-event debriefing" or "terminal debriefing") [21, 43]. The key distinction is whether the simulation continues from start to finish without interruption or if the facilitator pauses the simulation at various points to correct substandard performance or to acknowledge great work.

Facilitators often guide the post-event debriefing immediately after the simulated scenario [10, 21]. In this approach, the facilitator observes the simulation and identifies specific actions to discuss after the event. During the debriefing, the facilitator moderates the conversation as a "co-learner" or as a content expert with the aim of covering the main learning objectives [21, 29, 35]. Facilitators and learners discuss case aspects to explore why learners may or may not have performed specific actions. Through a process of seeking to understand learners' rationales for action

Table 8.3 Debriefing models

Technique	Description	Notes for use
Advocacy-inquiry [21, 22, 36–38]	Three-step conversational structure: *Observation* *Perspective* *Question*	Uses genuine curiosity to investigate the frame behind an action
Circular questioning [21, 32, 39]	Questioning technique in which the facilitator asks a third person to comment on the actions of two others in their presence	Effective for communication skills
Directive feedback [21, 31, 40]	Communication of information from facilitator to learner without engaging in discussion	Effective when learners are less experienced
Debriefing with good judgment [21, 27, 38]	Three-phase debriefing structure: *Reaction* *Analysis* *Summary*	Integrates a sense of curiosity and the conversational strategy to explore learners' frames of mind
Diamond debrief [21, 30]	Three-phase debriefing structure: *Description* *Analysis* *Application*	Basic debriefing model linked to a clear visual representation of debriefing structure
GAS [21, 33]	Three-phase debriefing structure: *Gather* *Analyze* *Summarize*	Debriefing structure with phases clearly aligned with function, namely gather feelings and facts, analyze the case, summarize learning points
Guided team self-correction [21, 41]	Two-phase debriefing structure: *A pre-specified model of relevant teamwork skills is discussed prior to the simulation scenario* *Critical and systematic self-analysis occurs after the simulation scenario*	Can be learner-directed Effective for teamwork skills
Healthcare simulation AAR [21, 29]	Seven-phase debriefing structure: *Define rules* *Explain learning objectives* *Benchmark performance* *Review expected actions* *Identify what happened* *Examine why things happened the way they did* *Formalize learning*	Based on the U.S. Army After Action Review (AAR) procedure. Allows for shared mental model and objective comparison of performance against an established standard
PEARLS [21, 31]	Four-phase debriefing structure: *Reactions* *Description* *Analysis* *Summary*	Can be learner-directed Hybrid tool that incorporates plus/delta, advocacy-inquiry and guided team self-correction
Plus/delta [21, 29, 31, 42]	Two-question technique or conversational structure: *What went well?* *What would you change?*	Can be learner-directed

Table 8.3 (continued)

Technique	Description	Notes for use
Team GAINS [21, 32]	Six-step debriefing structure: *Reactions* *Discuss clinical component* *Transfer from simulation to reality* *Discuss behavioral skills* *Summary* *Supervised practice of clinical skills, if needed*	Effective for clinical and behavioral skills Hybrid tool that incorporates advocacy-inquiry, circular questioning and guided team self-correction
3D model [21, 34]	Three-phase debriefing structure: *Diffusing* *Discovering* *Deepening*	Incorporates common elements of debriefing phases based on Kolb's experiential learning cycle

and how learner thinking may need modification, facilitators work through scenario objectives and target areas of improvement for the next practice round. Research shows that facilitator-guided post-event debriefing improves individual and team performance [10, 12, 21].

Within-event debriefing occurs during a scenario with or without a pause in the action [2, 21, 43, 44]. Such micro-debriefings comprise a key element of deliberate practice needed for SBML. Facilitators may pause the case, provide feedback, and discuss a focused performance aspect before asking learners to "rewind 10 seconds and try it again" [21, 43–45]. Alternatively, facilitators may pose questions or provide feedback during a scenario without pausing action. This prompts reflection-in-action [43]. Within-event debriefing allows learners to incorporate feedback and improve real-time performance [45]. This approach maximizes learner deliberate practice, just like a coach training an athlete [43, 45]. Within-event debriefing enhances pediatric resuscitation skill acquisition [46] and serves mastery learning goals for a variety of performance domains [21, 43–45].

Debriefing Adjuncts

Facilitators can also use adjuncts to support the debriefing conversation. A review on debriefing by Sawyer and colleagues identified three debriefing adjuncts: (a) co-debriefing, (b) a debriefing script, and (c) use of video [21].

Co-debriefing involves more than one facilitator during a debriefing [46]. Co-debriefing may be an effective approach because multiple facilitators bring added expertise and experience to a conversation and may complement each other's styles [21, 46]. Multiple observers also help provide different perspectives and identify additional discussion topics. The ratio of facilitators to learners should be considered because too many facilitators may be intimidating for a small group of learners. This may reduce the psychological safety needed for a quality debriefing session.

Facilitator use of a debriefing script may improve session effectiveness, particularly when employed by novices [21]. A debriefing script is a guide that provides the facilitator pre-formulated questions to ask during the session. These questions correspond to specific case objectives and can be written with alternate versions depending on learner actions. Research shows a knowledge acquisition improvement when the facilitator uses a debriefing script [21, 47].

The use of video in debriefing, also known as video-enhanced debriefing, is generally considered to be a useful and powerful adjunct. Video provides objective evidence about what transpired during the simulation as a source of content for the debriefing [21]. However, video-enhanced debriefing may give the learner too much data, leading to information overload [48]. Additionally, several studies have failed to show a benefit for video-enhanced debriefing, and a meta-analysis demonstrated that learning outcomes were similar whether or not video review was incorporated into debriefing [2, 21, 48, 49].

Feedback and Debriefing for SBML

In a SBML curriculum, learner performance is compared to a rigorously established, pre-determined mastery standard [43, 50]. Outcomes are uniform with all learners achieving the mastery standard in variable amounts of time [43, 50]. Deliberate practice and feedback promote learner skill acquisition and improvement and are essential for learners to move toward and achieve the mastery standard [43, 50].

The facilitated post-event debriefing is the most commonly used approach in health professions simulation. However, post-event debriefing does not promote deliberate practice or give learners an opportunity to apply newly gained knowledge or skills because it occurs after a simulated scenario has concluded [2, 21, 43]. In contrast, debriefing in a mastery learning curriculum should maximize opportunities for feedback and additional practice [43].

However, evidence about how educators should develop feedback and debriefing strategies for a SBML curriculum is limited. Within the context of SBML, Eppich and colleagues provide several recommendations about how to tailor feedback and debriefing. The main principles and recommendations include establishing a supportive yet challenging learning environment, maximizing opportunities for feedback and deliberate practice, and using within-event debriefing [43].

As discussed earlier, ensuring psychological safety and creating a safe, supportive learning environment are essential in simulation [22–24]. This is particularly true for deliberate practice-based approaches to prepare learners for effortful practice and regular feedback about their performance [43]. SBML adds another layer of challenge to this process. Integral to the design of SBML is the requirement that learners must demonstrate performance which meets or exceeds the minimum passing standard (MPS). This objective standard may create increased apprehension or stress for the learner going into the session. Recognizing that this occurs, and even acknowledging this during the pre-briefing process, will help ensure psychological safety. Explicitly reinforcing the notion that the goal of SBML is to ensure that all learners achieve the MPS by the end of training irrespective of the amount of time or practice that it may take also helps create a supportive learning environment. General strategies for establishing psychological safety have been addressed in this chapter, but there are five more approaches that may be useful within the mastery learning framework:

1. Identify from the outset that the goal is not perfection. Instead, the goal is learning through being challenged and ultimately achieving the MPS [43, 51].
2. Highlight the honest, nonthreatening nature of the feedback that will be provided [43, 52] which is similar to the way an athlete is coached [43, 45].
3. Discuss the specific details of how and when feedback will be provided to the learner [43].
4. If using a micro-debriefing strategy, inform learners that they may be interrupted during the simulation to receive feedback and reflect on performance [43].
5. Encourage peer-to-peer feedback, if appropriate to the session [43].

A SBML curriculum should be designed to maximize opportunities for learners to receive feedback and engage in deliberate practice [43]. Eppich and colleagues describe four ways to accomplish this:

1. If there are different phases of the educational intervention, such as a procedural skills component and a simulation scenario, incorporate feedback and opportunities for deliberate practice into each phase. For example, during deliberate skills practice, the learner practices a procedural skill while the facilitator provides hands-on feedback in real time. During the simulation scenario, within-event debriefing provides the learner with in-the-moment feedback, and a "pause and rewind" approach gives the learner the opportunity to try again when an error is made or performance falls short of the target [21, 43–45].
2. Encourage peer-to-peer feedback [43].
3. Keep scenarios and debriefings brief to devote the majority of the time to deliberate practice. The debriefing sessions are not about the facilitator but rather should be focused on guiding the learner to make connections and improve performance, moving toward the ultimate goal of achieving the MPS.
4. Incorporate core skills, such as chest compressions, into each case within a sequence of increasingly complex cases such that the time spent by the learner practicing and receiving feedback on performance of the core skill is maximized [43].

The within-event debriefing style is well suited to a SBML curriculum because it maximizes the time learners spend in deliberate practice on the key curricular topics [43, 45]. Within-event debriefing improves technical skills, increases adherence to resuscitation guidelines, and helps learners achieve mastery learning goals [21, 43–45].

Procedural Skills Curriculum

Chapter 13 discusses the application of SBML for procedural skills. A SBML curriculum on procedural skills can use many potential sources of feedback. When using *directive feedback from a facilitator*, the facilitator highlights good performance or an opportunity for improvement during a pause in the simulation scenario [21, 31, 40, 43]. For example, during a session on teaching bag-valve-mask ventilation, the facilitator could pause the session to provide the following feedback: "Instead of holding the bag valve mask with one hand, try holding it with both hands" [43]. Similarly, when teaching bag-valve-mask ventilation, *feedback from devices* could be used to directly quantify the degree of chest rise of the mannequin during each ventilation [5–9, 43]. A group of learners could provide *peer-to-peer feedback* to each other on bag-valve-mask technique as well [43].

Within-event debriefing strategies should be incorporated when designing a SBML curriculum on procedural skills. These strategies give learners maximum opportunities to perform deliberate practice and improve technical skills [21, 43]. *Deliberate practice with active hands-on faculty feedback* [43] should be integrated into the session to advance efficient coaching and improve learner-centered skills. *Rapid cycle deliberate practice,* another approach to within-event debriefing, is particularly useful for procedural skills debriefing. In rapid cycle deliberate practice for procedural training, fundamental core skills are integrated into the procedural training, and each step of the procedure builds upon the previous core skills and adds a new skill. Learners receive feedback through micro-debriefing. Learners do not progress to the next phase of the procedure until proficiency is achieved [43].

Table 8.4 summarizes sources of feedback and debriefing strategies for a simulation-based mastery learning curriculum on procedural skills, communication skills, and team-based resuscitation.

Communication Skills Curriculum

Chapter 10 discusses the application of SBML for communication skills. There are many potential sources of feedback to consider when designing a SBML curriculum on communication skills. *Directive feedback from the facilitator*, in which the facilitator highlights good performance or an opportunity for improvement during a pause in the simulation scenario, may be effective [21, 31, 40, 43]. For example, the facilitator may pause a scenario to highlight an excellent use of closed-loop communication [43]. *Video-enhanced debriefing* and *peer-to-peer feedback* may also be used. Unfortunately, literature in this domain is limited so the best approach remains unclear.

There are several debriefing approaches to consider when designing a SBML curriculum on communication skills. *Post-event debriefing* likely has benefit for social interactions, and there is evidence that learner-guided post-event debriefing may be just as effective as facilitator-guided post-event debriefing to improve behavioral skills [2, 21, 43]. Evidence is lacking to support the effectiveness of *video-enhanced debriefing* of communication skills but this approach makes sense for this application [2, 21, 43] (Table 8.4).

Algorithm Team-Based Resuscitation Curriculum

Chapter 3 discusses the application of SBML for algorithm team-based resuscitation. There are many potential sources of feedback to consider when designing a SBML curriculum on algorithm team-based resuscitation. *Directive feedback from the facilitator*, where the facilitator highlights good performance or an opportunity for improvement, is a useful strategy [21, 31, 40, 43]. Consider a team training for advanced cardiac life support (ACLS). The facilitator provides feedback that a pause in chest compressions lasted greater than 10 seconds, using that observation to guide the team discussion about why the overly long pause occurred and identify strategies about how to minimize pauses during chest compression [43]. In the same scenario, the facilitator may wish to use *feedback from devices*, such as a visual representation of CPR rate and depth during chest compressions [5–9, 43]. *Video-assisted debriefing*, particularly the use of selected video clips, may provide concrete imagery for learner refection [2, 21, 43, 48, 49]. Finally, while learning in groups, the participants may provide valuable *peer-to-peer feedback* to each other [43].

Within-event debriefing strategies should be incorporated when designing a simulation-based mastery learning curriculum on algorithmic team-based resuscitation. These strategies provide learners with maximum opportunities to perform deliberate practice and improve adherence to guidelines such as resuscitation algorithms [21, 43]. One strategy is to use *micro-debriefing with pause (reflection-on-action)*. Here, the scenario is paused by the facilitator to ask a question, prompt a discussion or provide directive feedback, and the rationale for why improvement is necessary ("pause and discuss") [21, 43]. After receiving specific feedback, learners may be asked to rewind 10 seconds and try it again ("pause and rewind") [21, 43–45]. For example, the facilitator may pause the case, provide feedback on an aspect of performance that needs improvement such as a long pre-defibrillation pause, and ask the learners to rewind 10 seconds and practice defibrillation again. This approach prompts learners to reflect on actions that have already occurred [43]. A second approach is *micro-debriefing without pause (reflection-in-action)*. When using this strategy, the facilitator can prompt real-time reflection-in-action without pausing the scenario. For example, the facilitator may ask the resuscitation team leader, "Are the chest compressions being performed right now adequate?" And, "If not, what needs to change to improve them?" [43]. Finally, consider using *rapid cycle deliberate practice*. In rapid cycle deliberate practice, a series of cases is sequenced with an increasing difficulty level. Fundamental core skills are integrated into the cases and each case builds upon the previous core skills and adds a new skill. Learners are provided with feedback through micro-debriefing. Learners do not progress to the next case until proficiency is achieved [43]. Rapid cycle deliberate practice improves pediatric resident resuscitation skills [45] (Table 8.4).

Table 8.4 Sources of feedback and strategies for debriefing in SBML

Type of SBML curriculum	Sources					Strategies						
	Directive feedback from facilitator	Peer-to-peer feedback	Feedback from devices	Feedback from video	Feedback from standardized patient	Micro-debriefing with pause (reflection-on-action)	Micro-debriefing without pause (reflection-in-action)	Rapid cycle deliberate practice	Deliberate practice with active hands-on faculty feedback	Facilitator guided post event debriefing	Learner-guided post event debriefing	Video Assisted debriefing
Procedure skills	X	X	X	X				X	X			
Communication skills	X	X		X	X					X	X	X
Algorithm team-based resuscitation	X	X	X	X	X	X	X	X	X	X	X	X

Coda

Feedback and debriefing are fundamental components of a SBML curriculum. Feedback and debriefing are essential to the core objective of guiding learners to achieve the MPS through deliberate practice. Rather than relying on traditional approaches to simulation, facilitators must align feedback and debriefing to specific performance domains. These targeted strategies include within-event debriefing or micro-debriefings to maximize deliberate practice so learners achieve mastery and the skills they need to provide excellent patient care.

References

1. van de Ridder JMM, Stokking KM, McGaghie WC, ten Cate OTJ. What is feedback in clinical education? Med Educ. 2008;42(2):189–97.
2. van de Ridder JMM, McGaghie WC, Stokking KM, ten Cate OTJ. Variables that affect the process and outcome of feedback, relevant for medical training: a meta-review. Med Educ. 2015;49(7):658–73.
3. Lefroy J, Watling C, Teunissen PW, Brand P. Guidelines: the do's, don'ts and don't knows of feedback for clinical education. Perspect Med Educ. 2015;4(6):284–99.
4. Hatala R, Cook DA, Zendejas B, et al. Feedback for simulation-based procedural skills training: a meta-analysis and critical narrative synthesis. Adv Health Sci Educ. 2014;19:251–72.
5. Kirkbright S, Finn J, Tohira H, et al. Audiovisual feedback device use by health care professionals during CPR: a systematic review and meta-analysis of randomised and non-randomised trials. Resuscitation. 2014;85(4):460–71.
6. Couper K, Kimani PK, Abella BS, et al. The system-wide effect of real-time audiovisual feedback and postevent debriefing for in-hospital cardiac arrest: the cardiopulmonary resuscitation quality improvement initiative. Crit Care Med. 2015;43(11):2321–31.
7. Yeung J, Meeks R, Edelson D, et al. The use of CPR feedback/prompt devices during training and CPR performance: a systematic review. Resuscitation. 2009;80(7):743–51.
8. Cheng A, Brown LL, Durr JP, et al. Improving cardiopulmonary resuscitation with a CPR feedback device and refresher simulations (CPR CARES Study): a randomized clinical trial. JAMA Pediatr. 2015;169(2):137–44.
9. Yeung J, Davies R, Gao F, Perkins GD. A randomized control trial of prompt and feedback devices and their impact on quality of chest compressions—a simulation study. Resuscitation. 2014;85(4):553–9.
10. Cheng A, Eppich W, Grant V, et al. Debriefing for technology-enhanced simulation: a systematic review and meta-analysis. Med Educ. 2014;48(7):657–66.
11. Raemer D, Anderson M, Cheng A, et al. Research regarding debriefing as part of the learning process. Simul Healthc. 2011;6(Suppl):S52–7.
12. Tannenbaum SI, Cerasoli CP. Do team and individual debriefs enhance performance? A meta-analysis. Hum Factors. 2013;55(1):231–45.
13. Kluger AN, DeNisi A. The effects of feedback interventions on performance: a historical review, a meta-analysis, and a preliminary feedback intervention theory. Psychol Bull. 1996;119(2):254–84.
14. Dine CJ, Gersh RE, Leary M, et al. Improving cardiopulmonary resuscitation quality and resuscitation training by combining audiovisual feedback and debriefing. Crit Care Med. 2008;36(10):2817–22.
15. Edelson DP, Litzinger B, Arora V, et al. Improving in-hospital cardiac arrest process and outcomes with performance debriefing. Arch Intern Med. 2008;168(10):1063–9.

16. Morgan PJ, Tarshis J, LeBlanc V, et al. Efficacy of high-fidelity simulation debriefing on the performance of practicing anaesthetists in simulated scenarios. Br J Anaesth. 2009;103(4):531–7.
17. Wolfe H, Zebuhr C, Topjian AA, et al. Interdisciplinary ICU cardiac arrest debriefing improves survival outcomes. Crit Care Med. 2014;42(7):1688–95.
18. Davis DA, Mazmanian PE, Fordis M, et al. Accuracy of physician self-assessment compared with observed measures of competence: a systematic review. JAMA. 2006;296(9):1094–102.
19. Kruger J, Dunning D. Unskilled and unaware of it: how difficulties in recognizing one's own incompetence lead to inflated self-assessments. J Pers Soc Psychol. 1999;77(6):1121–34.
20. Bowers C, Braun CC, Morgan BB. Team workload: its meaning and measurement. In: Brannick MT, Salas E, Prince C, editors. Team performance assessment and measurement: theory, methods, and applications. Mahwah: Erlbaum; 1997.
21. Sawyer T, Eppich W, Brett-Fleegler M, et al. More than one way to debrief: A critical review of healthcare simulation debriefing methods. Simul Healthc. 2016;11(3):209–17.
22. Ganley B, Linnard-Palmer L. Academic safety during nursing simulation: perceptions of nursing students and faculty. Clin Simul Nurs. 2012;8(2):49–57.
23. Rudolph JW, Raemer DB, Simon R. Establishing a safe container for learning in simulation: the role of the presimulation briefing. Simul Healthc. 2014;9(6):339–49.
24. Rosenbaum L. Cursed by knowledge—building a culture of psychological safety. N Engl J Med. 2019;380(8):786–90.
25. Edmondson A. Psychological safety and learning behavior in work teams. Adm Sci Q. 1999;44(2):350–83.
26. Kolbe M, Grande B, Spahn DR. Briefing and debriefing during simulation-based training and beyond: content, structure, attitude and setting. Best Prac Res Clin Anaesthesiol. 2015;29(1):87–96.
27. Rudolph JW, Simon R, Dufresne RL, Raemer DB. There's no such thing as "nonjudgmental" debriefing: a theory and method for debriefing with good judgment. Simul Healthc. 2006;1(1):49–55.
28. Der Sahakian G, Aliner G, Savoldelli G, et al. Setting conditions for productive debriefing. Simul Gaming. 2015;46(2):197–208.
29. Sawyer TL, Deering S. Adaptation of the U.S. Army's after-action review to simulation debriefing in healthcare. Simul Healthc. 2013;8(6):388–97.
30. Jaye P, Thomas L, Reedy G. "The diamond:" a structure for simulation debrief. Clin Teach. 2015;12(3):171–5.
31. Eppich W, Cheng A. Promoting excellence and reflective learning in simulation (PEARLS): development and rationale for a blended approach to healthcare simulation debriefing. Simul Healthc. 2015;10(2):106–15.
32. Kolbe M, Weiss M, Grote G, et al. TeamGAINS: a tool for structured debriefings for simulation-based team trainings. BMJ Qual Saf. 2013;22(7):541–53.
33. Phrampus P, O'Donnell J. Debriefing using a structured and supported approach. In: Levine A, DeMaria S, Schwartz A, Sim A, editors. The comprehensive textbook of healthcare simulation. New York: Springer; 2013.
34. Zigmont JJ, Kappus LJ, Sudikoff SN. The 3D model of debriefing: defusing, discovering, and deepening. Semin Perinatol. 2011;35(2):52–8.
35. Fanning RM, Gaba DM. The role of debriefing in simulation-based learning. Simul Healthc. 2007;2(2):115–25.
36. Senge P. The fifth discipline fieldbook: strategies and tools for building a learning organization. New York: Crown Business; 1994.
37. Rudolph JW, Simon R, Raemer DB, et al. Debriefing as formative assessment: closing performance gaps in medical education. Acad Emerg Med. 2008;15(11):1010–6.
38. Rudolph JW, Simon R, Rivard P, et al. Debriefing with good judgment: combining rigorous feedback with genuine inquiry. Anesthesiol Clin. 2007;25(2):361–76.
39. Kriz WC. A systematic-constructivist approach to the facilitation and debriefing of simulation and games. Simul Gaming. 2010;41(5):663–80.

40. Flanagan B. Debriefing: theory and techniques. In: Riley RH, editor. A manual of simulation in healthcare. New York: Oxford University Press; 2008.
41. Smith-Jentsch KA, Cannon-Bowers JA, Tannenbaum SI, et al. Guided team self-correction: impacts on team mental models, processes, and effectiveness. Small Group Res. 2008;39(3):303–27.
42. Ahmed M, Arora S, Russ S, et al. Operation debrief: a SHARP improvement in performance feedback in the operating room. Ann Surg. 2013;258(6):958–63.
43. Eppich WJ, Hunt EA, Duval-Arnould JM, et al. Structuring feedback and debriefing to achieve mastery learning goals. Acad Med. 2015;90(11):1501–8.
44. Van Heukelom JN, Begaz T, Treat R. Comparison of postsimulation debriefing versus in-simulation debriefing in medical simulation. Simul Healthc. 2010;5(2):91–7.
45. Hunt EA, Duval-Arnould JM, Nelson-McMillan KL, et al. Pediatric resident resuscitation skills improve after "rapid cycle deliberate practice" training. Resuscitation. 2014;85(7):945–51.
46. Cheng A, Palaganas J, Eppich W, et al. Co-debriefing for simulation-based education: a primer for facilitators. Simul Healthc. 2015;10:69–75.
47. Cheng A, Hunt EA, Donoghue A, et al. Examining pediatric resuscitation education using simulation and scripted debriefing: a multicenter randomized trial. JAMA Pediatr. 2013;167(6):528–36.
48. Savoldelli GL, Naik VN, Park J, et al. Value debriefing during simulated crisis management: oral versus video-assisted oral feedback. Anesthesiology. 2006;105(2):279–85.
49. Sawyer T, Sierocka-Casteneda A, Chan D, et al. The effectiveness of video-assisted debriefing versus oral debriefing alone at improving neonatal resuscitation performance: a randomized trial. Simul Healthc. 2012;7(4):213–21.
50. McGaghie WC, Issenberg SB, Barsuk JH, Wayne DB. A critical review of simulation-based mastery learning with translational outcomes. Med Educ. 2014;48(4):375–85.
51. Eppich WJ, O'Connor L, Adler MD. Providing effective simulation activities. In: Forrest K, McKimm J, Edgar S, editors. Essential simulation in clinical education. Chichester: Wiley-Blackwell; 2013.
52. Arora S, Ahmed M, Paige J, et al. Objective structured assessment of debriefing: bringing science to the art of debriefing in surgery. Ann Surg. 2012;256(6):982–8.

Faculty Development for Mastery Learning

9

Walter J. Eppich and David H. Salzman

Faculty development in the health professions historically involves knowledge and skill improvement in at least five domains: (a) professional development, (b) health professions education, (c) clinical and educational research, (d) professional communications, and (e) ethics—teaching and patient care [1]. Faculty development efforts can cover broad areas of professional practice. This chapter narrows the scope and addresses one of the five domains, faculty development for *health professions education*, with a specific focus on simulation faculty development. We use simulation-based mastery learning (ML) as a platform to address key concepts. However, the ML concepts readily apply to other areas of educational practice that also use mastery learning approaches.

Recent scholarship underscores the power of mastery learning (ML)-based educational interventions to achieve clinical proficiency [2]. A key ingredient for recreating similar successful interventions lies in expert educator-coaches, who require highly specific skills to design and implement ML curricula. Inadequate educator preparation jeopardizes the demonstrated benefits of mastery learning with potentially negative downstream effects on patients. Poor execution of key elements in the ML education bundle due to unprepared faculty will be, at best, ineffective and inefficient, and at worst, potentially harmful to learners and patients. While previously published frameworks for simulation faculty development provide guidance [3, 4], the simulation field requires more specificity for educators seeking to design and implement ML curricula. This chapter provides an introduction to approaches

W. J. Eppich (✉)
Northwestern University Feinberg School of Medicine, Departments of Pediatrics and Medical Education, Chicago, IL, USA
e-mail: w-eppich@northwestern.edu

D. H. Salzman
Northwestern University Feinberg School of Medicine, Departments of Emergency Medicine and Medical Education, Chicago, IL, USA

W. C. McGaghie et al. (eds.), *Comprehensive Healthcare Simulation: Mastery Learning in Health Professions Education*, Comprehensive Healthcare Simulation, https://doi.org/10.1007/978-3-030-34811-3_9

tailored to prepare simulation educators to use the ML framework. We focus on three areas: (a) healthcare simulation educator development in general; (b) specific learning needs for ML simulation educators including the knowledge, skills, and attitudes (KSAs) ML educators require; and (c) strategies that support educator development for ML. A coda summarizes key points.

Simulation Educator Competencies

Our field now recognizes the specialized skill set needed among health professions educators in general and simulation educators in particular. Faculty development programs to enhance this skill set have gained increasing recognition. Steinert defines faculty development as "all activities health professionals pursue to improve their knowledge, skills, and behaviors as teacher and educators, leaders and managers, and researchers and scholars, in both individual and group settings" [5]. Faculty development activities enhance individual educational practice and change culture at an organizational level [6–9]. In this chapter, we focus attention on "behaviors as teachers and educators" in our discussion of simulation faculty development.

Specialized educational skills require corresponding professional standards to which educators can aspire and provide shared understandings to guide faculty development. For example, the Academy of Medical Educators (AOM) in the United Kingdom advocates general overarching professional standards for medical educators that articulate core values and broad competency domains [10]. These apply to simulation educator development. The key competencies in the AOM framework include: (a) designing and planning learning; (b) teaching and facilitating learning; (c) assessment of learning; (d) educational research and scholarship; and (e) educational management and leadership. Professional simulation societies build on these standards and offer more specificity for simulation educators, such as the Society for Simulation in Healthcare (SSH) [11] and the International Nursing Association for Clinical Simulation and Learning (INACSL) Standards of Best Practice: Simulation^{SM} [12]. SSH provides criteria for professional certification and methods for assessing competence in the following domains [11]:

- Professional values and capabilities (e.g., integrity, motivation, leadership)
- Knowledge of educational principles, practice, and methodology in simulation (e.g., designing simulation education, managing issues of realism, using appropriate simulation methods, understanding feedback)
- Implementing, assessing, and managing simulation-based educational interventions (e.g., feedback and debriefing practices, simulation center operations)
- Scholarship in the spirit of inquiry and teaching

These simulation competency standards highlight the skill development domains simulation educators require and provide helpful general guidance about skill acquisition. For example, the SSH Standards uniformly emphasize creation of a supportive learning environment through explicit strategies that engender a sense of psychological safety, strategies that Rudolph and colleagues fully describe [13]. The SSH Standards also emphasize the important role of debriefing in simulation education. Peterson and colleagues take this one step further and describe a tiered approach to simulation faculty development [3] and outline a pathway to local certification across five progressively complex tiers of simulation faculty development. The tiers range from two entry-level "apprentice" tiers to three successive tiers of "simulation expert." Each of the five tiers is linked to (a) specific elements of simulation faculty development and (b) well-defined markers of achievement such as completion of learning activities or performance ratings from debriefing. The Peterson et al. faculty development elements address the spectrum of approaches to learning new skills [3]. The Peterson et al. faculty development elements are:

- Observation of educational activities to provide context and vicarious experiential learning;
- Didactic components covering core knowledge;
- Interactive learning experiences in small group activities, including simulation exercises;
- Practice for skill building and maintenance across a variety of capabilities;
- Expert feedback;
- Mentoring; and
- Networking for professional growth.

Peterson and colleagues' certification framework presents clear criteria for advancement from one tier to the next. Entry levels of achievement involve completing online modules and observation of simulation education events. Progressively expert tiers of achievement require increasing degrees of participation in a variety of activities, such as completing required and optional didactic modules, documentation of proficiency in debriefing using the Debriefing Assessment for Simulation in Healthcare (DASH) [14, 15] and regular involvement in simulation-based educational events. These tiers inform faculty development efforts and provide a clear path for advancement within simulation programs while also recognizing individual talents and interests. Such a developmental trajectory from novice to expert also corresponds to increasing institutional impact and recognition, which drive career development and academic promotion depending on the workplace setting [16].

We also see limitations in Peterson and colleagues' framework. While the framework outlines clear targets to advance from one tier to the next [3], it provides only a broad sense of the capabilities at each tier. However, since debriefings are context-specific and depend on learner group, performance domain, time available, and other factors [17, 18], excellent debriefing performance in one area, such as with undergraduate nursing students learning basic procedural skills, might not translate to performance with experienced interprofessional teams. In our view, debriefing skills for simulation curricula requires high specificity because structuring feedback and debriefing during deliberate practice for skill acquisition in communication, advanced life support, or invasive procedures demand unique educator abilities.

Standards from AOM, SSH, INACSL, and Peterson and colleagues' framework serve as valuable prerequisites for simulation educators but they lack detail about unique elements for ML curricula addressed in the next chapter section. For example, assessment features prominently in all phases of the ML education bundle and contributes to unique approaches to prompting deliberate practice which is a core component of ML. While the INACSL Standards of Best Practice: Simulation^{SM} touch on formative and summative assessment, the Peterson and colleagues' tiered model neglects capabilities in assessment which are not featured even at expert levels. Additionally, how simulation educator-coaches manage feedback and debriefing and structure deliberate practice specifically in ML environments fundamentally contributes to the success of these curricula [19].

The DASH criteria, which Peterson and colleagues use to document debriefing proficiency, were not designed to assess within-event micro-debriefings that characterize deliberate practice sessions. For example, the DASH authors advocate for broad applicability of their tool with a "wide range of educational objectives, from an exercise in suturing skills to one in disaster management for a whole hospital" and "in a variety of settings with various physical and time constraints" [14]. However, the DASH instrument does not address the iterative, repetitive, and deliberate cyclical nature of practice-feedback/debriefing-practice. Therefore, as they relate to facilitating the debriefing component of a simulation-based learning experience, general competency frameworks provide only non-specific and decontextualized direction, in part leading to simulation faculty development approaches that are similarly wide-ranging. This has led some to question the effectiveness of debriefing workshops and courses that may not be changing practice to the degree expected because everyday educators may fail to transfer key lessons when they return to their educational settings [20]. In our view, the absence of context represents the main obstacle for educators to translate lessons to their own educational settings. This lack of focused preparation for ML education, specifically the approaches to structuring feedback and debriefing during deliberate practice, threatens the integrity of the ML education bundle. To address this gap, we use these existing frameworks and tiered approaches to simulation faculty development to outline specific capabilities for educators using ML to design and implement educationally robust curricula. Then we propose approaches to faulty development to help ML education achieve these key capabilities.

Educator Competencies for Mastery Learning

Simulation-based education requires unique skills and expertise given its highly interactive nature. Eppich and Cheng [21] summarize key competencies simulation educators must acquire: (a) conducting an effective [pre]briefing, (b) delivering high-quality standardized simulation events, (c) attending to relevant realism issues, (d) integrating actors or simulated participants effectively when appropriate, (e) debriefing simulation events effectively, and (f) assessing learning outcomes [21]. As we have previously discussed, most simulation educator training courses seek to provide educators with a general skill set while leaving gaps. By contrast, the ML approach represents a comprehensive education bundle that integrates design and implementation with robust assessment of learning outcomes, placing additional demands on simulation educators. Education for ML requires active engagement by learners and teachers. Mastery learning is not at all passive. Further, rather than working in isolation, many ML simulation educators implement their curricula using teaching teams. Solid team composition produces high levels of competency in a number of areas. These broad competencies include (a) curriculum design and (b) curriculum delivery. See Table 9.1 for a snapshot. Other chapters in this book provide readers with additional details: curriculum design (Chap. 3), ML curriculum delivery (Chaps. 4 and 7), and ML assessment (Chap. 5).

Some ML educators may need added expertise in several areas. However, individual educators may not require equal levels of expertise in all ML competencies depending on the local context, personnel resources, and the curriculum scope. For example, some educators may primarily design curriculum and assessment instruments, while others deliver the curriculum and perform assessment. Expertise is shaped by degree of involvement, frequency of participation, interests, and career trajectory. A nursing simulation educator may design a ML curriculum for a particular skill, including robust assessment instruments to guide deliberate practice. To implement the curriculum for 100+ undergraduate nursing students, however, the nursing educator will need to recruit additional faculty to support curriculum delivery. While the lead educator may design the curriculum and direct the course, other faculty may deliver the curriculum by implementing scenarios, structuring deliberate practice as educator-coaches, and assessing learning outcomes.

Table 9.1 Key competencies for simulation faculty development for mastery learning

Key competencies	Description
Curriculum design	Designs curricula design using established principles and deliberately integrates elements of assessment and feedback throughout to maximize opportunities for deliberate practice
	Measures learner performance to provide the basis for formative feedback to guide learner improvement, including designing assessment instruments, setting performance standards, and training raters
Curriculum delivery	Oversees course implementation, including: Scheduling learners Recruiting and preparing educators Overseeing course schedule Preparing simulated patients Preparing simulated learning environments and managing simulation technology
	Serves as a simulation-educator coach, by implementing existing curricula, including Creating psychologically safe learning environments Enacting existing simulation scenarios Supporting deliberate practice through feedback and debriefing grounded in performance data derived from robust assessment

Simulation Educator-Coaches

Of the competencies we have outlined here, those required for a simulation educator-coach have unique characteristics for a ML environment and represent the most significant paradigm shift in healthcare education (Chap. 4). A majority of simulation educators conceptualize debriefing as part of the educational intervention that occurs after a simulated patient care episode. Mastery learning approaches and robust deliberate practice by simulation educators demand targeted use of post-simulation *and* within-simulation debriefing or "micro-debriefings" [19]. We now devote detailed attention to micro-debriefing or coaching here.

The concept of coaching is gaining traction in health professions education [22, 23]. Recent work emerging from surgery also highlights the potential for coaches to enhance residents' experiential learning in the operating room through structured coaching approaches that apply principles of feedback, debriefing, and behavioral modeling [24], although current surgical culture has been identified as a potential obstacle [25] (Chap. 21). Further, Watling and LaDonna [26] interviewed physicians, physicians with sports coaching experience, and business coaches and identified three core elements of coaching: (a) mutual engagement between coaches and learners who share an orientation toward growth and development, (b) reflection involving both coaches and learners, and (c) embrace of failure to drive learning [26]. Armson and colleagues further delineated key aspects of coaching and differentiate between process and content skills [27]. These skills include:

- Process skills: coach preparation, micro-communication skills to promote learner reflection and self assessment, coach flexibility;
- Content skills: specific content of feedback as part of a collaborative discussion with learners that includes goal setting.

These recent studies highlight that coaching is a highly active process, involves collaboration on the part of learners and coaches, and involves not only feedback and debriefing but also goal setting and structured and guided practice (Chap. 4). Lovell points out that coaches do not necessarily need subject matter expertise. Coaches must be skilled at drawing out ever better performance, which requires specific skills that can be learned [28]. This assertion underscores the recognition that physicians do not necessarily need to be trained by physicians (Chaps. 4 and 21). Instead, medical learners require simulation educator-coaches prepared to create learning environments to facilitate continued improvement toward mastery standards through structured deliberate practice. Powerful learning outcomes have been achieved by resident physicians through structured coaching by a non-physician simulation educator using the ML approach [29, 30].

Faculty Development for Mastery Learning

Simulation faculty development requires not only knowledge about key competencies but also specific faculty development initiatives to help educators acquire those competencies. Creating a faculty development program to address skills needed to direct or participate in a clinical ML course of study should follow the curriculum development principles given in Chap. 3. The only difference is that faculty, not students, are the clientele. Clear educational targets help make informed decisions about how to structure faculty development. These educational targets often depend on an educator's degree of involvement. We now outline categories of faculty development approaches. Then we propose stages of simulation faculty development that set levels of advancement with continued involvement. Finally, we consolidate these ideas and propose a blend of event-based and workplace-based approaches to develop key educator-coach behaviors and skills across stages of ML educator expertise.

Approaches to Faculty Development

Traditionally, simulation educator development has been viewed as formal and event-based, with new ML educators attending a range of educational events. The educational events extend from online courses or webinars, journal clubs, workshops, or even multi-day simulation educator courses [7, 31]. In particular, multi-day courses try to meet the needs of all participants by emphasizing universal principles of healthcare simulation that apply broadly. However, the general nature of these courses leaves individual educators to adapt course content and experiences to their own educational environments, with the risk that key messages get lost in translation [20]. For example, such general simulation educator courses may emphasize debriefing and insufficiently address assessment issues that are integral to ML. Some events may offer a specific focus, such as a conference workshop, journal clubs, or online webinars devoted to a particular aspect of simulation education such as assessment, although the challenges of translating lessons learned to educational practice remain. Longitudinal educator development programs can begin to bridge this gap because they offer greater integration of KSA acquisition and application [32]. Such longitudinal programs offer a significant added benefit to the learner community that beginning educators can rely on as an additional learning resource [33].

Complementary workplace-based approaches have recently emerged that embed educator development within authentic teaching experiences [8]. Such embedded approaches allow for peer coaching or mentoring from more experienced educators [8]. Workplace-based simulation educator development includes collaborative development of simulation curricula, co-teaching educational events, self-assessment of teaching, peer coaching and assessment, learner feedback, program evaluation, and scholarly production. These workplace-based approaches to simulation faculty development permit tighter linkages between expertise acquisition and its immediate application. Importantly, such close collaboration within educational teams enhances relationships and lines of communication that promote highly contextualized attainment of relevant KSAs [34]. In these educational communities of practice [35], more experienced educators nurture those less experienced during shared social experiences with the common goal of designing and implementing high-quality educational events. Role modeling [36] and peer coaching [37–39] feature prominently in workplace-based faculty development approaches. Ideally, simulation educator development includes both event-based and workplace-based approaches integrated in an individualized longitudinal plan. See Table 9.2 for several features, advantages, disadvantages, and examples of event-based and workplace-based approaches.

Stages of Simulation Faculty Development

As we have outlined, not all simulation faculty participating within ML curricula require equal levels of expertise in all the educator competencies because the faculty level of participation varies. We propose a staged approach to ML faculty development that describes developmental stages based on increasing degrees of participation. These stages logically align with specific faculty development initiatives, generally focusing first on curriculum delivery and later on curriculum design because most educators follow this developmental trajectory. However, some ML simulation faculty development educators may focus primarily on curriculum design and program leadership and less on curriculum delivery.

Table 9.2 Key types of simulation faculty development

Simulation faculty development approaches	Features	Advantages	Disadvantages	Examples

Event-based	Dedicated events designed primarily to develop educators	In-depth didactic inputs about key issues to ensure conceptual foundations
		Focused, dedicated time to skill develop core skills
		No risk to learners since faculty development is a distinct event
			Removed from learners
			Lacks context
			  Removed from curriculum to be taught
			  Removed from teaching team
				One-time or longitudinal events
				  One or multi-day courses
				  Workshops
				  Conferences
				  Webinars
				  Journal club

Workplace-based	Embedded within authentic teaching is designed primarily to prepare learners for clinical practice	Highly contextualized
		  Learning while enacting actual curriculum
		  Integrally linked to teaching team
		  Engagement with learners
		Integration with longitudinal educator development
			Limited didactic input to support theoretical understanding
			Need for close faculty supervision and peer coaching
			More risk to learners since faculty development occurs during authentic educational settings
				Procedural skills training
				Communications training
				Resuscitation training
				Team training
				Interprofessional/uniprofessional

The four stages of ML simulation educator development align competences with levels of participation and measured skill achievement (see Table 9.3). While a simulation educator may start at Stage 1 and find it relatively easy to achieve Stage 2, Stages 3 and 4 represent a significant commitment to ML simulation education.

Table 9.3 Stages of mastery learning simulation faculty development

Stage with brief description	Detailed description
Stage 1 *Infrequent participation and assessment* *Supports existing curricula with supervision* *Co-teaches sessions with experienced educators*	Contributes to a supportive learning environment but requires support Implements scenarios designed by others Structures the feedback and debrief for deliberate practice, yet requires support Requires technical support to manage simulation equipment Gives effective feedback Demonstrates expertise in the course content

Stage 2
Frequent participation and assessment
Supports existing curricula
Leads educational sessions independently
	All of the above, plus:
	Independently establishes a supportive learning environment
	  Creates and maintains psychological safety
	  Minimizes evaluation apprehension
	  Clarifies expectations and outlines how deliberate practice will be structured, how feedback and debriefing will occur
	Structures feedback and debriefing for deliberate practice independently
	Assesses performance using appropriate tools
	Demonstrates technical expertise with simulation equipment
	Integrates actors or simulated participants
	Manages difficult educational situations
	Uses advanced strategies applicable for performance domain
	Designs basic scenarios and matches simulation modality to type of learning objective

Stage 3
Regular participation and assessment
Designs and implements ML curricula
Directs courses
Local expert in ≥1 domain
Mentors other educators
	All above, plus:
	Serves as course director
	  Manages educational team and simulation staff
	  Schedules learners and faculty
	  Trains simulated patients for their roles
	Models key skills from stages 1 and 2, provides peer coaching, mentors other educators
	Use of technology effectively
	Designs assessment instruments such as checklists
	Performs standard setting procedures to determine mastery standards
	Trains raters to use assessment instruments
	Generates scholarship, such as workshops at regional/national meetings

Stage 4
Program leadership, sustained assessed excellence
Local/regional/national expertise
	Demonstrates sustained excellence in multiple domains
	  Faculty development
	  Curriculum development and integration within UME, GME
	  Program development & evaluation
	  Research
	Mentors other faculty

- Stage 1: Infrequent participation and assessment, requires support to deliver existing curricula
- Stage 2: Frequent participation and assessment, leads individual educational sessions independently
- Stage 3: Regular participation and assessment, designs and directs courses; mentors other educators
- Stage 4: Program leadership, sustained assessed excellence

These stages are based on a progression from infrequent to regular participation and assessment, along with potential leadership roles, and align with realities of an everyday delivery of simulation-based education. Ideally, all simulation educators would participate in multi-day simulation educator courses to serve as a foundation before engaging learners. However, time and financial constraints make this strategy infeasible for most. Therefore, a majority of ML simulation educators will benefit from faculty development strategies that prepare them specifically for the courses they teach.

Professional Consolidation

We advocate a hybrid approach that purposefully blends event-based and workplace-based simulation educator development for ML. As we have already noted, one size does not fit all. Faculty development plans need to be individualized based on current and anticipated level of participation, prior simulation and teaching experience, assessed educational competence, career trajectory, and faculty readiness.

For educator-coaches with infrequent participation several times per year, workplace approaches seem best suited if experienced simulation educators can support such endeavors. These might include teaching observations with role modeling and post-session explanation of educational strategies. Here the focus should lie in establishing psychologically safe learning environments, enacting existing scenarios, and supporting deliberate practice. As educators become more committed with regular involvement, workplace-based peer coaching combined with participation in simulation educator workshops, either locally or at simulation conferences, can accelerate skill development. Topics might include assessment, specific feedback and debriefing strategies, and ML curriculum design. Longitudinal faculty development programs are also beneficial because they purposefully blend such events as workshops with peer coaching during actual education sessions. As participation increases, collaboration in teaching teams during the design of new curricula also serve as powerful faculty development opportunities.

Some educators try to build a ML program without the benefit of experienced simulation educators to support and guide them. Here, we recommend an early multi-day simulation educator course that addresses basic skills. Ideally, such course would be focused on ML curriculum design and delivery. An example includes the 3-day Northwestern Simulation™ course on Designing and Implementing a Mastery Learning Curriculum. Simulation educators working in silos should try to build their team and foster collaborations with educators at other centers who can provide support as they plan and implement their own curricula.

As individual educators progress along the stages of development, some educators will naturally develop specific expertise in unique domains such as feedback and debriefing, assessment and rater training, curriculum design, program development, or educational research. Such domain expertise typically develops through particular individual interests that fuel additional reading, coursework, and scholarship. These educators can serve as valuable local resources to support ML educator and program development.

Coda

In this chapter, we provide an introduction to faculty development for mastery learning with a focus on simulation educator development. In doing so, we describe the current state of affairs in simulation faculty development in general and identify gaps in how educators prepare to design and implement ML curricula. We highlight unique capabilities for ML educators that require specific consideration. We offer key principles for simulation programs seeking to develop faculty to design and implement ML curricula. Creating a rigorous ML faculty development program should follow curriculum development protocols presented in Chap. 3 of this volume. We believe that by keeping these key considerations in mind, faculty developers can build on existing faculty development programming and provide targeted offerings for those educators devoting their attention to ML.

References

1. McGaghie WC, Frey JJ, editors. Handbook for the academic physician. New York: Springer Verlag; 1986.
2. McGaghie WC, Issenberg SB, Barsuk JH, Wayne DB. A critical review of simulation-based mastery learning with translational outcomes. Med Educ. 2014;48(4):375–85.
3. Peterson DT, Watts PI, Epps CA, White ML. Simulation faculty development: a tiered approach. Simul Healthc. 2017;12(4):254–9.
4. Sittner BJ, Aebersold ML, Paige JB, et al. INACSL standards of best practice for simulation: past, present, and future. Nurs Educ Perspect. 2015;36(5):294–8.
5. Steinert Y. Faculty development: core concepts and principles. In: Steinert Y, editor. Faculty development in the health professions. Dordrecht: Springer Netherlands; 2014.
6. Bligh J. Faculty development. Med Educ. 2005;39(2):120–1.
7. Leslie K, Baker L, Egan-Lee E, et al. Advancing faculty development in medical education: a systematic review. Acad Med. 2013;88:1038–45.
8. Steinert Y, Mann K, Anderson B, et al. A systematic review of faculty development initiatives designed to enhance teaching effectiveness: a 10-year update. BEME guide no. 40. Med Teach. 2016;15:1–18.
9. Jolly B. Faculty development for organizational change. In: Steinert Y, editor. Faculty development in the health professions. Dordrecht: Springer Netherlands; 2014.
10. Academy of Medical Educators. Professional standards. 2014. Available at: https://www.medicaleducators.org/write/mediamanager/AOME_professional_standards_2014.pdf.

11. Society for Simulation in Healthcare. Professional certification standards and elements. 2012. Available at: https://www.ssih.org/portals/48/certification/CHSE%20Standards.pdf.
12. INACSL Standards Committee. INACSL standards of best practice: simulation[SM]. Clin Simul Nurs. 2016;12(Suppl):S5–S50.
13. Rudolph JW, Raemer DB, Simon R. Establishing a safe container for learning in simulation: the role of the presimulation briefing. Simul Healthc. 2014;9(6):339–49.
14. Simon R, Raemer D, Rudolph JW. Debriefing assessment for simulation in healthcare (DASH) [Internet]. Boston; 2010. Available at: https://harvardmedsim.org/wp-content/uploads/2016/10/DASH_handbook_2010_Rev2.pdf.
15. Brett-Fleegler M, Rudolph J, Eppich W, et al. Debriefing assessment for simulation in healthcare: development and psychometric properties. Simul Healthc. 2012;7(5):288–94.
16. Thorndyke LE, Gusic ME, George JH, et al. Empowering junior faculty: Penn State's faculty development and mentoring program. Acad Med. 2006;81(7):668–73.
17. Eppich W, Cheng A. Promoting excellence and reflective learning in simulation (PEARLS): development and rationale for a blended approach to health care simulation debriefing. Simul Healthc. 2015;10(2):106–15.
18. Cheng A, Grant V, Dieckmann P, et al. Faculty development for simulation programs: five issues for the future of debriefing training. Simul Healthc. 2015;10(4):217–22.
19. Eppich WJ, Hunt EA, Duval-Arnould JM, et al. Structuring feedback and debriefing to achieve mastery learning goals. Acad Med. 2015;90(11):1501–8.
20. Krogh K, Chan A, McNaughton N. Another debriefing course! Who benefits? Adv Simul. 2018;3:26.
21. Eppich W, Cheng A. Competency-based simulation education: should competency standards apply for simulation educators? BMJ Stel. 2015;1(1):3–4.
22. Lovell B. What do we know about coaching in medical education? A literature review. Med Educ. 2017;52(4):376–90.
23. Gifford KA, Fall LH. Doctor coach: a deliberate practice approach to teaching and learning clinical skills. Acad Med. 2014;89(2):272–6.
24. Bonrath EM, Dedy NJ, Gordon LE, Grantcharov TP. Comprehensive surgical coaching enhances surgical skill in the operating room. Ann Surg. 2015;262(2):205–12.
25. Mutabdzic D, Mylopoulos M, Murnaghan ML, et al. Coaching surgeons: is culture limiting our ability to improve? Ann Surg. 2015;262(2):213–6.
26. Watling CJ, LaDonna KA. Where philosophy meets culture: exploring how coaches conceptualise their roles. Med Educ. 2019;53(5):467–76.
27. Armson H, Lockyer JM, Zetkulic M, et al. Identifying coaching skills to improve feedback use in postgraduate medical education. Med Educ. 2019;53(5):477–93.
28. Lovell B. Bringing meaning to coaching in medical education. Med Educ. 2019;53(5): 426–7.
29. Wayne D, Butter J, Siddall V, et al. Mastery learning of advanced cardiac life support skills by internal medicine residents using simulation technology and deliberate practice. J Gen Intern Med. 2006;21:251–6.
30. Wayne DB, Siddall VJ, Butter J, et al. A longitudinal study of internal medicine residents' retention of advanced cardiac life support skills. Acad Med. 2006;81(10 Suppl):S9–S12.
31. Steinert Y, Mann K, Centeno A, et al. A systematic review of faculty development initiatives designed to improve teaching effectiveness in medical education: BEME guide no. 8. Med Teach. 2006;28(6):497–526.
32. Gruppen LD. Intensive longitudinal faculty development programs. In: Steinert Y, editor. Faculty development in the health professions. Dordrecht: Springer Netherlands; 2014.
33. Steinert Y. Faculty development: from workshops to communities of practice. Med Teach. 2010;32(5):425–8.
34. O'Sullivan PS, Irby DM. Reframing research on faculty development. Acad Med. 2011;86(4):421–8.

35. Steinert Y. Learning from experience: from workplace learning to communities of practice. In: Steinert Y, editor. Faculty development in the health professions. Dordrecht: Springer Netherlands; 2014.
36. Mann KV. Faculty development to promote role-modeling and reflective practice. In: Steinert Y, editor. Faculty development in the health professions. Dordrecht: Springer Netherlands; 2014.
37. Cheng A, Grant V, Huffman J, et al. Coaching the debriefer: peer coaching to improve debriefing quality in simulation programs. Simul Healthc. 2017;12(5):319–25.
38. Mcleod PJ, Steinert Y. Peer coaching as an approach to faculty development. Med Teach. 2009;31(12):1043–4.
39. Boillat M, Elizov M. Peer coaching and mentorship. In: Steinert Y, editor. Faculty development in the health professions. Dordrecht: Springer Netherlands; 2014.

Part III

Mastery Learning in Action

Mastery Learning of Clinical Communication Skills

10

Julia H. Vermylen and Gordon J. Wood

Other chapters in this book have focused on introducing the mastery learning model and have explored issues of curriculum design including checklist development, setting a minimum passing standard (MPS), models of deliberate practice, and key elements of feedback and debriefing. There are also examinations of translational outcomes and modes of curriculum dissemination. Throughout this discussion, however, the majority of the examples presented and data reviewed have come from the application of mastery learning to procedural skills and team skills such as those needed for advanced cardiac life support. This chapter will focus on the relatively nascent field of mastery learning for communication skills with an emphasis on communication about serious illness because this is where much of the current work has occurred.

In recent years, a robust body of evidence has developed showing that how we communicate impacts patient outcomes. Communication interventions have been shown to improve clinical decision making [1, 2], trust in physicians [3], family satisfaction [4], caregiver psychological outcomes [5–8], physician well-being [9], and resource use [2, 10–13]. Recent data suggest that palliative care communication interventions focused on supporting specific coping strategies are associated with improved quality of life, and decreased depression [14]. These strategies, along with discussion to improve illness understanding, contribute to the prolonged survival demonstrated in patients who receive early integrated palliative care [15]. Because of all of these and other outcomes, communication is now identified in research agendas and lists of quality indicators [16–21] and has become the focus of

J. H. Vermylen (✉) · G. J. Wood
Northwestern University Feinberg School of Medicine,
Departments of Medicine and Medical Education, Chicago, IL, USA
e-mail: j-vermylen@northwestern.edu

W. C. McGaghie et al. (eds.), *Comprehensive Healthcare Simulation: Mastery Learning in Health Professions Education*, Comprehensive Healthcare Simulation, https://doi.org/10.1007/978-3-030-34811-3_10

numerous educational interventions [22]. "Interpersonal and communication skills" is also one of the 6 Accreditation Council on Graduate Medical Education (ACGME) core competencies [23]. Since mastery learning has been linked to improved patient outcomes in other domains [24] (Chap. 16), there is interest in applying mastery learning to communication skills training to see if similar results can be obtained.

This chapter begins with a review of the current state of communication skills training and then examines the degree to which these programs have been shown to change, or not change clinical outcomes. Mastery learning of communication skills will be introduced as a model that builds on and may augment other current models. We then review the evidence for mastery learning of communication skills and compare and contrast the various approaches to teaching communication skills with a mastery learning approach. In particular, we highlight how methods of small group role play with a simulated patient (SP) can be used in a mastery learning model with robust results. In these discussions, we highlight how mastery learning of communication skills is similar to mastery learning of procedural skills and how it also presents some unique challenges. We conclude with a discussion of future directions needed to aid in the development of the new field of mastery learning of communication skills.

Are Communication Skills Teachable?

There has long been a perception that you are either a good communicator or you are not. Learners are assumed to have an innate level of ability to communicate and relate to patients that they bring to a health professions education setting. Health professions education has traditionally focused more on clinical facts and procedural skills rather than on how to communicate with patients and their families. Many learners, especially senior learners across specialties and disciplines, report that they received no training in communication skills during their schooling [25–31]. Fortunately, there is now an abundance of evidence that shows communication skills are teachable and almost all training programs in the health professions have adopted some communication skills training as part of their curriculum [32].

Much of the best data that training can improve communication skills comes from studies of small group role play with SPs [33]. The paradigmatic study is from a National Cancer Institute-funded communication skills training program for oncology fellows called "Oncotalk" [34]. This 4-day residential workshop used small group role play with SPs with opportunities for deliberate practice. Attendees were videotaped before and after the workshop. Statistically significant improvements were seen in the frequency with which participants used various communication skills. The most telling result, however, is that more than 90% of the time blinded raters could accurately differentiate a pre- from a post-intervention video of a learner breaking bad news. Similar methods have been shown to improve skills among internal medicine residents after a one-day retreat [35]. Additionally, a focused, multimodal curriculum using deliberate practice, online modules, and self-reflection showed improved skills in code status discussions [36] and skills were retained 1 year later [37]. Multiple other studies, most involving some opportunity to practice and receive feedback, have shown varying degrees of improvement [38, 39]. Based on this robust body of evidence and positive changes seen with training programs around the world there is now consensus that communication skills are, in fact, teachable.

Does Communication Skills Training Change Clinical Outcomes?

If communication skills are teachable, the next question is whether the training programs can improve clinical outcomes. There are many examples of communication interventions that start a new conversation that was not happening before (e.g., an end-of-life family conference for patients dying in the ICU [6]) or a new communication structure that was not previously in place (i.e., a multidisciplinary meeting within 72 hours of admission to the ICU with follow-up meetings based on clinical milestones (1)). These interventions improve patient and family outcomes [2, 6, 11, 40]. It has been harder, however, to demonstrate that training in how to communicate more skillfully in a conversation that is already being done (i.e., breaking bad news) can result in improved patient-level outcomes [41–43]. Demonstrating these sorts of T3-level outcomes (see Chap. 16) has not been impossible, however, and there are some positive results in the literature. Communication skills training has been linked to multiple patient outcomes including increased patient trust in the clinician [44], improved patient and family satisfaction [9, 45–47], increased physician empathy and decreased burnout [9], increased likelihood of patients reporting feeling better after the visit [48], increased documentation of goals of care conversations, decreased desire for aggressive care, decreased mortality, and decreased readmissions [49].

Despite these positive trials there have been some negative trials. One study examined internal medicine residents and nurse practitioners who were trained in several serious illness communication tasks like giving bad news and responding to emotions [50]. The training used the same methods (small group role play with SPs) that had been previously shown to improve communication skills when comparing pre- and posttests [51]. This study, however, was not able to show improved patient and family ratings about the quality of communication or quality of end-of-life care and may have even been associated with some harm due to an increased rate of depression in the intervention group. Much has been written about what might account for these surprising results [52]. In examining from a mastery learning lens, there may have been two issues. First, it is not clear whether improved skills were documented in all learners. Second, the degree to which skills improved may not have been sufficient. In post-training evaluation, the majority of the skills were successfully performed by less than 50% of post-intervention trainees [51]. For example, one of the key skills in breaking bad news is to start by asking what the patient understands so you know where to begin. Before the training, only 22.8% of trainees performed this step, which improved to 39.3% after training. While this was a statistically significant improvement, the majority of trainees are still skipping this critical step after training which may explain the negative results of the study. One can easily imagine how much more robust the intervention might have been using a mastery model in which outcomes are uniform and only time of training varied.

Mastery Learning in Communication Skills Training

We are aware of three examples of simulation-based mastery learning of communication skills that have been reported. These studies are described in detail in Table 10.1. The first two studies build on each other and focus on code status discussions. The first study was part of a multi-faceted "boot-camp" for internal medicine residents [53]. The communication skills training portion used a mix of didactic teaching and demonstrations followed by one-to-one deliberate practice with a faculty member that was repeated until mastery was achieved. This resulted in a statistically significant improvement in skills with all residents eventually meeting the MPS. In the second study, a checklist developed for this intervention was modified and a similar training intervention with one-to-one deliberate practice with a faculty member was used in a randomized trial with a population of faculty physicians [54]. Statistically significant improvement in checklist scores was reached with multiple new skills used after the training and all of the hospitalists reached the MPS with 30% requiring one additional training session to reach the MPS.

The third application of mastery learning to communication skills reported in the literature focused on breaking bad news [55]. It differs from the first two because it used a small group model for deliberate practice rather than one-to-one training as was done in the code status discussion programs. This training was similar in other ways because it involved didactic teaching, a demonstration, and deliberate practice until a MPS was reached. The checklist for this intervention was different because, in addition to standard "done vs. not done" checklist items similar to those used in the prior two studies, the measure added three 5-point global rating scale items and three Likert-scale questions about communication quality. With this model there was again a significant skill improvement post-training.

To summarize, the reported literature on mastery learning of clinical communication skills is sparse yet promising. Studies have used one-to-one and group models of deliberate practice and checklist structures have varied but outcomes have been uniform and robust, giving hope that future studies may show better T3 and T4 outcomes. We are aware of several studies underway involving multiple different conversational tasks so we expect this literature to grow rapidly.

Curriculum Design: Mastery Learning of Communication Skills

Having described the background and evidence above, we will now begin to shift our focus to a discussion about how to design a mastery learning curriculum for communication skills, starting with a discussion about how mastery learning of

Table 10.1 Details on teaching, content, assessment for each of the published three communication skills mastery learning curricula

Reference	Participants	Teaching Method(s)	Simulator or model used	Skill(s) assessed	Outcome Measurement	Reliability coefficient of outcome score in prior publication
Cohen et al. [53]	47 first-year internal medicine residents	Didactic on code status discussion Demonstration of conversation between expert faculty member and standardized patient (SP) Deliberate skills practice: 15-minute role play for each student with 10-minute feedback from faculty Time involved: 4 hours of faculty time	One-to-one role play with trained standardized patient, 1 faculty member spends 20 minutes reviewing case and debriefing with student	Ability to initiate and complete a code status discussion with trained standardized patient. Skill assessed in three domains: 1. general patient-centered interviewing, 2. code status discussion skills, 3. responding to emotion	18-item checklist of communication skills	Kappa = 0.70
Sharma et al. [54]	10 faculty physicians	Didactic content Deliberate skills practice: One-to-one role play and feedback from a palliative care physician	One-to-one role play with trained standardized patient, 1 faculty member and 1 faculty physician	Same as above	19-item checklist of communication skills, modified version of above	Kappa = 0.70

(continued)

Table 10.1 (continued)

Reference	Participants	Teaching Method(s)	Simulator or model used	Skill(s) assessed	Outcome Measurement	Reliability coefficient of outcome score in prior publication
Vermylen et al. [55]	10 fourth-year medical students	Didactic content Demonstration of conversation between expert faculty member and SP Deliberate skills practice: small group roleplay with 6 cases Time involved: 4 hours	Small group role play with 6 cases using simulated patients, 6 students and 1 faculty member	Ability to complete a breaking bad news (BBN) conversation with a trained SP; skill assessed in three domains: 1. BBN skills 2. general patient-centered interviewing 3. qualitative assessment of the quality of responding to emotion and overall communication	15-item checklist of BBN skills, Three 5-point global rating scale questions assessing ability to respond to emotion and quality of communication Three Likert-scaled questions developed from data about patient preferences regarding receiving bad news	Kappa = 0.91 for the checklist Intraclass correlation (ICC) coefficient = 0.72 for the 3 global rating scale questions ICC = 0.63 for the three Likert-scale items

communication skills is similar to mastery learning of procedural skills and four issues that make mastery learning of communication skills unique. This discussion will lay the groundwork for the subsequent section which reviews key tasks in creating a mastery learning curriculum for communication skills.

Similarities in Mastery Learning of Communication and Procedural Skills

The essential elements of a mastery learning curriculum for communication skills are the same as for any mastery learning curriculum described in this book [56]. Similar to other mastery learning courses, a mastery learning communication course begins with a pretest to provide a baseline assessment of the skill at hand. This not only gives the learner a context to inform future learning, it also creates buy-in as learners struggle with parts of the conversation roadmap or particular skills they have yet to master. Following this crucial first step, there is a didactic teaching session including a demonstration of the conversation being taught. The learner then engages in an intense and focused deliberate practice session informed by pretest data. The deliberate practice can be performed in different ways. Last, the learner takes a posttest to see if she has acquired the skills necessary to achieve the MPS. If the standard is not met, there is further instruction and deliberate practice until the standard is reached. Having a posttest not only keeps the learner engaged during deliberate practice sessions knowing there will be an assessment at the end, but it also provides more feedback to the learner to inform future performance in the skill lab and with patients.

Unique Issues in Mastery Learning of Communication Skills

Although the overall structure of the curriculum is similar to mastery learning of other topics like procedural skills, there are four key issues that make mastery learning of communication skills unique: (a) data overload, (b) learner vulnerability, (c) learner exhaustion, and (d) variability in what is "right." The first key difference is that communication involves a plethora of data. In a 15-minute conversation, as one might have when breaking bad news, there may be hundreds or even thousands of words spoken. Each of these words is a potential teaching point. Not only are there the spoken words that have varying effects on patients, there is also tone, pace of conversation, and nonverbal communication that impact the quality of conversation. Thus, even in simple conversations, there are innumerable tweaks that a teacher may like to make on the learner's communication yet, if all of this feedback was given it would be overwhelming for both the learner and the teacher. This concept of data overload makes appropriate assessment and focused teaching challenging.

Second, there is increased learner vulnerability when it comes to communication skills training. When a learner comes to study a new procedure she has never performed, such as a central line, she likely knows and accepts procedural ineptness and is not embarrassed by making mistakes. When a student is learning how to communicate with patients, however, she often has a preconceived notion that she should excel at this skill. Although they may have never received formal training in advanced communication skills, many learners feel vulnerable and embarrassed when making mistakes. The importance of creating a safe learning environment is essential for learners to try new skills and be open to feedback.

Third, due to the emotional nature of the conversations and the vulnerable state of the learners, communication skills training may be more intense and emotionally draining than procedural skill training. It becomes increasingly important to make the feedback focused and actionable so that the learners feel they can apply this to future conversations. Additionally, it becomes imperative that the task at hand is at an appropriate level of difficulty for the learner. It is also necessary to consider the model of deliberate practice to allow learners time to process the flood of data they are receiving. Breaks may be needed so the learner does not become overwhelmed.

Fourth, in teaching communication skills, there is significant variability about what is "right." When teaching someone how to do a lumbar puncture, there are key steps that occur in a certain order and there is general agreement that, for example, you need to sterilize the field before inserting the needle. While there may be debate about some subtleties of the steps in a lumbar puncture, the variability of what is "right" within a complex conversation is much greater. Fortunately, there is a growing evidence base to support the various elements of conversations. For example, one research group had cancer patients watch videos of oncology fellows giving bad news to SPs and gave them an opportunity to pause and provide feedback about what they liked and did not like. From this study, we know that patients receiving serious news want their clinicians to recognize the impact of the moment, provide information and guidance, and be able to switch between attending to emotions and providing information based on the needs of the patient [57]. This evidence base is incomplete and experts generally agree that there is more than one way to approach many of the key steps. For example, when a patient's son is emotional, it may be appropriate to explore that emotion by saying, "Tell me more about what's going through your head right now." By contrast, it may be equally effective to name the emotion and say, "I can see how much you love your dad and how you wish things were different." This variability in what is "right" requires careful consideration in checklist development, rater training, and teacher flexibility during deliberate practice sessions.

Creating a Mastery Learning Communication Skills Curriculum

While the design of a mastery learning curriculum for communication skills should follow the same steps informed by the Thomas curriculum development model as described in Chap. 3, there are three tasks that deserve special attention when developing the educational strategies (step 4 in the Thomas model). The first task is to develop an appropriate assessment tool for the conversation at hand. The second task is to choose a deliberate practice model. The third task is to craft a method of bringing the learners to mastery.

TASK 1: Create an Assessment Tool

Developing an assessment tool for mastery learning of communication skills follows a similar framework as described in Chap. 5 for developing tools for procedural skills training. However, communication assessment also has some unique elements. The first step is to look for established models in the published literature. This is often challenging regarding communication tasks. Depending on the conversation, established models may be checklists or assessments previously used in research though the model may also come in the form of a framework used to teach the conversation without clear recommendations on how to assess the skill. If tools exist, they may not be well suited to mastery learning assessments.

If there is not an established gold standard that is applicable to mastery learning, we recommend convening content and education experts to create a new tool (See Fig. 10.1 for an example of an assessment tool for breaking bad news.) Given variability in what is "right," the experts must turn to the data when available and rely on expert opinion when it is not. Items must be written with variation in mind, emphasizing essential elements and allowing variability where it is reasonable, for example, in the order of some tasks. When creating a tool, similar to when considering procedural skills, the first task is usually to break a conversation down into key steps in as chronological a fashion as possible. This creates a stepwise roadmap for the conversation that is often also the focus of a didactic presentation. For a communication task, there are also key communication skills that need to be employed to successfully navigate the roadmap (e.g., avoids medical jargon) so these must also be included on the checklist.

Consider also different types of items to assess the quality of various skills involved in communication skills training. As discussed earlier, communication quality is affected not only by spoken words, but also by the tone of voice, nonverbal communication such as the use of silence or touch, and the ability to respond to patients' emotional cues. Depending on the communication task at hand it may be important to not only assess whether learners ask particular questions or say particular words but also to assess communication quality. One strategy is to use a mix of checklist items that evaluate whether learners know to ask particular questions or say particular words and then use scaled items to assess communication quality.

When both checklists and scaled items are used, the checklist can be written to be a rigid assessment of whether particular tasks are performed. For example, the first statement after giving bad news is an empathic statement: "DONE" or "NOT DONE." The checklist should be written with precise language giving careful attention to words such as "and" and "or." Vague terms such as "learner pauses" should be avoided unless they specify how long the pause should last. Scaled items can then be used to assess how well the learner completed specific tasks, for example, "verbally responded to emotion," where the quality of response is rated on a scale

Delivering Bad News:		Done (1 point)	Not Done (0 points)
1	Creates initial rapport when first walking into room. (Introduces self if 1st visit and acknowledges you prior to discussing medical information: e.g. "It's good to see you" or "how you are doing" etc.)		
2	Assesses patient/family's perception or understanding of medical situation (e.g. "tell me what you understand…", "what have the other doctors told you about…")		
3	Asks permission before giving the news (e.g. "I would like to discuss the results of your scan now. Is that OK?")		
4	Gives a clear and concise "warning shot" (e.g. "I have some serious news")		
5	Uses word "cancer" when giving bad news		
6	Waits 3+ seconds after delivering bad news		
7	Delivers bad news within the first few minutes of the conversation		
8	First statement after giving the news is an empathic statement (e.g. "I know this is not what you expected to hear today", "This is difficult news")		
9	Discusses plan only after patient asks to, or gives permission to discuss next steps.		
10	Suggests a plan for the next step		
General Patient-Centered Interviewing Skills:			
11	Uses summary statements to ensure understanding of patient/family's statements (e.g., "It sounds like…")		
12	Avoids medical jargon (uses technical language without clarifying what it means)		
13	Gives information in small chunks (no more than 1 chunk of information before allowing patients to process)		
14	Avoids giving information or discussing plan while patient/family very emotional		
15	Avoids providing reassurance as first response to patient/family's emotion (avoided saying something like "It's okay" or "Don't worry!")		

In the following questions, please indicate the level to which you agree on the following scale; 1 = Strongly Disagree, 2 = Disagree, 3 =Neither Agree nor Disagree, 4 = Agree, 5 = Strongly Agree.

	1	2	3	4	5
The doctor demonstrated that he or she was able to recognize the impact of this moment on me.					
The doctor was able to convey the information clearly and provide guidance on how we should proceed.					
During the conversation, the doctor was able to notice how I was doing and switch back and forth between providing information/guidance and acknowledging the impact of the news on me.					

Quality of Communication:

We would like to know, in as much detail as possible, how good the clinician is at talking with you about your illness. To help us improve communication between doctors and their patients, please be critical.

When talking with the clinician about important issues like bad news, how good is he/she at:

1. **Verbally responding to your emotion.** Examples include: Named an emotion; Expressed understanding of an emotion; Showed respect for, or praise of, you; Assured you of support throughout disease process; Asked questions about your emotions

1	2	3	4	5
No verbal response to my emotion or responses hampered my relationship with the physician (e.g. said something I found off-putting).	Little verbal acknowledgment of my emotion.	Intermittent verbal acknowledgment of my emotion and/or responses felt significantly awkward or not tailored to my needs.	Consistent verbal acknowledgement of my emotion though some responses may not have felt natural or tailored to my needs. (E.g. not able to make multiple empathic statements for a strong emotion).	Consistent verbal acknowledgment of my emotions that almost always felt natural and tailored to my needs.

2. **Non-verbally responding to your emotions.** Examples include: Used appropriate touch; Silence; Offered tissues if emotional; Used supportive body language.

1	2	3	4	5
No nonverbal response to my emotion or nonverbal actions hampered my relationship with the physician (e.g. inappropriate touch, uncomfortable silence, distracted body language, no eye contact)	Little nonverbal acknowledgment of my emotional state (e.g. neutral body posture, little or no silence).	Intermittent nonverbal acknowledgment of my emotion and/or responses felt significantly awkward or not tailored to my needs.	Consistent nonverbal acknowledgement of my emotion though some actions may not have felt natural or tailored to my needs. (e.g. uses silence but not long enough).	Consistent non verbal acknowledgment of my emotions that almost always felt natural and tailored to my needs.

3. **Overall, how would you rate this clinician's communication with you?**

1	2	3	4	5
The physician communicated in a way that was detrimental to our relationship.	The physician's communication was not overtly detrimental but he/she rarely said/did anything that I found particularly helpful.	The physician sometimes said/did things that I found particularly helpful and/or responses felt significantly awkward or not tailored to my needs.	The physician consistently said/did things that I found helpful but some responses/actions may not have felt natural or tailored to my needs.	The physician consistently said/did things that I found helpful and responses/actions that almost always felt natural and tailored to my needs.

Fig. 10.1 Breaking bad news assessment tool. (Reprinted from Vermylen et al. [55], with permission from Elsevier)

of 1–5. When developing the scaled items, provide anchors that can focus the assessor on specific behaviors and ideally have less than seven categories. Research shows it becomes difficult for assessors to distinguish more than six categories consistently [58].

Once the tool is created, it should be pilot tested to reveal issues not considered in the initial design. To illustrate, a small group of learners can be video recorded having a conversation with a SP before and after deliberate practice and key design team members can watch the conversations together and try out the tool. Raters should discuss how the assessment tool captures or does not capture relevant issues in the conversation and, where necessary, make adjustments until it covers key material. Ease of use by design team members is also important. The pilot test also expedites establishing inter-rater reliability as well as setting a MPS using the methods discussed in Chap. 6.

TASK 2: Choose a Deliberate Practice Model

There are two deliberate practice models reported in the literature as part of mastery learning of communication skills training. Each model has different ways to address communication skill acquisition. These models are shown in Fig. 10.2. There are no data comparing these two methods. Thus, it is important for different programs to evaluate their own resources, faculty time, and the conversation at hand when determining the most appropriate model of communication skills training.

One-to-One Deliberate Practice

The model first reported in the literature included a focused, mixed-method intervention for a discussion of a patient's code-status. In this approach, learners engage with the teacher individually to review their videos, study their checklist assessments, and then practice with a SP until learners feel comfortable repeating the assessment. Learners are free to choose when they have had enough practice to move to the next step. One of the greatest strengths of this model is that it allows focused deliberate practice with a faculty member. The learner can choose how much to practice before attempting the post-assessment conversation and thus can gauge her own level of exhaustion. Additionally, the learner is able to learn in a one-to-one fashion with the faculty member and thus does not need to worry about peer criticism in this sensitive skill. Finally, the learner is able to practice an entire conversation while receiving feedback.

This approach, however, also comes with some trade-offs. Since the learner is practicing the entire conversation, she may need to learn multiple new skills in a relatively short period of time. This runs the risk of causing data overload to the learner and may make the learning less efficient. Additionally, the learner often only experiences one case example and this lack of variation may lead to increased difficulty applying the conversation to future patients. Finally, this model requires significant faculty time and does not allow the learner to receive peer-feedback which can be a powerful motivator for individual learning.

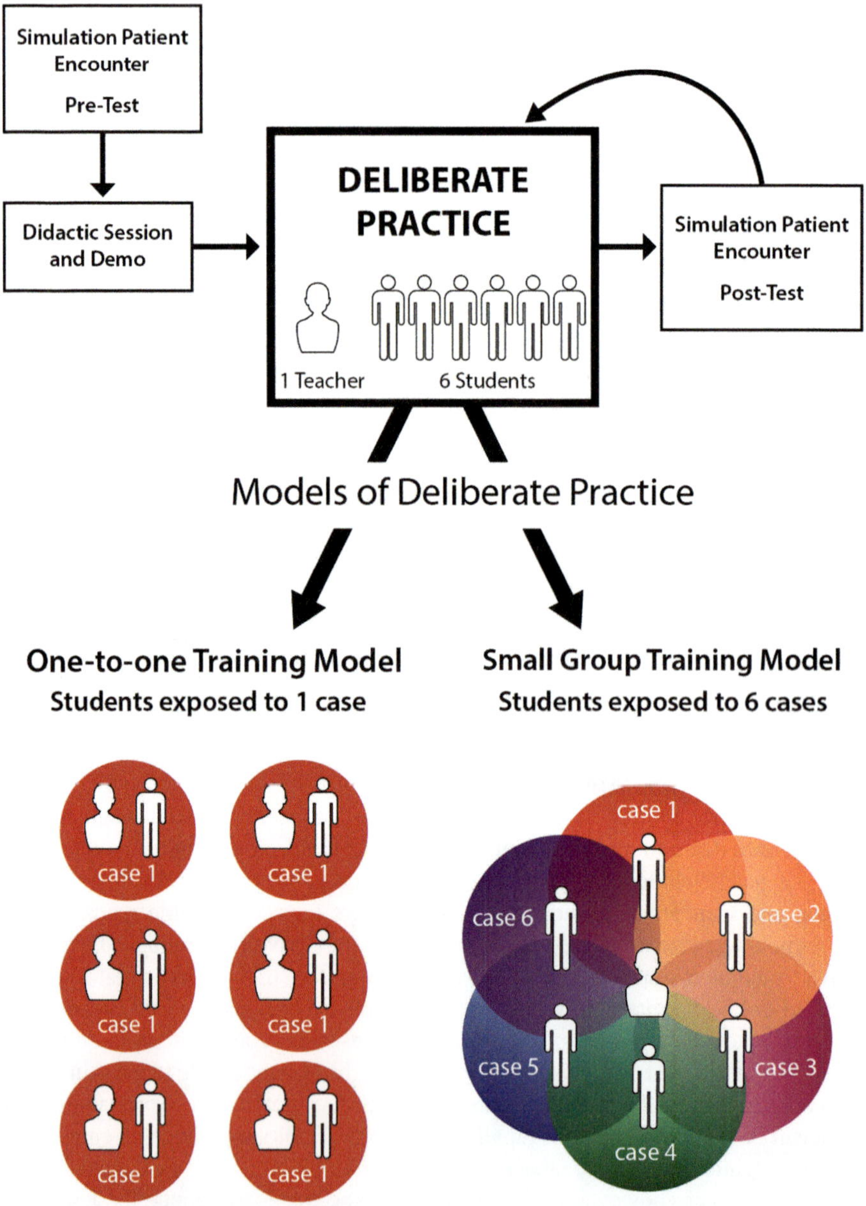

Fig. 10.2 Models of communication skills mastery learning curricula

Small Group Role Play

The other model for deliberate practice as part of mastery learning of communication skills is small group role play with SPs. This approach has been widely used outside of mastery learning and has solid evidence that it can result in a change in learner behavior. Several nonprofit organizations now teach approaches to running small group role play, including VitalTalk and the Academy of Communication in Healthcare (ACH). Such training can be helpful if these approaches are intended for use in a mastery learning curriculum. The model discussed here adapts the approach presented by VitalTalk (both JV and GW have attended and taught VitalTalk or VitalTalk-related courses). This is our favored approach for complex, serious illness conversations because it facilitates behavior change and addresses communication challenges.

Teachers using the VitalTalk model work with groups of four to six learners, going through a series of cases with different SPs all focused on the same communication task. In the reported example, the task was "breaking bad news." Practice involved six cases over one half-day. Before the practice starts, the teacher and learners study pretest results and set goals for each learner for the session. With each case, two learners participate in completing part of the conversation by taking turns conversing with the SP. During each turn, the teacher helps the learner define the deliberate practice focus for that case before the learner talks to the SP. The rest of the group takes careful notes concurrently about what was said on a guided note-taking template that maps to key elements of the checklist. The learner or teacher may call a time-out for a discussion about what the learner did well and brainstorming with the group about how to address a challenge. The teacher then places the learner and SP back in the conversation at a moment where a new approach can be tried. After the learner sees the response to what she said, another time-out is called so the effect of the new approach can be highlighted and the learner can leave with a single take-home point. A second learner then takes the conversation forward to work on a separate skill in the same conversation. Thus, in a half day, the small group sees multiple cases and each person practices several times before completing the session and moving to the posttest.

This model meets all of the key elements of deliberate practice in a mastery learning model [59, 60]. Learners are highly motivated to succeed with good concentration because of the opportunities for improvement highlighted by the pretest and because they are being watched by peers. The reality of the simulation provided by well-trained SPs also maintains engagement as does the fact that a time-out occurs when the learner is stuck and is therefore invested in becoming unstuck. Learners have a well-defined objective informed by pretest data which is evaluated with a carefully created checklist (see below) and helps inform identification of learning goals from discussion with the teacher. Practice occurs at an appropriate level of difficulty that can be titrated by the teacher who can call a "time-out" if the learner is unable to navigate a challenge in the conversation or pause and refocus the encounter if the learner is challenged insufficiently. Learners engage in focused repetitive practice from exposure to multiple cases either as the one talking to the SP or as part of the small group where they are involved in active feedback and brainstorming with peers. Practice leads to rigorous precise measurements through the specific words recorded by the small group on the guided note-taking template that aligns with the checklist. This allows the learner to receive informative feedback from their peers, the teacher, and from their responses to learner behaviors by the

SPs. Trainees monitor their learning experience and identify where they want to practice before the encounter and where they want to brainstorm during the timeout. Each of these guides more deliberate practice. Although learners do not complete the entire conversation at any given moment, they are exposed to multiple cases that allow them to work on the various aspects of the complicated tasks. Similar to other models of procedural based mastery learning, this is an excellent example of rapid cycle deliberate practice where individuals report gradual improvement of specific aspects of a complex task (see Chap. 3, Fig. 3.3).

This model also addresses many of the challenges of mastery learning of communication skills. First, it addresses the data overload problem. Teachers help the learner identify a single focus for deliberate practice before the encounter which gives the group and teacher guidance about what to watch for during the session. A "time-out" occurs within the first 3–5 minutes, often by the learner because she is stuck, providing an additional limit to the data. The teacher then focuses on identifying a single topic on which the group can brainstorm and helps the learner identify a single take-home point from a SP encounter. All of these steps help to minimize data overload and focus deliberate practice where it is needed most.

This model also attends to learner vulnerability. Before practice begins, the teacher spends time doing introductions, often using an ice breaker to increase comfort level. The teacher then discusses what is hard about role play and why and how role play is done and sets grounds rules including "what happens here, stays here." The teacher then gets a volunteer to talk to the SP and this learner identifies what specific element from the checklist they want to practice before the encounter, giving the learner some control. After a time-out, the discussion first focuses on what went well which builds up the learner's self-esteem and gives her time to settle down if the conversation was difficult or emotional. The learner then chooses, with guidance from the teacher, where to focus the brainstorming and receives the option of either trying her own idea or turning to the group for help. The fact that group input is sought directly around the learner's self-identified stuck point also minimizes vulnerability by avoiding the general and wide-ranging criticism that may be received if the group input was less focused.

Learner exhaustion is limited because the time talking to the SP is short and they are able to get breaks while they take on different roles within the small group. Scheduling formal breaks during the session is also critical.

This model helps with issue of variability in what is "right" by giving each learner multiple opportunities to practice, receive feedback, and try new approaches to see how they work. If there is debate about how best to approach a particular task, the teacher can redirect the discussion toward practicing with the (well-trained) SP and the outcomes of different approaches can be analyzed. The teacher can then highlight the key principles that produced successful results. Watching others, taking notes, and providing specific feedback can also help identify alternative approaches. Finally, this approach allows the learners to see several different cases that can be designed to present unique challenges requiring unique responses.

The small group practice model presents several advantages for more complex conversations. It allows learners to see multiple cases and variations of the conversation. It breaks the conversation into small chunks. The small group practice model also allows peer feedback and an opportunity to observe others. The amount of practice time each learner experiences can also be increased without increasing faculty time.

A potential weakness of this model is that learners do not practice the entire conversation in any one moment. Although data suggests that most learners are able to synthesize the individual skills into a larger conversation, some learners may struggle as they attempt to perform the entire conversation in the post-assessment and later with patients. Additionally, it is important for the teacher to create a safe learner environment where learners feel comfortable making mistakes and working on a new skill before peers. This model may also be more expensive in terms of SP costs because multiple cases are used and most SPs are booked for a half-day independent of how long they actually work. We have minimized this by having three cases with two parts to each case so only three SPs are needed.

TASK 3: Bring Learners to Mastery

The third and final task in creating a mastery learning communication skills curriculum is developing a plan for how to bring learners to mastery. If the learner does not meet the MPS, further deliberate practice and posttesting are needed, and how this is achieved depends on the model of deliberate practice chosen in Task 2.

If the curriculum uses one-to-one deliberate practice, a posttest can be performed in real time with the SP as the teacher observes. If the MPS is not met, the teacher can review the opportunities for improvement and have the learner practice them with the SP until she feels ready to attempt the posttest again. This may extend the duration of the session so this will need to be considered when scheduling teacher and learner training time. Alternatively, the teacher, learner, and SP could schedule another time to return for more deliberate practice and posttesting.

With the small group role play model, designing the curriculum to bring all learners to mastery can be more challenging. This is because in most situations only one or two learners out of a group of 4–6 will not reach the MPS after the initial deliberate practice time. The result is that this leaves too few learners to do immediate deliberate practice in the small group setting. If the training involves multiple simultaneous small groups, each run by a separate teacher, the learners who do not reach the MPS on the first posttest can be reassembled in one or more new small groups for more deliberate practice. A different approach is needed if the training involves just one small group with one teacher. One option for the breaking bad news training is to develop a system of ongoing monthly training sessions. Learners who need more practice can join a later small group training session and repeat sessions until the MPS is met. Alternatively, a mixed model could be used where the initial training is done in a small group setting and any further deliberate practice is scheduled separately in a one-to-one model.

Other Considerations

Simulated Patient Training

Continuous SP training is essential throughout the communication skills training program. This ensures that SPs understand the case and respond appropriately to trainee behavior. Emotion laden cases provide an opportunity to titrate stress and ensure that the SP changes when the learner addresses the emotion skillfully. We typically devote about an hour of training per SP before a course and repeat the training if more than a month has passed. Busy SPs are occupied during the interim and may have forgotten the earlier training. SP training on the test cases should focus on response consistency and how to behave over an entire encounter. Training for the deliberate practice cases should focus on ensuring the SP understands the teaching model and can present common challenges and show different responses when the skills are used.

Rater Training

Just like procedural skills training, it is important to devote time to rater training to ensure inter-rater reliability. Raters should watch conversations together and perform assessments at the same time to compare their data [61–64]. This may reveal key subtleties in the tool and ensure that all raters interpret the items consistently. Given the volume of communication data, it is common for assessors to notice and record different cues from the patient and learner. Discussing these differences openly allows raters to reach consensus when using the rating instrument.

Depending on resources, it may also be helpful to train the SPs to assess learners to minimize faculty time in video review. Of course, this requires establishing inter-rater reliability among the SPs, a challenge if the SP pool is large and changes over time.

Costs

Costs for communication skills training curricula may be high, and costs for mastery learning communication curricula may be even higher due to testing and retraining of those who did not meet the MPS. Additionally, it is important to note that conversations may be long and complicated requiring extensive faculty time and there are ongoing SP costs. This is in contrast with a single upfront cost for a simulator to practice and master a procedural skill. While costs warrant close attention, if skill acquisition and retention is high due to the rigorous educational intervention of using SBML methods, institutions may save on costs in the end. Collecting data to show training impact can be persuasive to ensure stable funding. Fortunately, most health professions schools recognize the value of SPs and the task may be more one of redesigning how SPs are used.

Future Directions

Although promising, the field of mastery learning for communication skills is still currently in its infancy. To date, there are no head-to-head trials assessing various education techniques and methods of deliberate practice for communication skills training to guide future curriculum development. Additionally, most research has focused on serious illness communication for physicians. There are many other health professions where communication skills could be mastered including nursing, social work, and hospital chaplains. Interdisciplinary communication, patient education, and many other difficult conversations such as early or late goals of care discussions or family meetings at the end of life could also benefit from the application of a mastery learning model. Finally, although T1 outcomes have shown promising improvements in clinician communication behavior, to date there have been no patient-level T2 or T3 outcomes reported as a result of communication skills mastery learning. Next steps should include assessment of patient-level outcomes to support this cost- and labor-intensive training.

Coda

This chapter has described in detail the exciting and relatively new field of mastery learning for communication skills. There is a growing body of evidence showing that how we communicate affects patient outcomes and that communication skills are teachable. Mastery learning is poised to extend this strong foundation by providing a structure that allows deliberate practice until all learners can perform communication skills at a high level. Early research suggests that mastery learning can be just as effective in achieving "excellence for all" in communication skills as in procedural skills. We look forward to new studies evaluating the impact of this robust training to see if mastery learning can help us all communicate more effectively and achieve better outcomes for patients, families, the healthcare system, our colleagues, and ourselves.

References

1. Majesko A, Hong SY, Weissfeld L, White DB. Identifying family members who may struggle in the role of surrogate decision maker. Crit Care Med. 2012;40(8):2281–6.
2. Lilly CM, De Meo DL, Sonna LA, et al. An intensive communication intervention for the critically ill. Am J Med. 2000;109(6):469–75.
3. Hutchison PJ, McLaughlin K, Corbridge T, et al. Dimensions and role-specific mediators of surrogate trust in the ICU. Crit Care Med. 2016;44(12):2208–14.
4. Kirchhoff KT, Song MK, Kehl K. Caring for the family of the critically ill patient. Crit Care Clin. 2004;20(3):453–66. ix-x.
5. Nunez ER, Schenker Y, Joel ID, et al. Acutely bereaved surrogates' stories about the decision to limit life support in the ICU. Crit Care Med. 2015;43(11):2387–93.
6. Lautrette A, Darmon M, Megarbane B, et al. A communication strategy and brochure for relatives of patients dying in the ICU. N Engl J Med. 2007;356(5):469–78.
7. Wall RJ, Engelberg RA, Gries CJ, Glavan B, Curtis JR. Spiritual care of families in the intensive care unit. Crit Care Med. 2007;35(4):1084–90.
8. Wall RJ, Curtis JR, Cooke CR, Engelberg RA. Family satisfaction in the ICU: differences between families of survivors and nonsurvivors. Chest. 2007;132(5):1425–33.
9. Boissy A, Windover AK, Bokar D, et al. Communication skills training for physicians improves patient satisfaction. J Gen Intern Med. 2016;31(7):755–61.

10. Dowdy MD, Robertson C, Bander JA. A study of proactive ethics consultation for critically and terminally ill patients with extended lengths of stay. Crit Care Med. 1998;26(2):252–9.
11. Lilly CM, Sonna LA, Haley KJ, Massaro AF. Intensive communication: four-year follow-up from a clinical practice study. Crit Care Med. 2003;31(5 Suppl):S394–9.
12. Norton SA, Hogan LA, Holloway RG, et al. Proactive palliative care in the medical intensive care unit: effects on length of stay for selected high-risk patients. Crit Care Med. 2007;35(6):1530–5.
13. Lamba S, Murphy P, McVicker S, Harris Smith J, Mosenthal AC. Changing end-of-life care practice for liver transplant service patients: structured palliative care intervention in the surgical intensive care unit. J Pain Sympton Manage. 2012;44(4):508–19.
14. Geer JA, Jacobs JM, El-Jawahri A, et al. Role of patient coping strategies in understanding the effects of early palliative care on quality of life and mood. J Clin Oncol. 2018;36(1):53–60.
15. Irwin KE, Greer JA, Khatib J, Temel JS, Pirl WF. Early palliative care and metastatic non-small cell lung cancer: potential mechanisms of prolonged survival. Chronic Resp Dis. 2013;10(1):35–47.
16. Rubenfeld GD, Curtis JR. End-of-life care in the ICUWG. End-of-life care in the intensive care unit: a research agenda. Crit Care Med. 2001;29(10):2001–6.
17. Mularski RA, Curtis JR, Billings JA, et al. Proposed quality measures for palliative care in the critically ill: a consensus from the Robert Wood Johnson Foundation Critical Care Workshop. Crit Care Med. 2006;34(11 Suppl):S404–11.
18. Nelson JE, Mulkerin CM, Adams LL, Pronovost PJ. Improving comfort and communication in the ICU: a practical new tool for palliative care performance measurement and feedback. Qual Saf Health Care. 2006;15(4):264–71.
19. Clarke EB, Curtis JR, Luce JM, et al. Quality indicators for end-of-life care in the intensive care unit. Crit Care Med. 2003;31(9):2255–62.
20. Nelson JE, Puntillo KA, Pronovost PJ, et al. In their own words: patients and families define high-quality palliative care in the intensive care unit. Crit Care Med. 2010;38(3):808–18.
21. Halpern SD, Becker D, Curtis JR, et al. An official American Thoracic Society/American Association of Critical-Care Nurses/American College of Chest Physicians/Society of Critical Care Medicine policy statement: the Choosing Wisely (R) top 5 list in critical care medicine. Am J Respir Crit Care Med. 2014;190(7):818–26.
22. Tulsky JA, Beach MC, Butow PN, et al. A research agenda for communication between health care professionals and patients living with serious illness. JAMA Intern Med. 2017;177(9):1361–6.
23. ACGME Common Program Requirements 2017. Available from https://www.acgme.org/Portals/0/PFAssets/ProgramRequirements/CPRs_2017-07-01.pdf.
24. Barsuk JH, McGaghie WC, Cohen ER, et al. Simulation-based mastery learning reduces complications during central venous catheter insertion in a medical intensive care unit. Crit Care Med. 2009;37(10):2697–701.
25. Hebert HD, Butera JN, Castillo J, Mega AE. Are we training our fellows adequately in delivering bad news to patients? A survey of hematology/oncology program directors. J Palliat Med. 2009;12(12):1119–24.
26. Adler DD, Riba MB, Eggly S. Breaking bad news in the breast imaging setting. Acad Radiol. 2009;16(2):130–5.
27. Eggly S, Afonso N, Rojas G, et al. An assessment of residents' competence in the delivery of bad news to patients. Acad Med. 1997;72(5):397–9.
28. Schellenberg KL, Schofield SJ, Fang S, et al. Breaking bad news in amyotrophic lateral sclerosis: the need for medical education. Amyotroph Lateral Scler Frontotemporal Degener. 2014;15(1–2):47–54.
29. Lamba S, Nagurka R, Offin M, Scott SR. Structured communication: teaching delivery of difficult news with simulated resuscitations in an emergency medicine clerkship. West J Emerg Med. 2015;16(2):344–52.
30. Buss MK, Lessen DS, Sullivan AM, et al. Hematology/oncology fellows' training in palliative care: results of a national survey. Cancer. 2011;117(18):4304–11.

31. Holley JL, Carmody SS, Moss AH, et al. The need for end-of-life care training in nephrology: national survey results of nephrology fellows. Am J Kidney Dis. 2003;42(4):813–20.
32. Makoul G. Communication Skills Education in Medical School and Beyond. JAMA. 2003;289(1):93.
33. Fryer-Edwards K, Arnold RM, Baile W, et al. Reflective teaching practices: an approach to teaching communication skills in a small-group setting. Acad Med. 2006;81(7):638–44.
34. Back AL, Arnold RM, Baile WF, et al. Efficacy of communication skills training for giving bad news and discussing transitions to palliative care. Arch Intern Med. 2007;167(5):453–60.
35. Szmuilowicz E, el-Jawahri A, Chiappetta L, et al. Improving residents' end-of-life communication skills with a short retreat: a randomized controlled trial. J Palliat Med. 2010;13(4):439–52.
36. Szmuilowicz E, Neely KJ, Sharma RK, et al. Improving residents' code status discussion skills: a randomized trial. J Palliat Med. 2012;15(7):768–74.
37. Wayne DB, Moazed F, Cohen ER, et al. Code status discussion skill retention in internal medicine residents: one-year follow-up. J Palliat Med. 2012;15(12):1325–8.
38. Chung HO, Oczkowski SJ, Hanvey L, et al. Educational interventions to train healthcare professionals in end-of-life communication: a systematic review and meta-analysis. BMC Med Educ. 2016;16:131.
39. Moore PM, Rivera Mercado S, Grez Artigues M, Lawrie TA. Communication skills training for healthcare professionals working with people who have cancer. Cochrane Database Syst Rev. 2013; Cd003751.
40. Wood GJAR. What is the evidence that advance care plans change patient outcomes? In: Goldstein NEMR, editor. Evidence-based practice of palliative medicine. Philadelphia: Elsevier Saunders; 2017. p. 270–4.
41. Barth J, Lannen P. Efficacy of communication skills training courses in oncology: a systematic review and meta-analysis. Ann Oncol. 2011;22(5):1030–40.
42. Schoenthaler A, Kalet A, Nicholson J, Lipkin M Jr. Does improving patient-practitioner communication improve clinical outcomes in patients with cardiovascular diseases? A systematic review of the evidence. Patient Educ Couns. 2014;96(1):3–12.
43. Uitterhoeve RJ, Bensing JM, Grol RP, et al. The effect of communication skills training on patient outcomes in cancer care: a systematic review of the literature. Eur J Cancer Care. 2010;19(4):442–57.
44. Tulsky JA, Arnold RM, Alexander SC, et al. Enhancing communication between oncologists and patients with a computer-based training program: a randomized trial. Ann Intern Med. 2011;155(9):593–601.
45. Shaw DJ, Davidson JE, Smilde RI, et al. Multidisciplinary team training to enhance family communication in the ICU. Crit Care Med. 2014;42(2):265–71.
46. Sullivan AM, Rock LK, Gadmer NM, et al. The impact of resident training on communication with families in the intensive care unit: resident and family outcomes. Ann Am Thorac Soc. 2016;13(4):512–21.
47. Stein T, Frankel RM, Krupat E. Enhancing clinician communication skills in a large healthcare organization: a longitudinal case study. Patient Educ Couns. 2005;58(1):4–12.
48. Stewart M, Brown JB, Hammerton J, et al. Improving communication between doctors and breast cancer patients. Ann Fam Med. 2007;5(5):387–94.
49. Orford NR, Milnes S, Simpson N, et al. Effect of communication skills training on outcomes in critically ill patients with life-limiting illness referred for intensive care management: a before-and-after study. BMJ Support Palliat Care. 2019;9(1):e21.
50. Curtis JR, Back AL, Ford DW, et al. Effect of communication skills training for residents and nurse practitioners on quality of communication with patients with serious illness: a randomized trial. JAMA. 2013;310(21):2271–81.
51. Bays AM, Engelberg RA, Back AL, et al. Interprofessional communication skills training for serious illness: evaluation of a small-group, simulated patient intervention. J Palliat Med. 2014;17(2):159–66.
52. Curtis JR, Back AL, Engelberg RA. Training for effective patient communication—reply. JAMA. 2014;311(13):1356–7.

53. Cohen ER, Barsuk JH, Moazed F, et al. Making July safer: simulation-based mastery learning during intern boot camp. Acad Med. 2013;88(2):233–9.
54. Sharma RK, Szmuilowicz E, Ogunseitan A, et al. Evaluation of a mastery learning intervention on hospitalists' code status discussion skills. J Pain Symptom Manage. 2017;53(6):1066–70.
55. Vermylen JH, Wood GJ, Cohen ER, Barsuk JH, McGaghie WC, Wayne DB. Development of a simulation-based mastery learning curriculum for breaking bad news. J Pain Symptom Manag. 2019;57(3):682–7.
56. Barsuk JH, Cohen ER, Wayne DB, et al. Developing a simulation-based mastery learning curriculum; lessons from 11 years of advanced cardiac life support. Simul Healthc. 2016;11(1):52–9.
57. Back AL, Trinidad SB, Hopley EK, et al. What patients value when oncologists give news of cancer recurrence: commentary on specific moments in audio-recorded conversations. Oncologist. 2011;16(3):342–50.
58. Beckstead J. On measurements and their quality. Paper 4: verbal anchors and the number of response options in rating scales. Int J Nurs Stud [Internet]. 2014;51(5):807–14.
59. Ericsson KA. Deliberate practice and the acquisition and maintenance of expert performance in medicine and related domains. Acad Med. 2004;79(10 Suppl):S70–81.
60. McGaghie WC, Siddall VJ, Mazmanian PE, Myers J. Lessons for continuing medical education from simulation research in undergraduate and graduate medical education: effectiveness of continuing medical education: American College of Chest Physicians Evidence-Based Educational Guidelines. Chest. 2009;135(3 Suppl):62S–8.
61. Mahmood O, Dagnaes J, Bube S, et al. Nonspecialist raters can provide reliable assessments of procedural skills. J Surg Educ. 2018;75(2):370–6.
62. George BC, Teitelbaum EN, DaRosa DA, et al. Duration of faculty training needed to ensure reliable performance ratings. J Surg Educ. 2013;70(6):703–8.
63. Adler MD, Vozenilek JA, Trainor JL, et al. Comparison of checklist and anchored global rating instruments for performance rating of simulated pediatric emergencies. Simul Healthc. 2011;6(1):18–24.
64. Eppich W, Nannicelli AP, Seivert NP, et al. A rater training protocol to assess team performance. J Contin Educ Heal Prof. 2015;35(2):83–90.

Mastery Learning of Team Skills

11

Aashish K. Didwania, Erin D. Unger, Debi L. Mitra,
and William C. McGaghie

The Apollo 13 space mission launched on April 11, 1970, intended to be the third moon landing. The initial launch, rise to space, and early mission course were smooth and uneventful. But without warning, an oxygen tank exploded 2 days into the mission, crippling the spacecraft and jeopardizing the lives of the three astronauts. The lunar landing was aborted. Despite hardships due to low power, loss of cabin heat, water shortage, and the urgent need to perform makeshift repairs to the carbon dioxide removal system, the crew returned safely to earth on April 17, 1970, 6 days after departure.

Mission commander Captain James Lovell, played by Tom Hanks in the hit Hollywood movie *Apollo 13*, faced a life-threatening situation never seen before in human history. Ingenuity under extreme pressure was required from the crew, flight controllers, and support personnel to achieve a safe return. Their tools inside the spacecraft included plastic bags, cardboard, duct tape, and a slide rule. Handheld computers and cell phones were not yet invented. Lovell, working with the other astronauts and ground control team, brought the flight back to earth safely against all odds. Survival of the Apollo 13 crew was considered "miraculous." Years later,

A. K. Didwania (✉)
Northwestern University Feinberg School of Medicine,
Departments of Medicine and Medical Education, Chicago, IL, USA
e-mail: aashish@northwestern.edu

E. D. Unger · D. L. Mitra
Northwestern University Feinberg School of Medicine, Department of Medicine,
Chicago, IL, USA

W. C. McGaghie
Northwestern University Feinberg School of Medicine, Departments of Medical Education
and Preventive Medicine, Chicago, IL, USA

W. C. McGaghie et al. (eds.), *Comprehensive Healthcare Simulation: Mastery Learning in Health Professions Education*, Comprehensive Healthcare Simulation, https://doi.org/10.1007/978-3-030-34811-3_11

Lovell called the Apollo 13 mission a "successful failure" due to safe return of the astronauts but the aborted lunar landing [1].

On Tuesday, January 30, 2018, 48 years after the Apollo 13 mission, our writing team was privileged to meet with Captain James Lovell, then 90 years of age, to recount his National Aeronautics and Space Administration (NASA) training experiences and enjoy his wisdom. The 2-hour interview was fun and informative.

"Failure is not an option," said actor Ed Harris in the movie *Apollo 13*, playing the role of flight director Gene Kranz. Lovell explained this order was barked at him repeatedly by Kranz during his earlier Gemini mission. Captain Lovell reported the keys to team success were repetitive practice, hardnosed feedback, and having a positive attitude. Lovell explained the crew outlook was always about problem-solving despite hazards or the likelihood of failure. As we address team skill acquisition later in this chapter, we will show how this frame of mind can lay the foundation for mastery learning of teamwork principles.

Captain Lovell noted other features that lead to successful teamwork, starting with selecting the right crew members. Lovell described how each astronaut on his three space missions had clearly defined and specialized roles, yet each had an understanding of the other members' duties so they could be interchangeable.

When it came to Apollo 13 team training in the late 1960s, the three-member crew of James Lovell, Fred Haise, and Jack Swigert recognized the importance of practicing together and working with ground control personnel. They understood that for excellence to become habit, they needed to practice in unison, over and over, until flying to the moon became second nature. Team practice enabled the crew to function with what Lovell called "telepathic communication." (Today this is called a shared mental model.) Days before the Apollo 13 launch, one of the frontline crew members, Ken Mattingly, was diagnosed with German measles. Consequently, Mattingly was scrubbed from the mission and replaced by Jack Swigert. Captain Lovell issued a soft protest noting that he and Mattingly had achieved telepathic communication, stating "We knew what each other was thinking at all times without even talking." Lovell relented about the crew change acknowledging the concern for Mattingly's measles exposure and because a core part of their team training was backup behavior, the ability to have team members substitute for one another. The astronaut team understood Mattingly's health was a flight risk and Swigert had trained just as hard.

The most distinguishing features of NASA team training that apply to the idea of mastery learning for healthcare teams are training rigor and intensity. NASA training before 1970 did not have a pretest or a mastery posttest with a minimum passing standard (MPS) to certify competence for space flight. However, Captain Jim Lovell described training to the point of exhaustion and, most critical, constant assessments for team improvement and readiness. When asked about how his team trained to address conflict and emergencies, Captain Lovell praised team training in a simulation lab. Flight directors presented countless unexpected scenarios for the astronauts to solve. The pilots tested different solutions to figure out which answer was best. The team worked through "lots of mishaps and died many times" in the NASA simulation laboratory. Failure was OK in the simulation lab. Feedback and debriefing about simulated failures were a foundation for team skill improvement. Deliberate practice with feedback (before these terms were articulated) from flight directors allowed the astronauts to perfect team skills. Captain Lovell summed up the interview by saying "The simulators were the savior of the program. We could simulate almost everything about going to the moon. By the time of Apollo 13 (1970) when we were ready to go to the moon, there was nothing in the flight that was unusual or unexpected…except seeing the Earth!"

This chapter addresses history, definitions, concepts, and potential applications of mastery learning to acquire and maintain team skills in health professions education. Throughout the chapter, we present illustrations to amplify Captain Lovell's NASA training that allowed his team to dodge space flight catastrophe and become a signature event in American space history. The chapter has four more sections: (a) the history and evolution of team training; (b) effective healthcare teams; (c) team training for effective healthcare—curriculum, instruction, and assessment; and (d) coda.

History and Evolution of Team Training

Origins of Team Training

Our interview with Captain Lovell was also a lesson in the origins of team training science. Team training really came into focus as the aviation and aerospace industry sought to improve flight safety. In the early 1970s, a series of devastating airplane crashes drew widespread attention. Crash investigations revealed that human error, not mechanical issues, contributed to a majority of aircraft incidents and accidents. Most revealing was that the airline crashes were not the result of individual deficiencies in crew technical abilities but from a lack of leadership and teamwork [2]. In a sentinel 1979 NASA-sponsored workshop, representatives from academia, the airline industry, and the government met to discuss how to improve airline safety. Team training became a central tenet to achieve safety goals. The workshop gave birth to cockpit resource management training later referred to as crew resource management (CRM) [3]. The aim of CRM is to train all flight crew members to effectively use available resources including people, information, and equipment and to optimize interpersonal activities to reduce error. The central focus of CRM is crew performance as a team, not the performance of individuals. CRM has evolved since its inception, but the core curriculum includes concepts of communication, workload management, situation awareness, problem-solving and decision-making, leadership and followership, and stress reduction [4, 5].

The Federal Aviation Administration required CRM training in 1995 for all commercial airlines though most had been using CRM training since the 1980s. CRM has overall had a positive effect on the aviation industry with formal evaluation during full mission simulation showing improved crew coordination [6]. The celebrated 2009 "Miracle on the Hudson" occurred when Captain Chelsea "Sully" Sullenberger successfully landed U.S. Airways Flight 1549 in the Hudson River following engine failure due to a bird strike. Captain Sully credited his crew's performance to CRM [7]. CRM training changed the aviation industry. Team training concepts from CRM are now the foundation of team training in medicine.

Team Training in Medicine

Using simulation models in medical education to improve skills and reduce errors parallels that of the space and aviation programs. Driven by an understanding that many errors were at least partially attributable to human error, Drs. Judson Denson and Stephen Abrahamson developed the first full-body mannequin simulator, aptly named "Sim One," in the late 1960s for use in anesthesia training [8, 9]. Sim One was rudimentary, yet novel—it had a heartbeat, could be ventilated, and responded to medical interventions with immediate feedback for trainees. Sim One allowed individual trainees to experience "real-world" scenarios and even make medical errors without putting real patients at risk.

In the 2000s, use of simulators in medical education expanded from individual training to address medical team training. A series of medical education and evaluation research studies on the acquisition and maintenance of advanced cardiac life support (ACLS) team skills conducted at Northwestern University and Northwestern Memorial Hospital illustrates this work. The first report of this series described the development, implementation, and evaluation—via a randomized controlled trial—of a simulation-based ACLS team curriculum featuring deliberate practice and rigorous outcome measurement [10]. Simulation-based training increased residents' ACLS competencies measured in the laboratory by 38% [10]. A follow-up cohort study addressing real in-hospital cardiac arrests, or "codes," showed that resident teams trained in the simulation laboratory delivered higher quality code responses than resident teams that had not received simulation training [11]. The simulation-based ACLS team training curriculum was subsequently transformed to a mastery learning program that has produced powerful short-run results [12] that are retained over a 12-month time interval [13].

At the University of Manitoba in Winnipeg, Ziesmann et al. applied team skill training in the Simulated Trauma and Resuscitative Team Training (S.T.A.R.T.T.) study [14]. Course leaders combined traditional classroom teaching with four 15-minute simulations completed by teams of surgical residents, nurses, and respiratory therapists. While satisfaction among trainees was very high, the impact on patient outcomes was not evaluated [15]. Physicians at Frankfurt University leveraged simulation training to develop a stroke team to coordinate rapid and efficient care for patients suffering a stroke [16]. By using simulation-based training for a newly established stroke team, door-to-needle times improved significantly from 43 to 31 minutes, and more patients received thrombolysis within the goal time of 30 minutes of presentation [16].

One of the most well-studied simulation training programs is for the treatment of shoulder dystocia in obstetric deliveries. While rare, shoulder dystocia is an obstetric emergency and requires fast action [17–19]. Using the NOELLE birthing simulator, investigators from the United Kingdom developed an integrated didactic and team-based simulation curriculum for residents using simulated deliveries on a model. Residents trained using the simulator had better overall performance and better performance of specific maneuvers than those trained with the standard didactic curriculum [20]. Croft and colleagues later demonstrated that training with high-fidelity simulation was associated with higher rates of successful delivery compared to low-fidelity simulation [21]. The simulation-based training programs emphasized teamwork skills and showed improved communication among team members.

These examples highlight the role for team-based simulation training particularly in critical situations that require a rapid response. However, to our knowledge, only one program [12] incorporates mastery learning as a rigorous teaching method. Chapter 3 describes development of a simulation-based mastery curriculum in ACLS. This curriculum is the first formally designed simulation-based mastery learning program in the health professions that addresses team training [12]. In the following sections of this chapter, we further define team skills and healthcare training concepts that came from CRM and then discuss team-based curriculum development in medical education.

Effective Healthcare Teams

Definition

Modern healthcare teams vary in many ways. Healthcare teams may be hierarchical like a surgeon leading a clinical team on morning rounds with military efficiency [22] or egalitarian such as primary care teamlet "huddles" where doctors, nurses, pharmacists, social workers, and many other professionals talk frequently during the day about patient care details [23]. Healthcare teams can be small, nimble, and stable over time like an emergency medical service (EMS) crew or have a large pool of individuals that turn over frequently as in a medical intensive care unit (MICU) [24]. Healthcare teams also vary by purpose. Some teams are defined by disease, such as a cystic fibrosis care team that manages patients in the clinic or when they are admitted to the hospital. Continuity and expertise define such a team's success. Other healthcare teams are shaped by emergency situations such as cardiac arrest and trauma where speed and technical skills are crucial.

There are also less acute team structures in healthcare. In teaching hospitals, for example, a general medicine inpatient team usually makes rounds every morning, 7 days/week. The general medicine team has senior and junior physicians and students and frequently includes nurses, pharmacists, and social workers. Outpatient clinical settings across specialties, from pediatrics to surgery, often have well-defined team structures where individual team members are rarely in the same physical space. Physicians appear at the front line with clinic patients, a triage nurse handles phone calls and emails using patient charts, and team members communicate closely with social workers and clinic schedulers. Teams are now dominant in healthcare because no one works alone any more.

Team research psychologist Eduardo Salas and his colleagues define a team as "… a distinguishable set of two or more people who interact, dynamically, interdependently, and adaptively toward a common and valued goal/objective/mission, who have each been assigned specific roles or functions to perform, and who have a limited life-span of membership" [25]. Salas and colleagues amplify the team definition by pointing out that "… task completion requires: (a) a dynamic exchange of information and resources among team members, (b) coordination of task activities (e.g., active communication, back-up behaviors), (c) constant adjustments to task demands, and (d) some organizational structuring of members" [25].

There is wide diversity among healthcare teams, yet there are fundamental team elements that distinguish thriving teams versus teams that struggle. Effective teams have clear goals, structure, measurement, feedback, and accountability. Goals govern the team and each team member. Structure comes from leadership and team communication. Salas and colleagues state elsewhere that "… teams have meaningful task interdependencies, hold shared and valued objectives, use multiple information sources, possess adaptive mechanisms, and perform through intensive communication processes. The key characteristic of a team is task interdependency. The team members must not only communicate but they must also coordinate actions and cooperate so that they can accomplish a task" [26].

The fundamental metrics for a healthcare team are always patient focused. Process measures of patient care practices can vary from team adherence to an algorithm like cardiac arrest, to measures of efficiency at managing a large patient volume in clinic or on the inpatient wards. Patient outcomes due to effective healthcare team interventions range from reduced hospital-acquired infections to fewer birth complications for newborn infants and their mothers in the maternity suite [27].

Born in the era of quality improvement and patient safety, team skills and team training have been emphasized in medical education. The Accreditation Council for Graduate Medical Education (ACGME) issued a set of new requirements for resident duty hours in 2002 [28]. The ACGME later identified six competencies as key outcomes for graduate medical education including classic qualities such as medical knowledge acquisition but also system-based practice (SBP). SBP is an awareness of and responsiveness to the larger context of healthcare and the ability to effectively use system resources to provide optimal care. The 2012 ACGME competency framework presents a granular definition of SBP by expecting doctors to "work effectively within an inter-professional team" [29]. Additionally, the core competency of interpersonal and communication skills (ICS) states trainees should "communicate effectively in inter-professional teams" with an aspirational goal to have trainees "role model and teach collaborative communication with the team to enhance patient care, even in challenging settings with conflicting team member opinions." The ACGME laid the foundation for medical education to address team skills rigorously by setting milestones for trainees within this competency framework.

Science of Team Science

The science of team science is a new scholarly concentration born from the recognition that twenty-first-century scientific and professional advancements are achieved by teams, not individuals working alone. Thus team formation, composition, training, turnover, morale, evaluation, and many other variables are the focus of study because they all affect team productivity. As described throughout this chapter, team science research is now underway in a host of industries and professions including healthcare, business, military, nuclear power, space exploration, advanced particle physics, and many others because the stakes are high and the potential return on investment is great [30–33]. Measurement and evaluation of team processes and outcomes are also being approached with much improved precision and professionalism [34–36].

A research synthesis published by Eduardo Salas and his team in 2005 presented a model of teamwork that was supported by scientific data and had practical relevance. The framework has five core components, termed the "big five," that promote team effectiveness and three coordinating mechanisms that enable a team to weave each of the core components together [37]. The "big five" of teamwork and the three coordinating mechanisms are presented in Table 11.1. The table identifies and defines each core component and coordinating mechanism and includes a set of behavioral markers for each item.

In retrospect, it is evident that each of the "big five" teamwork components and the three coordinating mechanisms were in operation during Apollo 13 crew training and flight even though they were never voiced.

Table 11.1 The "big five" and the three coordinating mechanisms of teamwork

Big five core components	Definition	Behavioral markers
Team leadership	Ability to direct and coordinate the activities of other team members; assess team performance; assign tasks; develop team knowledge, skills, and abilities; motivate team members; plan and organize; and establish a positive atmosphere	Facilitate team problem-solving Provide performance expectations and acceptable interaction patterns Synchronize and combine individual team member contributions Seek and evaluate information that affects team functioning Clarify team member roles Engage in preparatory meetings and feedback sessions with the team
Mutual performance monitoring	Ability to develop common understandings of the team environment and apply appropriate task strategies to accurately monitor teammate performance	Identifying mistakes and lapses in other members' actions Providing feedback regarding team member actions to facilitate self-correction
Backup behavior	Ability to anticipate other team members' needs through accurate knowledge about their responsibilities. This includes the ability to shift workload among members to achieve balance during high periods of workload or pressure	Recognition by potential backup provider that there is a workload distribution problem in their team Shifting of work responsibilities to underutilized team members Completion of the whole task or parts of tasks by other team members

(continued)

Table 11.1 (continued)

Big five core components	Definition	Behavioral markers
Adaptability	Ability to adjust strategies based on information gathered from the environment through the use of backup behavior and reallocation of intrateam resources. Altering a course of action or team repertoire in response to changing conditions (internal or external)	Identify cues that a change has occurred, assign meaning to that change, and develop a new plan to deal with the changes Identify opportunities for improvement and innovation for habitual or routine practices Remain vigilant to changes in the internal and external environment of the team
Team orientation	Propensity to take other's behavior into account during group interaction and the belief in the importance of team goals over individual members' goals	Taking into account alternative solutions provided by teammates and appraising that input to determine what is most correct Increased task involvement, information sharing, strategizing, and participatory goal setting
Three coordinating mechanisms		
Shared mental models	An organizing knowledge structure of the relationships among the task the team is engaged in and how the team members will interact	Anticipating and predicting each other's needs Identify changes in the team, task or teammates and implicitly adjusting strategies as needed
Mutual trust	The shared belief that team members will perform their roles and protect the interests of their teammates	Information sharing Willingness to admit mistakes and accept feedback
Closed-loop communication	The exchange of information between a sender and a receiver irrespective of the medium	Following up with team members to ensure message was received Acknowledging that a message was received Clarifying with the sender of the message that the message received is the same as the intended message

Adapted from Salas et al. [37]. Reprinted by permission of SAGE Publications

Evidence-Based Team Training Principles

Using the "big five" core components of team effectiveness and their three coordinating mechanisms as foundation ideas, the Salas research group sought to further distill healthcare team training knowledge into a set of basic principles. To reach this goal, the Salas group performed a quantitative synthesis and a specific qualitative review and content analysis of team training research reports implemented in healthcare. In an article published in 2008, the Salas research group states "Based on this review, we offer eight evidence-based principles for effective planning, implementation, and evaluation of team training programs specific to health care" [26].

Table 11.2 presents the eight evidence-based principles for team training derived by the Salas research team. Each team training principle is illustrated by a concrete example from the health professions education team training literature.

Given the eight evidence-based team training principles derived by the Salas research team from science and scholarship [26], the question becomes "How can

Table 11.2 Eight evidence-based principles for team training [26]

Principles	Examples
1. Identify teamwork competencies; use these as a focus for training content	Use established crew resource management (CRM) principles and their derivatives for curriculum development [26]
2. Emphasize teamwork over taskwork; design for teamwork to improve team processes	Combat trauma teams undergo team training, not task training, at the U.S. Army Ryder Trauma Training Center in Miami [38]
3. One size does not fit all; let the team-based learning outcomes desired, and organizational resources, guide the process	In situ simulation improves patient safety in a labor and delivery ward [39]
4. Task exposure is not enough; provide guided, hands-on practice	Internal medicine residents acquire ACLS skills to mastery standards from simulation-based (SB) team training with deliberate practice [12]
5. The power of simulation; ensure training relevance to transfer environment	SB obstetrical team training on shoulder dystocia management transfers to actual clinical care and patient outcomes [40]
6. Feedback matters; it must be descriptive, timely, and relevant	Debriefing with good judgment is an essential feature of SB healthcare education [41]
7. Go beyond reaction data; evaluate clinical outcomes, learning, and behaviors on the job	SB team training on obstetrical emergencies improves neonatal Apgar scores and reduces neonatal brain injury [42]
8. Reinforce desired teamwork behaviors; sustain through coaching and performance evaluation	Interdisciplinary SB in situ team training is an effective strategy to improve perinatal safety [43]

the team training principles be transformed into concrete team training strategies?" We now move to the "whys" and "hows" of turning team training principles into practical education strategies.

Team Training for Effective Healthcare

From Principles to Strategies

The synthesis of team concepts and the big five principles of teamwork provide a working plan of action about observation and assessment of routine clinical work which is highlighted in teams under stress.

Weaver, Dy, and Rosen used the Salas team's evidence-based team training principles from 2008 and a narrative synthesis of the literature updated to 2014 to produce a set of healthcare team training strategies including best practices [44]. These authors assert "…team training is a systematic methodology for optimizing the communication, coordination, and collaboration of healthcare teams that combines specific content with opportunities for practice, formative feedback and tools to support transfer of training to the daily care environment" [44].

A summary of these team training strategy best practices is presented in Table 11.3. The tabular entries identify and define six broad team training strategies ranging from assertiveness training to cross-training, error management training, guided team self-correction, metacognition training (situation awareness), and team adaptation and coordination training. Each of the six team training strategies is then broken down into the primary teamwork competencies targeted. The competencies can serve as learning objectives. Best education practices used to help trainee teams achieve the teamwork competencies are also listed. Table 11.3 provides the foundation of a blueprint for team training curriculum development (Chap. 3), instruction (Chap. 4), and assessment (Chap. 5) in the healthcare professions.

Another expression of healthcare team training best practices is embodied in the Team Strategies and Tools to Enhance Performance and Patient Safety (TeamSTEPPS™) program, a curriculum developed jointly by the U.S. Department of Defense (DoD) and the U.S. Agency for Healthcare Research and Quality (AHRQ) to integrate healthcare teamwork into practice [45]. TeamSTEPPS™ is a packaged curriculum, available "off the shelf," that contains modules that focus on four healthcare teamwork core competencies: (a) leadership, (b) situation monitoring, (c) mutual support, and (d) communication. TeamSTEPPS™ is delivered according to a carefully developed implementation and sustainment plan that has three phases:

- Phase I: Assessment—set the stage
- Phase II: Planning, training, and implementation—decide what to do and make it happen
- Phase III: Sustainment—make it stick

Table 11.3 Team-training strategies

Team training strategy	Definition	Primary teamwork competencies targeted	Best practices
Assertiveness training	Dedicated to developing communication strategies that support task-relevant and team-performance-relevant assertiveness	Backup behavior Closed-loop communication Conflict management Mutual trust Psychological safety Team leadership	Clearly define training objectives around task-relevant and team performance assertiveness rather than general assertive behaviors and differentiate from aggressive behaviors Compare and contrast effective and ineffective assertive behaviors Provide opportunities to practice appropriate assertiveness that include feedback. Practice should also strive to include realistic time pressures or other stressors to allow practice using and reacting to appropriate assertiveness under such conditions
Cross-training	Team members learn the roles that comprise the team, as well as the tasks, duties, and responsibilities fulfilled by fellow team members	Accurate and shared mental models (SMMs) of team roles and responsibilities	Include information about the roles and responsibilities of other team members and how they operate to achieve these Explain the why—clarify who members depend on for information Provide opportunities to shadow another role if possible Provide feedback during cross-training that facilitates the formation of reasonable expectations of one another
Error management training	Participants are encouraged to make errors during training scenarios, analyze these errors, and practice error recognition and management skills	Collective efficacy Cue-strategy associations SMMs Team adaptation	Ensure trainees understand the purpose of this training strategy is to encounter errors and to have the opportunity to practice managing them in a safe environment Frame errors as positive opportunities for learning Embed the opportunity to make errors into training scenarios by providing minimal guidance during the scenario Follow the scenario with immediate feedback and discussion to facilitate learning

(continued)

Table 11.3 (continued)

Team training strategy	Definition	Primary teamwork competencies targeted	Best practices
Guided team self-correction	Strategy designed around a cycle of facilitated briefings and debriefings that occur around a training scenario or live event	Backup behavior Collective orientation Closed-loop communication Cue-strategy associations Mission analysis Mutual trust SMMs Team adaptation Team leadership	Define the team self-correction skills to be trained prior to team self-correction training Record positive and negative examples of teamwork dimensions during team performance episode Classify and prioritize observations, diagnose strengths and weaknesses, and identify goals for improvement before beginning debrief Set the stage for team participation, and solicit examples of teamwork behavior during debrief
Metacognition training	Focuses on developing cognitive aspects of team performance by teaching strategies dedicated to analyzing, updating, and aligning mental models of the task, coordination strategy, and contingencies	Cue-strategy associations Mission analysis SMMs Team adaptation	Develop training objectives around cognitive processes such as planning, monitoring, and reanalysis. Structure metacognitive practice tasks around a subject that trainees have preexisting knowledge about
Team adaptation and coordination training	Focuses on how to effectively use all available resources (i.e., people, information, etc.) through effective team communication, coordination, and cooperation. Crew or Crisis Resource Management is a form of TACT	Backup behavior Closed-loop communication Cue-strategy associations Mission analysis Mutual performance monitoring Leadership Shared mental models	Develop training objectives that address around transportable teamwork competencies for ad hoc teams (no history or future) Training team-specific competencies can also be incorporated for intact teams Train intact teams together if possible Create opportunities for both guided and unguided practice Develop feedback mechanisms that engage self-reflection and team self-correction following practice opportunities Develop tools that support effective teamwork, but recognize that tools alone (e.g., checklists) cannot optimize team performance (and alone may negatively impact performance)

Reproduced from Ref. [44] with permission from BMJ Publishing Group Ltd.

TeamSTEPPS™ has been employed widely in a variety of health professions to boost team performance, communication, and morale. Examples include improving nurse-to-nurse patient handoffs in a multihospital setting [46] and advancing team performance and communication openness at an academic medical center's pediatric and surgical intensive care units (ICUs) [47]. However, a the TeamSTEPPS™ curriculum has never been used to educate healthcare teams to a mastery learning standard.

Team Training in Operation

Two basic concepts that underlie health professions team training principles and strategies need to be made plain because they are very different from usual education approaches in the health professions: (a) unit of training and evaluation and (b) teamwork vs. taskwork.

In team training for effective healthcare, the unit of training and evaluation is the group, not individual persons—leaders and co-workers—who make up the team. This is similar but not identical to training for a team athletic (e.g., soccer or football) or a choral music ensemble competition. The group, not individual persons, is the focus of instruction and assessment. This is very different from the way that health professionals have been educated and assessed traditionally with an emphasis on individual achievement compared to other learners cast on a normal curve [48].

The second basic concept that underlies team training for effective healthcare is the distinction between teamwork and taskwork. Healthcare teamwork addresses the goal of efficient and seamless patient care practices by a provider group. Healthcare taskwork involves the particular skills and competencies among healthcare team members (e.g., airway management by a respiratory therapist) that need to be orchestrated to deliver first-rate care. Healthcare taskwork is a necessary but not a sufficient condition for healthcare teamwork.

A common assumption is that healthcare taskwork competence has been measured and assessed among team members before team training exercises are undertaken.

A close approximation to a mastery learning healthcare team training model is seen in educating U.S. Army forward surgical teams (FSTs) at the Army Trauma Training Center at the University of Miami Ryder Trauma Center [38]. FSTs are elite healthcare units composed of general and orthopedic surgeons, nurse anesthetists, nurses, operating room (OR) technicians, emergency medical technicians (EMTs), and administrative staff. "The mission of the FST is to provide resuscitative and damage control surgery for the stabilization of life-, limb-, and eyesight-threatening injuries in austere environments" [38].

The FST curriculum embodies three main goals: "(a) provide basic and advanced trauma refresher training, (b) teach combat trauma unique concepts and skills, and (c) develop the group into a strongly functioning team to improve patient outcomes on the battlefield" [38]. The third goal, teamwork, receives much more training emphasis than taskwork. Education activities include lectures, single team-building exercises, clinical skills exercises, combat surgery and mass casualty (MASCAL) exercises, and other events.

The FST curriculum capstone event is a situational training exercise (STX) involving live tissue, moulaged standardized patients (SPs), trauma mannequins, and high-fidelity human trauma simulators. "The FST is simultaneously presented with increasing numbers of 'patients' with multiple traumatic injuries, and then finally a MASCAL, to evaluate their implementation of advanced trauma life support protocols, use of current (trauma treatment protocols), proper triaging and management of patients to the OR, intensive care unit, or stabilization for transport to the closest combat support hospital, while managing other tactical, logistical, and administrative activities" [38]. The STX is clearly a complex, engaging training and assessment exercise. The STX approximates a mastery learning experience because U.S. Army medical educators report "… student (teams) must *perform above a certain standard for successful completion of Phase 1 of the course*" (emphasis added). In addition, "… student [teams] must successfully handle the patient load and any adverse situations. Instructors remain silent and solely observant, grading the students on their performance" [38].

Lifespan of Healthcare Team Training

The team training principles given in Table 11.2 and team training strategies pointed out in Table 11.3 are bedrock ideas about how to design, implement, manage, and evaluate a team training program in health professions education. The principles and strategies guide us about what healthcare team training should address and offer a roadmap about how team training should be done. We now focus on what Salas, Reyes, and Woods call the "lifespan of team training," the origins, operations, and aftermath of team training in healthcare organizations [49]. This section aims to present practical tips about how to design, manage, and evaluate a robust team training program in a busy healthcare clinical environment.

Table 11.4 lays out the lifespan of healthcare team training as three connected phases: (a) before, (b) during, and (c) after team training events. The tabular entries point out that the lifespan of healthcare team training is a continuum which produce sequential, translational effects where (team training) "… learning outcomes lead to transfer outcomes, which improve results" [49].

Leaders responsible for healthcare team training know that this is not easy work. Team training requires careful curriculum planning; tight management due to hospital shift and schedule complexities; acknowledging and tackling evaluation apprehension among doctors, nurses, and other healthcare providers [50, 51]; and the tough job of collecting, analyzing, and using follow-up data to determine if team training really works. Imposition of a mastery learning minimum passing standard (MPS) for team training episodes (Chap. 6), with opportunities for improvement for teams in training who do not meet the MPS in the short run, adds a layer of complexity to the enterprise.

Table 11.4 Lifespan of healthcare team training [49]

Before team training	During team training	After team training
Needs assessment (Chaps. 3 and 15) Local problem recognition Incentive to improve	Instruction and assessment (Chaps. 4 and 5) Education plans Assessment united with instruction	Does the training program work? (Chaps. 7, 16 and 19) T1 (education setting) T2 (patient care practices) T3 (patient outcomes) T4 (skill retention, collateral effects, ROI, refresher training)
Curriculum development (Chap. 3) Problem identification and general needs assessment Targeted needs assessment Goals and objectives Education strategies Implementation Evaluation and feedback	What does the team training program look like? Training schedule Training frequency Training resources Training staff Learner morale Faculty incentives	Is the team training program maintained over time? Rigorous measurement of team training program effects Continuous outcome evaluation planning Vigilant attention to team training decay
Organizational readiness Team assembly/formation Team composition Team member interchangeability	How will the team training be delivered? Pretest Information Demonstration Deliberate practice Assessment Feedback Improvement to team MPS T1 outcomes (Chap. 16)	Will the training last? Supportive transfer climate Continued feedback Refresher training

Data from Salas et al. [49]

Events before team training include needs assessment, curriculum development, and preparing one's organization for insertion and management of team training activities into an already packed schedule. Organizational awareness should also grow about the importance of team assembly and formation, team composition, and team member interchangeability.

Management of people and events during team training requires careful planning, scheduling, control of training delivery events, staff preparation, and outcome measurement. Delivery of team training is similar, but not identical, to presenting a health professions curriculum focused on individual learners (Chap. 7). Team training is more complex than individual training because group units are more difficult to educate, evaluate, and keep together than person units.

Measuring and evaluating team training effectiveness is the principal duty after the program is completed. Did team training achieve short-run goals and are training outcomes resistant to decay? Are team training outcomes measureable only in the education setting (T1) or also as translational "downstream" effects including better patient care practices (T2), patient outcomes (T3), or as a variety of collateral effects (T4) (Chap. 16)? Team training outcome measurement warrants detailed and continuous attention to ensure that results are robust and sustained.

Challenges and Future Directions

One of the major challenges in team training is creating an assessment tool that reflects or emphasizes teamwork in addition to more traditional perceived clinical skill. Team performance assessment and measurement have been studied extensively by Eduardo Salas and colleagues. They document the need for measures which are derived from research, accurately represent the team dynamic, reflect the input of trained observers, represent the specific environment, yield reliable data when used by well-trained judges, and demonstrate content and construct validity. Loughry and colleagues developed a theory-based assessment of team member effectiveness based on the work of Salas and others. The short version of the Comprehensive Assessment of Team Member Effectiveness (CATME) is a 33-item instrument designed to apply to any context in which teamwork is used [35]. Assessment tools will need to get at the granular characteristics of a team such as "identifying oneself as the team leader" and team members "practicing closed-loop communication" and "taking corrective actions." More experience is needed to build assessment tools that measure and standardize such team behaviors.

With the history and evidence at hand, and the mandate by medical education accreditation boards, team training must expand at the undergraduate and graduate levels. Training must include the development of curricula, assessment tools, and mastery standards and involve interdisciplinary teams in a variety of healthcare settings.

Coda

Healthcare today is a team sport. Nurses, doctors, pharmacists, physical and occupational therapists, midwives, social workers, dentists, and other health professionals rarely work alone anymore. Strong evidence from a recent meta-analysis on healthcare team training shows without doubt that rigorous team education saves lives [52]. To date, the downstream outcomes of mastery learning of team skills have not been studied. We believe that taking healthcare team training to "the next level" of mastery learning will boost its power and utility.

References

1. Lovell JA. Houston, we've had a problem. In: Cartright EM, editor. Apollo expeditions to the moon, SP-350. Washington, DC: National Aeronautics and Space Administration, Scientific and Technical Information Office; 1975.
2. Helmreich RL, Foushee HC. Why crew resource management? Empirical and theoretical bases of human factors training in aviation. In: Weiner EL, Kanki BG, Helmreich RL, editors. Cockpit resource management. San Diego: Academic Press; 1993.
3. Cooper GE, White MD, Lauber JK, editors. Resource management on the flightdeck: proceedings of a NASA/industry workshop (NASA CP-2120). Moffett Field: NASA-Ames Research Center; 1980.

4. Flight Safety Foundation (FSF) Editorial Staff. Top 10 safety issues. AeroSafety World. Dec. 2014–Jan. 2015. Front page.
5. Wilson D. Failure to communicate. AeroSafety World. Nov. 2016. Front page.
6. Helmreich RL, Merritt AC, Wilhelm JA. The evolution of crew resource management training in commercial aviation. Int J Aviat Psychol. 1999;9(1):19–32.
7. Sullenberger C. Highest duty: my search for what really matters. New York: Harper; 2009.
8. Denson JS, Abrahamson S. A computer-controlled patient simulator. JAMA. 1969;208(3):504–8.
9. Abrahamson S, Denson JS, Wolf RM. Effectiveness of a simulator in training anesthesiology residents. J Med Educ. 1969;44:515–9.
10. Wayne DB, Butter J, Siddall VJ, et al. Simulation-based training of internal medicine residents in advanced cardiac life support protocols: a randomized trial. Teach Learn Med. 2005;17(3):210–6.
11. Wayne DB, Didwania A, Feinglass J, et al. Simulation-based education improves quality of care during cardiac arrest team responses at an academic teaching hospital: a case-control study. Chest. 2008;133:56–61.
12. Wayne DB, Butter J, Siddall VJ, et al. Mastery learning of advanced cardiac life support skills by internal medicine residents using simulation technology and deliberate practice. J Gen Intern Med. 2006;21:251–6.
13. Didwania A, McGaghie WC, Cohen ER, et al. Progress toward improving the quality of cardiac arrest medical team responses at an academic teaching hospital. J Grad Med Educ. 2011;3:211–6.
14. Ziesmann MT, Widder S, Park J, et al. S.T.A.R.T.T.: development of a national, multidisciplinary trauma crisis resource management curriculum—results from the pilot course. J Trauma Acute Care Surg. 2013;75(5):753–8.
15. Gillman L, Brindly P, Paton-Gay J, et al. Simulated trauma and resuscitation team training course—evolution of a multidisciplinary trauma crisis resource management simulation course. Am J Surg. 2016;212(1):188–93.
16. Tahtali D, Bohmann F, Kurka N, et al. Implementation of stroke teams and simulation training shortened process times in a regional stroke network—a network-wide prospective trial. PLoS One. 2017;12(12):e0188231. https://doi.org/10.1371/journal.pone.0188231.eCollection2017.
17. Deering S, Rowland J. Obstetric emergency simulation. Semin Perinatol. 2013;37:179–88.
18. Smith S. Team training and institutional protocols to prevent shoulder dystocia complications. Clin Obstet Gynecol. 2016;59:830–40.
19. Shaddean A, Deering S. Simulation and shoulder dystocia. Clin Obstet Gynecol. 2016;59:853–8.
20. Deering S, Poggi S, Macedonia C, et al. Improving resident competency in the management of shoulder dystocia with simulation training. Obstet Gynecol. 2004;104:634–5.
21. Crofts J, Bartlett C, Ellis D, et al. Training for shoulder dystocia: a trial of simulation using low-fidelity and high-fidelity mannequins. Obstet Gynecol. 2006;108:1477–85.
22. Shoham DA, Harris JK, Mundt M, McGaghie WC. A network model of communication in an interprofessional team of healthcare professionals: a cross-sectional study of a burn unit. J Interprof Care. 2016;39(5):661–7.
23. Fiscella K, McDaniel SH. The complexity, diversity, and science of primary care teams. Am Psychol. 2018;73(4):451–67.
24. Ervin JN, Kahn JM, Cohen TR, Weingart LR. Teamwork in the intensive care unit. Am Psychol. 2018;73(4):468–77.
25. Salas E, Dickinson TL, Converse SA, Tannenbaum SI. Toward an understanding of team performance and training. In: Swezey RW, Salas E, editors. Teams: their training and performance. Norwood: Ablex; 1992.
26. Salas E, DiazGranados D, Weaver SJ, King H. Does team training work? Principles for health care. Acad Emerg Med. 2008;15(11):1002–9.
27. McGaghie WC. Medical education research as translational science. Sci Transl Med. 2010;2(19):19cm8.
28. Philibert I, Friedmann P. Williams WT for the members of the ACGME work group on resident duty hours. New requirements for resident duty hours. JAMA. 2002;288(9):1112–4.

29. Nasca TJ, Philibert I, Brigham T, Flynn TC. The next GME accreditation system—rationale and benefits. N Engl J Med. 2012;366(11):1051–6.
30. Börner K, Contractor N, Falk-Krzesinski HJ, et al. A multi-level systems perspective for the science of team science. Sci Transl Med. 2010;2(49):49cm24.
31. Falk-Krzesinski HJ, Börner K, Contractor N, et al. Advancing the science of team science. Clin Transl Sci. 2010;3(5):263–6.
32. Hall KL, Vogel AL, Huand GC, et al. The science of team science: a review of the empirical evidence and research gaps on collaboration in science. Am Psychol. 2018;73(4):532–48.
33. Driskell JE, Salas E, Driskell T. Foundations of teamwork and collaboration. Am Psychol. 2018;73(4):334–48.
34. Baker DP, Salas E. Principles for measuring teamwork. In: Brannick MT, Salas E, Prince C, editors. Team performance assessment and measurement: theory, methods and applications. Mahwah: Lawrence Erlbaum Associates; 1997.
35. Loughry ML, Ohland MW, Moore DD. Development of a theory-based assessment of team member effectiveness. Educ Psychol Meas. 2007;67:505–34.
36. Grand JA, Pearce M, Rench TA, et al. Going DEEP: guidelines for building simulation-based team assessments. BMJ Qual Saf. 2013;22(5):436–48.
37. Salas E, Sims DE, Burke CS. Is there a "Big Five" in teamwork? Small Group Res. 2005;36(5):555–99.
38. Allen CJ, Straker RJ, Murray CR, et al. Recent advances in forward surgical team training at the U.S. Army Trauma Training Department. Mil Med. 2016;181(6):553–9.
39. Hamman WR, Beaudin-Seiler BM, Beaubien JM, et al. Using in situ simulation to identify and resolve latent environmental threats to patient safety: case study involving labor and delivery ward. J Patient Saf. 2009;5:184–7.
40. Draycott TJ, Crofts JF, Ash JP, et al. Improving neonatal outcome through practical shoulder dystocia training. Obstet Gynecol. 2008;112:14–20.
41. Rudolph JW, Simon R, Rivard P, et al. Debriefing with good judgment: combining rigorous feedback with genuine inquiry. Anesthesiol Clin. 2007;25:361–76.
42. Draycott T, Sibanda T, Owen L, et al. Does training in obstetric emergencies improve neonatal outcome? BJOG. 2006;113:177–82.
43. Miller KK, Riley W, Davis S, Hansen HE. In situ simulation: a method of experiential learning to promote safety and team behavior. J Perinat Neonatal Nurs. 2008;22(2):105–13.
44. Weaver SJ, Dy SM, Rosen MA. Team training in healthcare: a narrative synthesis of the literature. BMJ Qual Saf. 2014;23:359–72.
45. King HB, Battles J, Baker DP, et al. TeamSTEPPS: team strategies and tools to enhance performance and patient safety. In: Henriksen K, Battles JB, Keyes MA, Grady ML, editors. Advances in patient safety: new directions and alternative approaches, vol. 3: performance and tools. Rockville: Agency for Healthcare Research and Quality; 2008.
46. Thomas L, Donohue-Porter P. Blending evidence and innovation: improving intershift handoffs in a multihospital setting. J Nurs Care Qual. 2012;27(2):116–24.
47. Mayer CM, Cluff L, Lin W-T, et al. Evaluating efforts to optimize TeamSTEPPS implementation in surgical and pediatric intensive care units. Jt Comm J Qual Patient Saf. 2011;37(8):365–74.
48. Rosenbaum L. Divided we fall. N Engl J Med. 2019;380(7):684–8.
49. Salas E, Reyes DL, Woods AL. Team training in organizations: it works—when done right. In: Argote L, Levine JM, editors. The Oxford handbook of group and organizational learning. New York: Oxford University Press; 2015.
50. McGaghie WC. Evaluation apprehension and impression management in clinical medical education. Acad Med. 2018;93(5):685–6.
51. Rosenbaum L. Cursed by knowledge—building a culture of psychological safety. N Engl J Med. 2019;380(8):786–90.
52. Hughes AM, Gregory MC, Joseph DL, et al. Saving lives: a meta-analysis of team training in healthcare. J Appl Psychol. 2016;101(9):1266–304.

Mastery Learning of Surgical Skills

12

Ezra N. Teitelbaum, Katherine A. Barsness, and Eric S. Hungness

Since the early twentieth century, procedural learning during surgical residency has followed a model developed by Dr. William Halsted at Johns Hopkins University [1]. In the past century, there has been little deviation from this "see one, do one, teach one" model where surgical residents learn about operations by first watching attending surgeons or senior residents perform surgeries, later doing operations under supervision of a senior surgeon, and finally teaching a junior trainee. Although this process allows for one-on-one training, it does not ensure a surgical trainee is competent in their skills before completion of training and is completely at the mercy of the type of surgical cases with which trainees participate during residency. Surgical trainees traditionally have little opportunity to practice surgical skills, let alone whole operations, outside of the operating room (OR) without putting patients at risk. Recent restrictions on resident duty hours, an increasing focus on patient safety, and medicolegal considerations have also limited resident operative autonomy [2–4]. This has added greater concern that current surgical trainees are not prepared to operate independently and safely upon residency graduation and has led an increasing number of graduates to pursue post-residency fellowship training [5–8].

Simulation and mastery learning have emerged as a potential solution to these issues by preparing surgical residents to operate effectively and learn in a simulated

E. N. Teitelbaum (✉)
Northwestern University Feinberg School of Medicine, Department of Surgery, Chicago, IL, USA
e-mail: e-teitelbaum@northwestern.edu

K. A. Barsness · E. S. Hungness
Northwestern University Feinberg School of Medicine, Departments of Surgery and Medical Education, Chicago, IL, USA

W. C. McGaghie et al. (eds.), *Comprehensive Healthcare Simulation: Mastery Learning in Health Professions Education*, Comprehensive Healthcare Simulation, https://doi.org/10.1007/978-3-030-34811-3_12

OR [9]. Many aspects of a simulation-based mastery learning (SBML) model appear uniquely suited to address the educational needs of surgical trainees. Surgical residencies are no longer based on a "pyramid" structure where some residents are not allowed to progress. In the current training environment, all residents that begin a program as interns are expected to graduate in the same number of years and function as independent general surgeons. Mastery learning acknowledges that these learners will not all progress at the same pace because it requires that all learners reach a fixed endpoint of operative safety and autonomy. Use of simulation provides a low-stakes learning environment where trainees are permitted to make mistakes and learn from them without the consequences of practicing on patients. A SBML model also encourages training using deliberate practice with immediate feedback from expert instructors, in contrast to the Halstedian approach which is completely reliant on the cases in which a trainee participates during residency. Adding mastery learning to existing surgical training offers the potential to better prepare residents before they enter the OR. This allows surgery residents to still take advantage of the unique educational opportunities (e.g., variations in patient anatomy or dealing with complications) that only occur in the OR while permitting surgical faculty to more quickly advance residents to supervised and safe operative autonomy.

Mastery Learning of Surgical Skills

Simulation-based learning has assumed an increasing role in surgical training over the past decade. The most influential step in the codification of simulation into residency training was development of the Fundamentals of Laparoscopic Surgery (FLS) curriculum and exam [10]. Laparoscopic (i.e., minimally invasive) surgery gained prominence in the late 1980s and early 1990s with the introduction of laparoscopic cholecystectomy (gallbladder removal) and quickly was adopted for a range of abdominal operations. Use of a laparoscopic approach with smaller incisions dramatically decreased pain and convalescence after surgery while also lowering complication rates such as wound infections and hernia formation. However, with these advantages came the difficulty of teaching a completely new skill to residents and practicing surgeons. Many practicing surgeons participated in weekend courses where they performed laparoscopic cholecystectomy for the first time in animal models and then returned to their home institutions to perform the operation in actual patients and teach residents the very next week. This was not a safe approach to learning such a novel and fundamentally different set of surgical skills. As a result, the rate of common bile duct injury, the most serious complication of cholecystectomy, increased in the period of initial adoption of laparoscopy [11].

In response to this problem, a group of surgical educators from a collaboration of surgical societies and organizations developed the FLS curriculum and exam. FLS was created to address the difficulty of teaching and learning laparoscopic surgical skills and to ensure that graduating surgical residents reached proficiency in these skills (mastery learning) [10, 12]. Learners who do not "pass" the exam can retake

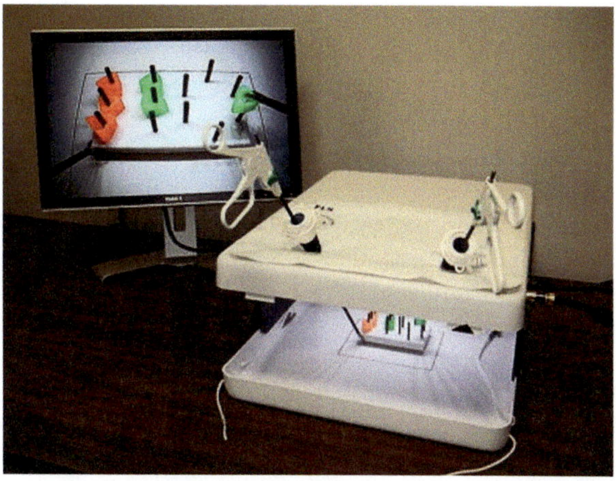

Fig. 12.1 The Fundamentals of Laparoscopic Surgery (FLS) box trainer allows learners to practice basic laparoscopic surgical tasks. Pictured here is the peg transfer task in which triangular pegs are transferred from one side of a peg board to another using laparoscopic graspers. (Figure from Vassiliou et al. [34]. Reprinted with permission from Elsevier)

it at a later time after further practice. FLS has two parts: (a) a series of online modules designed to teach the conceptual and factual knowledge required to perform laparoscopic surgery, and (b) a simulator-based component with five surgical tasks. The surgical tasks (peg transfer, circle cut, suture loop ligation, intracorporeal knot tying, and extracorporeal knot tying) are performed in a simple "box trainer" model of laparoscopic surgery (Fig. 12.1).

After completing the FLS curriculum, learners take a high-stakes summative exam having both a multiple-choice written portion and simulator-based test composed of the five FLS tasks. This form of simulation does not have a high degree of "face validity" because the FLS simulation environment does not look like the inside of the human abdomen, there are no simulated organs, and the learner performs simple tasks rather than an entire operation. However, the power of this form of simulator-based education and testing lies in the teaching of fundamental principles and skills that underlie complex laparoscopic operations. This is reinforced by construct validity evidence that supports FLS. A number of studies have shown that clinical laparoscopic surgical experience results in superior performance on the FLS exam, that FLS exam scores predict actual operative performance, and that undergoing the FLS curriculum improves surgical skills when they are applied clinically [10, 13, 14]. Given this evidence, in 2010, the American Board of Surgery required passing the FLS exam to earn board certification in surgery. This was the first evaluation of technical skills to be included in the board certification process, illustrating the revolutionary influence of FLS on surgical education in the United States.

Based on the success of the FLS curriculum and examination, a similar program, Fundamentals of Endoscopic Surgery (FES), was developed to teach and evaluate flexible endoscopic skills (e.g., upper endoscopy, colonoscopy) [15, 16]. Passing FES is now also required for board certification in surgery. Due to the high-stakes nature of this assessment and the intentional difficulty of the exam, there has been considerable interest on the part of surgical educators in preparing residents to perform endoscopy and pass the FES exam. One study found an experience threshold of 105 prior endoscopies to be predictive of passing the manual skills portion of the FES exam [17]. However, many surgical residents do not perform that many endoscopies during training.

To bridge this educational gap and accelerate resident learning outside of the patient care context, one residency program designed a SBML curriculum to teach flexible endoscopic skills and prepare trainees for the FES examination [18]. Although this curriculum was designed to teach a specific set of endoscopy skills, it can serve as a model for the use of SBML to teach basic and fundamental surgical skills more generally. The curriculum was tested on 17 junior surgical residents (postgraduate years 1 and 2) who had limited experience with flexible endoscopy (<10 prior patient endoscopies). Following the mastery learning model, trainees all took a pre-curriculum exam, consisting of the hands-on component of the FES exam. The trainees then participated in deliberate practice on an endoscopic simulator. They received individualized instruction and feedback from expert endoscopists initially but were then allowed to perform independent practice on the simulator once they demonstrated skill with proper technique. These practice sessions were limited to 90 minutes and two sessions per day to ensure a distributed and deliberate training regimen.

Practice sessions were performed using a different simulator than the one used for the FES exam (Fig. 12.2). The FES exam uses a virtual reality (VR) testing platform, and the actual test modules are not publicly available to ensure test security. The VR platform used for the exam is very expensive (GI Mentor, 3D SYSTEMS, Littleton, CO), limiting the capability for residency programs to include it in training curricula. For these reasons, the designers of the SBML endoscopy curriculum chose a non-VR model called Endoscopic Training System (ETS) to serve as the training platform. The ETS model was designed to cover the same domains of basic flexible endoscopy as FES and has previously demonstrated validity evidence for measuring core endoscopic skills [19, 20]. During the curriculum, residents performed a mean of 48 repetitions on the ETS model over the course of five training sessions.

After completing this simulator-based training, the residents took a posttest consisting of the same FES exam as the pretest. The impact of the curriculum on resident performance was striking. Only 3 trainees out of 17 (17.6%) passed the pretest, whereas 14/14 (100%; 2 participants did not take the posttest, 1 did not complete the training sessions) passed the posttest. Mean scores increased from 50.4 (SD = 16) to 74.0 (SD = 8; $p < 0.0001$) with an effect size of 2.4 (Fig. 12.3). When curriculum participant scores on the posttest were compared with those of senior residents and attending surgeons, their mean was in the range of clinicians who had performed 150–300 endoscopies [18].

These results illustrate several key points regarding SBML curricula for fundamental surgical skills. First, participants do not need to have extensive clinical experience before curriculum participation. In fact, it is likely best to position SBML for surgical skills at the beginning of residency training to allow interns and junior

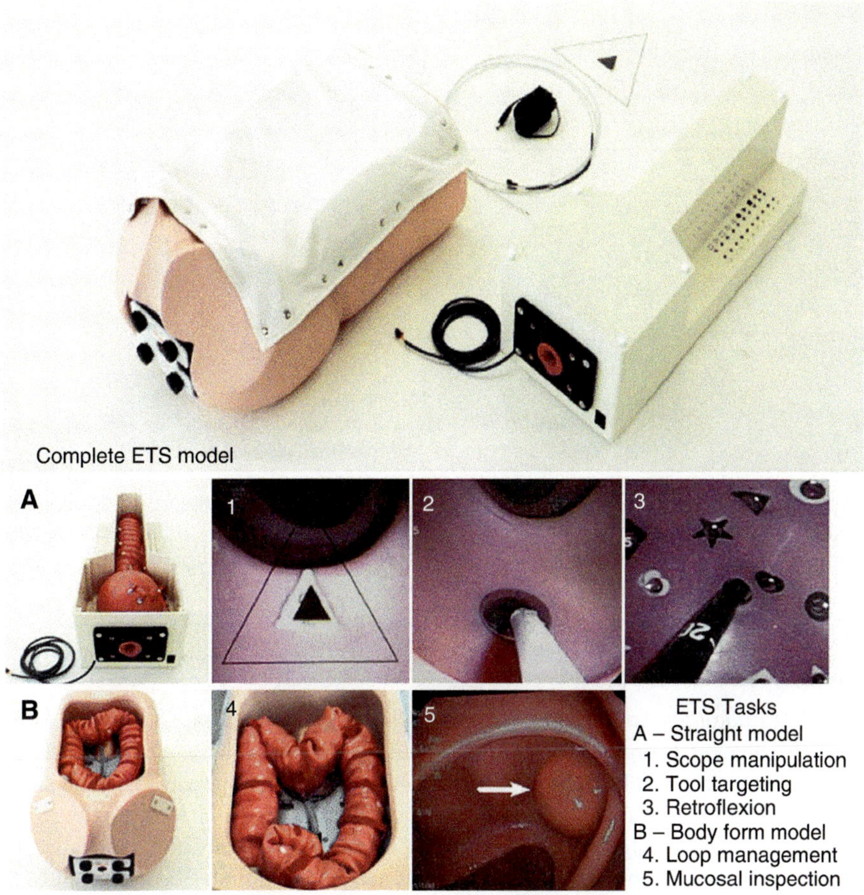

Fig. 12.2 The Endoscopic Training System (ETS) is a simulator designed to practice the basic skills of flexible endoscopy. It allows for learners to practice both (**A**) upper endoscopy and (**B**) colonoscopy and various skills within each of those modalities (1–5). (Figure from Ritter et al. [18]. Reprinted with permission from Springer Nature)

residents to develop these skills before using and practicing them in the OR. Second, SBML curricula can use training models that are different from the models used for high-stakes examinations. If curricula teach to the same domains as those being tested and are supported by validity evidence, less expensive and more practical training simulators can be highly effective. Third, a relatively brief curriculum intervention using SBML can produce significant improvement in surgical skills equal or superior to the more time-intensive traditional "see one, do one, teach one" experiential learning format. As described above, the FES SBML curriculum with an average of five training sessions produced posttest scores equivalent to those from physicians who had performed 150–300 endoscopies [18].

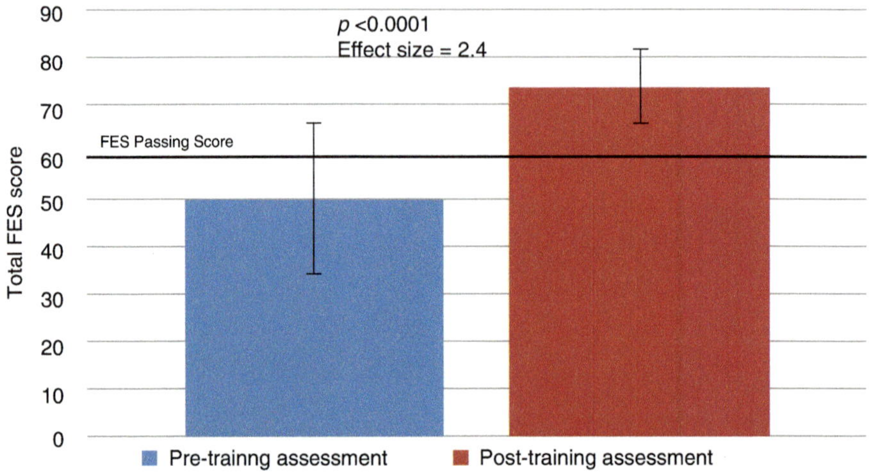

Fig. 12.3 A simulation-based mastery learning curriculum for flexible endoscopy resulted in significantly improved scores on the Fundamentals of Endoscopic Surgery (FES) technical skill exam. (Figure from Ritter et al. [18]. Reprinted with permission from Springer Nature)

Mastery Learning of Surgical Operations

It follows naturally from the principles of SBML that this model can be used to teach fundamental surgical skills (i.e., FLS, FES). Such techniques can be simulated in simple models, can be taught and practiced in short training sessions, and can be evaluated using simulator-based exams with objective metrics. However, when transitioning from teaching basic surgical skills to entire operations, the application of SBML becomes much more complex. Surgeries have multiple steps that can each require very different techniques. The surgeon must have an advanced understanding of anatomy and anatomical variation, advanced technologies and instruments, how to avoid complications, and how to manage emergent situations if problems occur. Understanding of preoperative evaluation, diagnosis, and preparation, as well as postoperative management and treatment of complications, is also essential. All these components and considerations make the application of SBML to complete operations challenging. However, by working in a stepwise manner to create a focused simulator model, curriculum, and exam, SBML can be translated to complex, multistep procedures. The remainder of this chapter discusses the development and implementation of curriculum for two such procedures—laparoscopic common bile duct exploration (LCBDE) and laparoscopic inguinal hernia repair—and examines the effect of those curricula on trainee performance and subsequent patient outcomes.

Development of any medical education curriculum should begin with a needs assessment to identify educational gaps and focus its goals and objectives (Chap. 3). It is helpful to follow a structured approach to this process so that educators are not left to "reinvent the wheel" when developing each new curriculum. When setting out to develop a SBML curriculum for the LCBDE operation, our group at Northwestern University Feinberg School of Medicine used a six-step approach to curriculum development, as described by Thomas, Kern, and colleagues [21]:

1. Problem identification and general needs assessment
2. Targeted needs assessment
3. Goals and objectives
4. Educational strategies
5. Implementation
6. Evaluation and feedback

The six-step approach begins with a *problem identification and general needs assessment*, which targets a clinical or educational problem on a broad level. In our case, the problem identification focused on patients with choledocholithiasis (i.e., gallstones that have migrated into the common bile duct from the gallbladder). Such patients can be treated using one of two care pathways: (a) a two-stage approach in which they undergo an endoscopic retrograde cholangiopancreatography (ERCP) to clear stones from the common bile duct and then a laparoscopic cholecystectomy is performed to remove the gallbladder and prevent recurrence, or (b) they undergo a single procedure during which an LCBDE is performed to clear the common duct at the time of laparoscopic cholecystectomy. Although multiple randomized controlled trials have demonstrated the clinical advantages of LCBDE over the two-stage approach [22, 23], the procedure remains significantly underused in the United States [24]. This is largely due to a lack of exposure and training in the operation during surgical residency [25]. This unmet educational need formed the basis for development of a SBML curriculum.

We next moved to the second step of the Thomas curriculum development model, conducting a *targeted needs assessment* focused on the educational needs and deficiencies of the intended learners. We planned to implement the curriculum for senior surgical residents at our institution, so we set out to evaluate their current exposure, knowledge, and technical capabilities with LCBDE. For a residency program with five residents per graduating class, an average of only one to two LCBDE procedures per year were being performed *in total* in the entire medical center. The next step was to determine the baseline technical abilities of the learners. With minimal LCBDE case volume, it would be difficult to assess resident performance during actual operations. Therefore, we set out to design an LCBDE-specific procedural simulator as a means of both performing a needs assessment of baseline aptitude and later developing a SBML curriculum to improve performance [26, 27].

Before designing a simulator and SBML curriculum for such a complex operation as LCBDE, it was necessary to understand the technical and cognitive steps that are required to perform the procedure successfully and safely. Thus our first step in

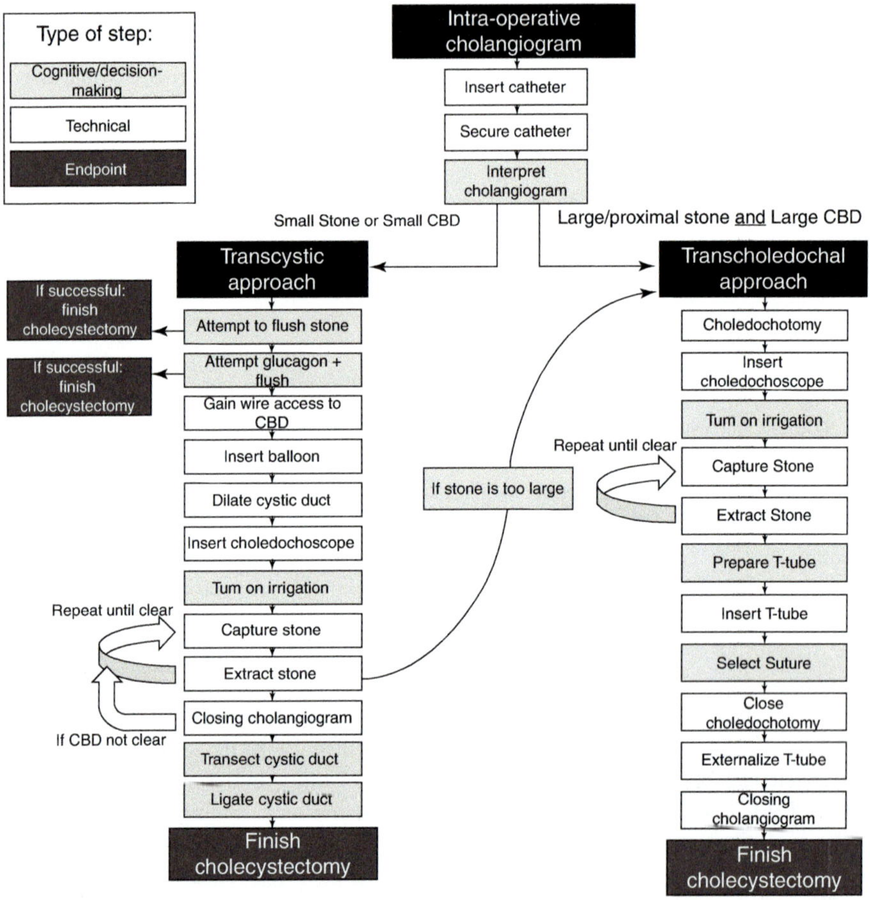

Fig. 12.4 A procedural algorithm for the laparoscopic common bile duct exploration (LCBDE) operation. The algorithm served as the basis for the design of an LCBDE-specific procedural simulator and mastery learning curriculum. (Figure from Santos et al. [26]. Reprinted with permission from Springer Nature)

the simulator development process was to create a procedural algorithm specifying the critical steps of the operation (Fig. 12.4). It was important to include cognitive decision-making points (e.g., choice of suture size and material), as well as purely technical maneuvers (e.g., suture closure of the common bile duct). With this algorithm as a guide, we then designed and constructed an LCBDE simulator where a learner could practice (and be evaluated on) each of the required steps (Fig. 12.5). The simulator was housed in a standard laparoscopic box trainer constructed of low-cost synthetic materials. It was designed to allow the trainee to use actual instruments to perform an LCBDE procedure from start to finish. In addition to the simulator, an LCBDE-specific procedural rating scale was created to assess performance on each of the key steps of the operation, both technical and cognitive.

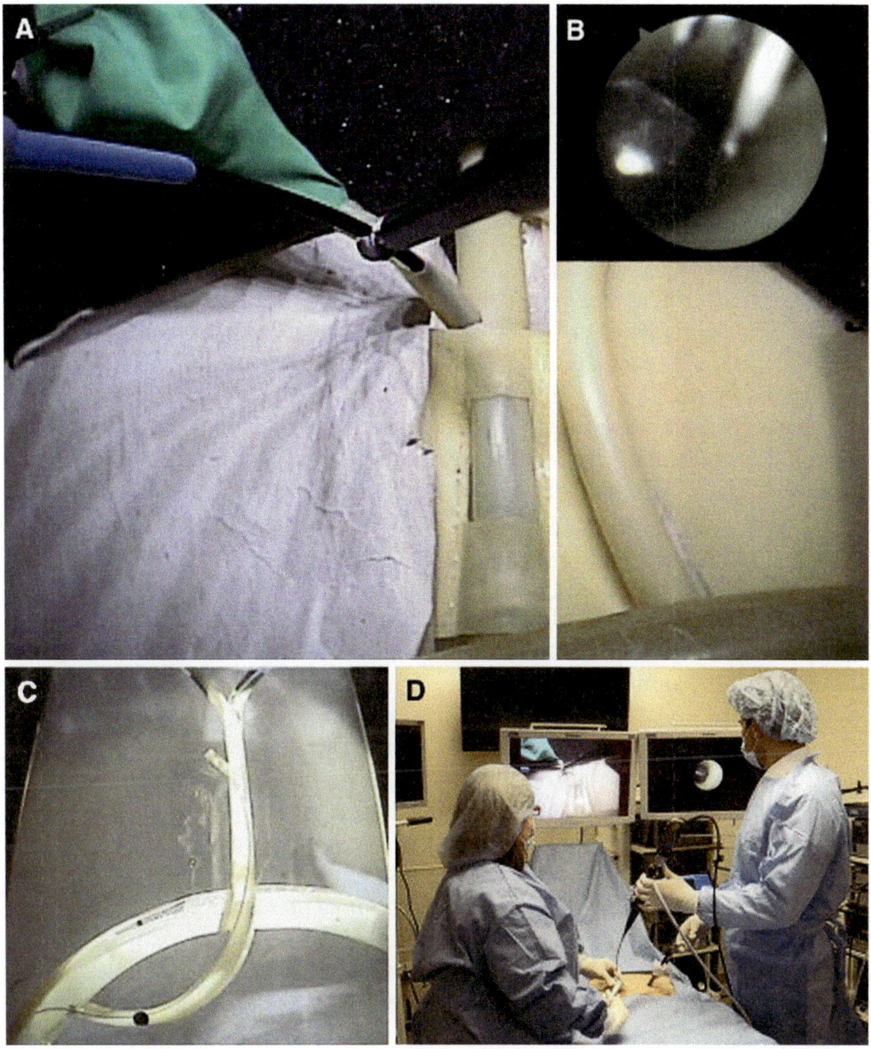

Fig. 12.5 The procedural simulator used for training in a mastery learning curriculum for laparoscopic common bile duct exploration (LCBDE). The simulator replicates the three imaging modalities used during LCBDE: (**A**) laparoscopy, (**B**) flexible choledochoscopy, and (**C**) fluoroscopy. (**D**) An external view of the simulator in use during training is shown. (Figure from Teitelbaum et al. [27]. Reprinted with permission from Elsevier)

We then set out to test inexperienced residents ($n = 15$) and an attending surgeon ($n = 1$) (without prior LCBDE experience) and compared their performance on the simulator to attending surgeons with prior LCBDE experience ($n = 5$) to acquire validity evidence for the simulator and associated rating scale. We found that attending surgeons with prior LCBDE experience had vastly superior overall scores (mean 32.8 (SD = 1.6) vs. 19.6 (SD = 3.3), scale 0–45; $p < 0.01$) and had significantly better performance on 8 of the 12 individual steps of the procedure compared to inexperienced residents [26]. The rating scales also demonstrated good internal consistency and inter-rater reliability (Cronbach's alpha = 0.76; intra-class correlation = 0.92). These data suggested that the LCBDE simulator-based exam produced reliable data that allowed for valid decisions when evaluating procedural performance. The results also guided the *targeted needs assessment* for curriculum development by identifying the specific individual steps of LCBDE that the residents performed poorly.

The next steps were to set *goals and objectives* for the curriculum and then develop *educational strategies* to achieve those goals. The overall goal of the curriculum was to train surgery residents to perform LCBDE effectively and safely. Therefore, since we had already created a procedural algorithm for the operation, the specific curriculum objectives followed the steps of that algorithm. A SBML model was chosen as the educational strategy for the curriculum for several reasons: (a) Using a standardized pre- and posttest enabled tracking of resident progression and ensured a uniform final performance standard; (b) frequent, but relatively short, sessions of deliberate simulator-based practice fit the busy schedules of surgery residents; and (c) SBML allowed for variable pace of progress toward the mastery standard based on individual resident ability.

The final curriculum has didactic written and video-based instructional materials followed by weekly hour-long deliberate practice sessions using the LCBDE-specific simulator. During these sessions, residents deliberately practice multiple iterations of each procedural step while receiving immediate feedback from an expert instructor. The training sessions are bookended by a simulator-based pre- and posttest, with a mastery standard that had been determined by expert faculty using the Angoff standard setting approach described in Chap. 6. For the *implementation* step in the Thomas development model, the curriculum was added as a mandatory component of residents' 10-week minimally invasive surgery rotation. Training sessions were built into a preexisting half-day of "protected" educational time to minimize interference and distractions from clinical responsibilities. Residents performed between three and five practice sessions and took a posttest when they felt confident they could achieve the mastery standard.

All 10 of the senior residents participating in the curriculum were unable to meet the minimum passing standard on the pretest, and all 10 passed the posttest on the first attempt. Mean scores using the LCBDE-specific procedural rating scale doubled from a pretest mean of 20 (SD = 4) to a posttest of 41 (SD = 2; scale 0–45), with a reduced variation (SD) demonstrating more uniformity in final performance (Fig. 12.6) [27]. Additionally, when measured with an objective attitude survey, residents demonstrated increased confidence in their ability to independently and safely perform LCBDE. These results were an encouraging step in the integration of SBML methodology into the curriculum of a general surgery residency. They showed that SBML can be used beyond basic technical skills training with successful application to the teaching of complex, multistep operations.

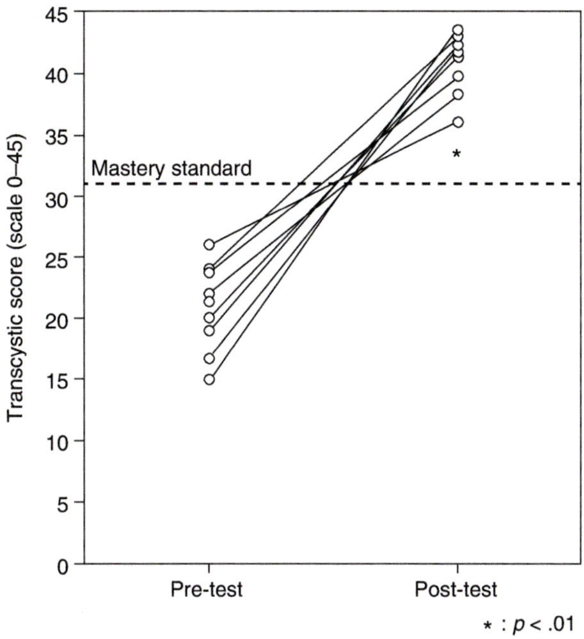

Fig. 12.6 A simulation-based mastery learning curriculum for the laparoscopic common bile duct exploration operation resulted in significantly increased scores when pre- and posttests were compared. All ten residents participating in the curriculum did not meet the minimum passing standard during the pretest, and all ten passed the posttest with little variation in posttest scores. (Figure from Teitelbaum et al. [27]. Reprinted with permission from Elsevier)

Clinical Impact

As seen in the LCBDE curriculum described above, it is important to demonstrate that SBML improves performance on simulator-based exams. However, the ultimate goal of any SBML surgical curriculum is to produce downstream translational science goals such as improved clinical performance and better patient outcomes [28]. Implementation of SBML in surgical education is still in its infancy, but some emerging data demonstrate a "real-world" effect (Chap. 16).

In another study, our research group examined the impact of the LCBDE SBML curriculum on clinical practice at Northwestern Memorial Hospital (NMH), a large tertiary care hospital in Chicago, Illinois [29]. We found that in the years preceding introduction of the curriculum, a mean of 1.7 LCBDE operations was performed annually at the entire institution. After implementation of the SBML training program for residents, this rate increased to 8.4 per year with a peak of 13 LCBDEs during the third year after implementation [29]. Interestingly, in the post-curriculum period, attending surgeons with no prior LCBDE experience were more likely to perform the procedure when assisted by a senior resident who had completed the SBML program. This finding provides evidence that the resident training drove changes in attending surgeon practice at NMH.

When treatment pathways for patients with choledocholithiasis during this period were compared, we found that those treated with LCBDE had a decreased hospital length of stay (mean 2.5 days (SD = 1.8) vs. 4.3 days (SD = 2.2) with LCBDE plus

ERCP; $p < 0.0001$) and lower mean total hospital costs by $2035 ($p = 0.01$, effect size 0.51). Assuming the SBML curriculum was responsible for this increase in clinical use of LCBDE, the curriculum produced a 3.8 to 1 return on investment for NMH. In addition to improving clinical outcomes, evidence demonstrating that SBML curricula reduced overall costs is essential to proving value to healthcare systems administrators and regulators. Without durable funding from institutions, SBML curricula run the risk of becoming "one-off" projects without staying power (see Chap. 19). To prevent this, we subsequently developed a "train the trainers" structure for the LCBDE curriculum in which chief residents who had mastered the SBML training in the prior year then served as instructors for more junior residents. The goal was to produce a self-sustaining curriculum that can function independent of the availability of the few faculty members with LCBDE-specific expertise.

Laparoscopic inguinal hernia repair (LIHR) is another appealing candidate for implementation of a SBML for several reasons. Inguinal hernia repair is one of the most common operations performed by general surgeons making it a focus of residency training. Multiple randomized control trials have demonstrated that a laparoscopic approach to the operation results in decreased pain and faster recovery when compared with traditional open surgery. However, inexperience with LIHR has been clearly linked to adverse outcomes including hernia recurrence rate. One prominent randomized trial defining a threshold of 250 LIHRs is necessary to achieve satisfactory outcomes [30]. This number is much larger than the clinical experience obtained during residency training, during which residents perform a median of 10 LIHR cases [3].

To address these issues, a SBML curriculum for LIHR was designed by Zendejas and colleagues for surgical residents at the Mayo Clinic in Rochester, Minnesota [31]. Its initial component had text- and video-based modules followed by a multiple-choice examination. Only residents who passed this initial written examination were allowed to progress to the simulator-based training portion of the curriculum. Hands-on training was performed on a commercially available LIHR-specific procedural simulator (Limbs and Things, Ltd. Bristol, UK). Residents performed supervised one-on-one training with immediate feedback from an expert instructor. Practice was confined to a single session, and residents trained until they achieved a mastery standard, defined as performing the simulated operation in less than 2 minutes without error.

Fifty surgical residents in the Mayo Clinic surgical residency program were randomized to undergo either (a) the SBML curriculum ($n = 26$) or (b) traditional clinical instruction in LIHR ($n = 24$). Patient outcomes for operations performed by both groups after the training period were then measured. LIHRs performed by the residents randomized to the SBML curriculum had shorter operative times and higher performance ratings when evaluated by attending surgeons who were blinded to group assignment. Intraoperative complications such as tears in the peritoneum, bladder injury, and vessel injury occurred less frequently in the SBML group (7% vs. 29% of patients; $p < 0.01$). Similarly, postoperative complications including urinary retention and surgical site infection were less common in the curriculum group (9% vs. 26%; $p < 0.02$) [31].

This study was the first to demonstrate that a SBML curriculum for a surgical operation resulted in improved patient outcomes. The outcomes are even more striking given the limited amount of time and resources spent on the curriculum. Residents participated in a single session, practicing LIHR on a relatively low-cost synthetic model. However, this practice period led to improved clinical performance and shorter operative times. Remarkably, the SBML curriculum reduced overall postoperative complications by an odds ratio of 0.17 (95% CI, 0.04–0.74) [31]. These results provide strong evidence for further development of procedure-specific SBML in surgical residency training.

Future Directions

While SBML curricula have demonstrated excellent results when applied to medical procedures, the translation of this educational approach to entire surgical operations is still in its infancy, and many hurdles must be overcome to achieve widespread adoption and dissemination. As discussed previously, the implementation of a SBML model in surgery is complex and requires significant resources for curriculum development, simulators, surgical equipment, instruments, and, most importantly, the time of the learners and expert instructors. Organizing frequent deliberate practice sessions for residents and faculty trainers can be difficult in the confines of unpredictable clinical schedules. Several potential strategies may help break down these barriers and pave a pathway to generalizability of SBML within surgical training.

One solution is consolidation of SBML curricula into shorter, more intensive sessions that reach a larger number of learners. Natural venues for such a model are surgical academic conferences and single or multiday courses for residents, fellows, and surgeons in practice. These events make possible simultaneous training of large numbers of highly motivated learners during time protected from competing clinical responsibilities. Such an approach was pilot tested during a simulator-based training course for pediatric surgery fellows [32]. Fellows from programs across the United States participated in a 2-day advanced minimally invasive surgery course where they underwent simulator-based training in LCBDE and other complex pediatric surgical procedures at Northwestern. Over 90% of participants reported an improvement in cognitive and technical skills for the majority of the operations covered. In a separate study evaluating the utility of simulator-based training for LCBDE, pediatric surgery fellows rated the training and simulator as a highly valuable addition to their traditional clinical educational experiences [33].

Another potential avenue for integration of SBML curricula for surgical procedures is their use in continuing medical education or maintenance of certification. Healthcare systems have much to gain from providing their practicing surgeons with opportunities to improve technical and cognitive skills and learn new procedures. By implementing SBML on a system-wide scale, healthcare organizations have the potential to decrease operative times and complications and improve patient outcomes and satisfaction while decreasing costs.

Coda

SBML has proven to be an extremely effective tool for medical education, especially in the realm of teaching procedural and technical skills. It follows that surgical education should be a prime domain for introduction of such curricula. While research into the application of SBML for surgical skills and complex operations is still in its infancy, current results are promising. The examples presented show that implementation of SBML in the surgical arena results in rapid skill acquisition and that groups of learners, including residents and practicing physicians, are able to achieve uniformly high-performance standards. Such curricula for residents have already demonstrated translational effects in terms of improved patient outcomes and increased use of procedures on a hospital-wide scale. Looking to the future, surgical educators must focus on creating sustainable and wide-reaching curricula for an increasing number of skills and procedures.

References

1. Osborne MP. William Stewart Halsted: his life and contributions to surgery. Lancet Oncol. 2007;8(3):256–65.
2. Bilimoria KY, Chung JW, Hedges LV, Dahlke AR, Love R, Cohen ME, et al. National cluster-randomized trial of duty-hour flexibility in surgical training. N Engl J Med. 2016;374(8):713–27.
3. Bell RH Jr, Biester TW, Tabuenca A, Rhodes RS, Cofer JB, Britt LD, et al. Operative experience of residents in US general surgery programs: a gap between expectation and experience. Ann Surg. 2009;249(5):719–24.
4. Malagoni MA, Biester TW, Jones AT, Klingensmith ME, Lewis FR Jr. Operative experience of surgery residents: trends and challenges. J Surg Educ. 2013;70(6):783–8.
5. Mattar SG, Alseidi AA, Jones DB, Jeyarajah DR, Swanstrom LL, Aye RW, et al. General surgery residency inadequately prepares trainees for fellowship: results of a survey of fellowship program directors. Ann Surg. 2013;258(3):440–9.
6. Klingensmith ME, Cogbill TH, Luchette F, Biester T, Samonte K, Jones A, et al. Factors influencing the decision of surgery residency graduates to pursue general surgery practice versus fellowship. Ann Surg. 2015;262(3):449–55.
7. Coleman JJ, Esposito TJ, Rozycki GS, Feliciano DV. Early subspecialization and perceived competence in surgical training: are residents ready? J Am Coll Surg. 2013;216(4):764–73.
8. Napolitano LM, Savarise M, Paramo JC, Soot LC, Todd SR, Gregory J, et al. Are general surgery residents ready to practice? A survey of the American College of Surgeons Board of Governors and Young Fellows Association. J Am Coll Surg. 2014;218(5):1063–72.
9. Schwab B, Hungness E, Barsness KA, McGaghie WC. The role of simulation in surgical education. J Laparoendosc Adv Surg Tech A. 2017;27(5):450–4.
10. Peters JH, Fried GM, Swanstrom LL, Soper NJ, Sillin LF, Schirmer B, et al. Development and validation of a comprehensive program of education and assessment of the basic fundamentals of laparoscopic surgery. Surgery. 2004;135(1):21–7.
11. Strasberg SM, Hertl M, Soper NJ. An analysis of the problem of biliary injury during laparoscopic cholecystectomy. J Am Coll Surg. 1995;180(1):101–25.
12. Fraser SA, Klassen DR, Feldman LS, Ghitulescu GA, Stanbridge D, Fried GM. Evaluating laparoscopic skills: setting the pass/fail score for the MISTELS system. Surg Endosc. 2003;17(6):964–7.
13. McCluney AL, Vassiliou MC, Kaneva PA, Cao J, Stanbridge DD, Feldman LS, et al. FLS simulator performance predicts intraoperative laparoscopic skill. Surg Endosc. 2007;21(11):1991–5.

14. Sroka G, Feldman LS, Vassiliou MC, Kaneva PA, Fayez R, Fried GM. Fundamentals of laparoscopic surgery simulator training to proficiency improves laparoscopic performance in the operating room – a randomized controlled trial. Am J Surg. 2010;199(1): 115–20.
15. Poulose BK, Vassiliou MC, Dunkin BJ, Mellinger JD, Fanelli RD, Martinez JM, et al. Fundamentals of endoscopic surgery cognitive examination: development and validity evidence. Surg Endosc. 2014;28(2):631–8.
16. Vassiliou MC, Dunkin BJ, Fried GM, Mellinger JD, Trus T, Kaneva P, et al. Fundamentals of endoscopic surgery: creation and validation of the hands-on test. Surg Endosc. 2014;28(3):704–11.
17. Gardner AK, Scott DJ, Willis RE, Van Sickle K, Truitt MS, Uecker J, et al. Is current surgery resident and GI fellow training adequate to pass FES? Surg Endosc. 2017;31(1): 352–8.
18. Ritter EM, Taylor ZA, Wolf KR, Franklin BR, Placek SB, Korndorffer JR Jr, et al. Simulation-based mastery learning for endoscopy using the endoscopy training system: a strategy to improve endoscopic skills and prepare for the fundamentals of endoscopic surgery (FES) manual exam. Surg Endosc. 2018;32(1):413–20.
19. Ritter EM, Cox TC, Trinca KD, Pearl JP. Simulated colonoscopy objective performance evaluation (SCOPE): a non-computer-based tool for assessment of endoscopic skills. Surg Endosc. 2013;27(11):4073–80.
20. Trinca KD, Cox TC, Pearl JP, Ritter EM. Validity evidence for the simulated colonoscopy objective performance evaluation scoring system. Am J Surg. 2014;207(2): 218–25.
21. Thomas PA, Kern DE, Hughes MT, Chen BY. Curriculum development for medical education: a six-step approach. 3rd ed. Baltimore: Johns Hopkins University Press; 2016.
22. Cushieri A, Lezoche E, Morino M, Croce E, Lacy A, Toouli J, et al. E.A.E.S. multicenter prospective randomized trial comparing two-stage vs single-stage management of patients with gallstone disease and ductal calculi. Surg Endosc. 1999;13(10):952–7.
23. Noble H, Tranter S, Chesworth T, Norton S, Thompson M. A randomized, clinical trial to compare endoscopic sphincterotomy and subsequent laparoscopic cholecystectomy with primary laparoscopic bile duct exploration during cholecystectomy in higher risk patients with choledocholithiasis. J Laparoendosc Adv Surg Tech A. 2009;19(6):713–20.
24. Wandling MW, Hungness ES, Pavey ES, Stulberg JJ, Schwab B, Yang AD, et al. Nationwide assessment of trends in choledocholithiasis management in the United States from 1998 to 2013. JAMA Surg. 2016;151(12):1125–30.
25. Helling TS, Khandelwal A. The challenges of resident training in complex hepatic, pancreatic, and biliary procedures. J Gastro Surg. 2008;12(1):153–8.
26. Santos BF, Beif TJ, Soper NJ, Nagle AP, Rooney DM, Hungness ES. Development and evaluation of a laparoscopic common bile duct exploration simulator and procedural rating scale. Surg Endosc. 2012;26(9):2403–15.
27. Teitelbaum EN, Soper NJ, Santos BF, Rooney DM, Patel P, Nagle AP, et al. A simulator-based resident curriculum for laparoscopic common bile duct exploration. Surgery. 2014;156(4):880–7, 90–3.
28. McGaghie WC. Medical education research as translational science. Sci Transl Med. 2010;2:19cm8.
29. Schwab B, Teitelbaum EN, Barsuk JH, Soper NJ, Hungness ES. Single-stage laparoscopic management of choledocholithiasis: an analysis after implementation of a mastery learning resident curriculum. Surgery. 2018;163(3):503–8.
30. Neumayer L, Giobbie-Hurder A, Jonasson O, Fitzgibbons R Jr, Dunlop D, Gibbs J, et al. Open mesh versus laparoscopic mesh repair of inguinal hernia. N Engl J Med. 2004;350(18): 1819–27.
31. Zendejas B, Cook DA, Bingener J, Huebner M, Dunn WF, Sarr MG, et al. Simulation-based mastery learning improves patient outcomes in laparoscopic inguinal hernia repair: a randomized controlled trial. Ann Surg. 2011;254(3):502–11.

32. Gause CD, Hsiung G, Schwab B, Clifton M, Harmon CM, Barsness KA. Advances in pediatric surgical education: a critical appraisal of two consecutive minimally invasive pediatric surgery training courses. J Laparoendosc Adv Surg Tech A. 2016;26(8):663–70.
33. Schwab B, Rooney DM, Hungness ES, Barsness KA. Preliminary evaluation of a laparoscopic common bile duct simulator for pediatric surgical education. J Laparoendosc Adv Surg Tech A. 2016;26(10):831–5.
34. Vassiliou, et al. FLS and FES: comprehensive models of training and assessment. Surg Clin North Am. 2010;90(3):535–48.

Mastery Learning of Bedside Procedural Skills

13

Jeffrey H. Barsuk, Elaine R. Cohen, and Diane B. Wayne

Mr. Campbell is a 57-year-old male with a history of diabetes and hypertension. He presented to the emergency department with a 2-day history of fever, cough, and shortness of breath. His chest x-ray showed findings consistent with a right lower lobe pneumonia. His vital signs (hypotension, tachycardia, and fever) and laboratory results (acute kidney injury) suggested sepsis. A clinical decision was made to insert a large intravenous (IV) line (central venous catheter (CVC)) into his right internal jugular vein to measure pressures and oxygenation in his central venous system and infuse vasopressor drugs. The attending physician inserted the CVC, but the carotid artery was cannulated instead of the intended vein. Mr. Campbell's care was delayed due to a lack of central venous access. He also required an invasive surgical procedure to remove the catheter safely. This is a common example used to highlight patient safety regarding bedside procedures. Mr. Campbell's case highlights the problem that variable skills among caregivers have important downstream effects on patient care quality.

Hospitals, professional boards, and government agencies certify and license clinicians to perform patient care competently [1]. Organizations such as the Accreditation Council for Graduate Medical Education (ACGME), the American Board of Internal Medicine (ABIM), the American Board of Surgery (ABS), and many others in nursing, pharmacy, physical therapy, and other health professions continue to require fulfillment of time-based training, often including an arbitrary, fixed number of procedures [2–4]. Individual hospitals may also ground physician procedure privileging decisions on clinical experience numbers. For example, to

J. H. Barsuk (✉) · D. B. Wayne
Northwestern University Feinberg School of Medicine, Departments of Medicine and Medical Education, Chicago, IL, USA
e-mail: jbarsuk@northwestern.edu; dwayne@northwestern.edu

E. R. Cohen
Northwestern University Feinberg School of Medicine, Department of Medicine, Chicago, IL, USA

W. C. McGaghie et al. (eds.), *Comprehensive Healthcare Simulation: Mastery Learning in Health Professions Education*, Comprehensive Healthcare Simulation, https://doi.org/10.1007/978-3-030-34811-3_13

obtain hospital privileges to perform CVC insertion, a physician may have to document five or ten procedures performed during residency. A step above this is the requirement, often used in nursing, that clinical skills are assessed at regular intervals. An example of this would be annual assessment of CVC maintenance skills among ICU nurses. Direct observation is more rigorous than reliance on procedure numbers alone, but only rigorous, reliable assessments should be used to make high-stakes decisions. Use of competency-based health professions education with reliance on rigorous measurement has increased dramatically over the past decade. However, more attention is needed to change healthcare systems to ensure that clinical experience alone is never used as a proxy for actual competence. Clinical skills measured precisely and compared to a high standard will contribute to safe patient care with the lowest possible rate of preventable errors.

Research reveals the consequences of a lack of rigorous assessment of procedural competence among healthcare providers. Many studies show that nurses, medical residents, fellows, and attending physicians demonstrate uneven performance in a variety of clinical skills despite significant patient care experience. This finding is consistent across procedures such as CVC insertion, CVC maintenance, lumbar puncture, and thoracentesis [5–11] despite completion of more than the minimum number of procedures required by specialty boards and licensing bodies.

A majority of studies covered in a systematic review by Choudhry and colleagues showed that highly experienced physicians provided lower-quality care than less experienced physicians [12]. Another recent study evaluated video-recorded polypectomies performed by gastroenterologists with at least 3 years of practice experience who had performed at least 150 screening colonoscopies in the prior year [13]. Despite clinical experience, the investigators reported wide variation in clinical skill. Only 64% of the polypectomies were graded as satisfactory. A recent research synthesis noted only a weak positive association between resident physician self-reported experience and simulated procedure performance [14]. However, overall performance was poor even among the most experienced residents.

Clinical experience is not a proxy for skill even though some studies suggest with weak data that completion of a larger number of procedures is correlated with safer care and fewer complications. Suggested numbers are more than 50 CVC insertions [15], 80 screening colonoscopies [16], and more than 1000 for complex procedures such as laparoscopic bariatric surgery [17]. Such procedure numbers are difficult to reach during training, and supervising physicians have little confidence that the numbers arbitrarily set accurately measure competence [18]. Taken together, the literature shows that clinical experience is not a skill proxy and that rigorous assessment of competence is needed to ensure patient safety.

Self-confidence is used occasionally as a surrogate for clinician skill acquisition. Multiple studies also show that procedural self-confidence does not predict performance [8–11] and should not be used as a competence surrogate [18]. In one study, attending physicians were extremely confident inserting internal jugular CVCs [6]. However, rigorous assessment showed the use of full sterile barrier and ultrasound imaging were often performed incorrectly. CVC incompetence may be due to the absence of post-residency refresher training which prevents practicing physicians from using newer techniques such as ultrasound. Practicing providers can be falsely confident about their procedural skills because they are not familiar with new best practices.

Simulation-based mastery learning (SBML) makes documenting procedural competence easy, consistent, and reliable. In SBML, trainees must meet or exceed a set minimum passing standard (MPS) in a simulated environment before performing a clinical procedure on patients [19]. Evidence shows that SBML is a more effective strategy than traditional clinical education alone [20–22], and use of this model ensures healthcare providers consistently meet competency standards for the procedures they perform [5, 8–10, 23, 24].

The rest of this chapter reviews published research using SBML to document bedside procedural skill competence. The chapter focuses on the patient care, communication, diagnostic, and physical examination skills needed to perform bedside procedures. In addition to covering past research, we use the four Ts of translational science [25–27] to review evidence about the effectiveness of SBML for bedside procedural skills and how its use improves patient care (Chap. 16).

Table 13.1 shows that SBML interventions have been used for many bedside procedures and linked to downstream translational patient outcomes. This chapter will focus on a subset of procedures shown in Table 13.1 (thoracentesis, CVC insertion and maintenance, and paracentesis) that have been evaluated and linked to T1–T4 translational science outcomes (see Chaps. 3 and 16). T1 outcomes show improvements in learner skills and attitudes demonstrated in the simulation laboratory due to powerful SBML interventions; T2 outcomes demonstrate SBML improvements in patient care practices; T3 results link SBML programs with patient outcomes; and T4 outcomes demonstrate unanticipated effects from powerful SBML interventions. We developed all of the SBML training for the above procedures using the Thomas and Kern curriculum development framework.

General Considerations

Studies that demonstrate improved bedside procedural skill acquisition share two common themes: (a) mastery learning (ML) and (b) deliberate practice (DP) [41]. When engaged in ML with DP, learners work hard on a focused task, while their coach or teacher provides actionable feedback that learners can use to improve (Chap. 4). Trainees are expected to learn and accomplish each clinical procedure from start to finish. Procedure components are practiced repetitively as needed. DP allows for mindful focus and incorporation of individualized feedback [41, 42]. In addition to DP, other core components of SBML interventions include standardized curricula, a set MPS derived by an expert panel, and debriefing. Another core principle of mastery learning is that learners who do not meet the MPS at posttest return to the skills laboratory or another educational setting for additional skills practice and retesting until the MPS is reached. Multiple studies show that the rigorous education provided in SBML is a powerful quality improvement strategy that leads to improved patient care outcomes [7, 8, 31, 35, 40].

Table 13.1 Bedside procedural skill training using SBML and translational science outcomes (T1–T4). CLABSI = Central Line-Associated Bloodstream Infection; IR = Interventional Radiology

Procedure	T1 outcomes	T2 outcomes	T3 outcomes	T4 outcomes
Cardiac auscultation	SBML-trained medical students performed better than traditionally trained students in the simulation lab [28]	SBML-trained students performed better than traditionally trained students with real patients [28]	–	–
Central venous catheter	SBML-trained internal medicine and emergency medicine residents' scores improved from pre- to posttest in the simulation lab [7, 8]	SBML-trained residents reported fewer needle passes, arterial punctures, and line adjustments compared to traditionally trained residents [7, 8]	Fewer CLABSIs in ICU after SBML-trained residents entered compared to both the same unit prior to training and a comparison ICU [29]	Cost savings from reduction in CLABSIs compared to cost of SBML intervention (7:1 return) and successful dissemination of SBML intervention with similar results [30, 31]
Spinal anesthesia	SBML-trained anesthesia residents had a greater pre- to posttest improvement compared to traditionally trained residents in the simulation lab [32]			
Forceps delivery	SBML-trained obstetrics and gynecology residents' scores improved from pre- to posttest in the simulation lab [33]	–	Reduction in severe perineal laceration among women delivered by residents who had completed SBML [33]	–
Laryngoscopy	SBML-trained emergency medicine residents performed better than traditionally trained residents in the simulation lab [34]	–	–	–
Lumbar puncture	SBML-trained first-year internal medicine residents performed better than traditionally trained neurology residents in the simulation lab [10]	–	–	–

Table 13.1 (continued)

Procedure	T1 outcomes	T2 outcomes	T3 outcomes	T4 outcomes
Paracentesis	SBML-trained internal medicine residents' scores improved from pre- to posttest in the simulation lab [23]	Unnecessary platelet and fresh frozen plasma transfusions were less common in patients undergoing procedures by SBML-trained residents [35]	Paracentesis procedures performed at the bedside by SBML-trained residents resulted in equal or better patient outcomes than procedures in IR [35]	Costs incurred for an IR paracentesis procedure were more than the cost of a bedside paracentesis performed by SBML-trained residents [36]
Melanoma screening	SBML-trained primary care physicians performed better than traditionally trained physicians in the simulation lab [37]	–	–	–
Temporary hemodialysis catheter	SBML-trained first-year nephrology fellows improved from pre- to posttest in the simulation lab and performed better than traditionally trained graduating fellows [5]	SBML-trained fellows scored similarly during 6-month THDC insertions on actual patients and immediate posttest [38]	–	–
Thoracentesis	SBML-trained internal medicine residents' scores improved from pre- to posttest in the simulation lab [11]	SBML-trained residents were more likely to perform bedside thoracenteses compared to traditionally trained residents and hospitalist physicians [39]	SBML-trained residents performed thoracenteses with lower rates of clinically meaningful complications compared to traditionally trained residents and referred procedures [40]	Potential savings in extra costs and hospital days [40]

Thoracentesis

Thoracentesis is a diagnostic and therapeutic bedside procedure in which a large needle is used to drain abnormal fluid from the space between the chest wall and lung. Serious complications such as pneumothorax (damaging the lung and releasing air into the chest) and bleeding can occur if thoracentesis is performed incorrectly. In a series of studies at Northwestern University Feinberg School of Medicine, we evaluated T1 outcomes (skills and knowledge) [11, 39], T2 outcomes (patient care) [39], T3 outcomes (clinical patient outcomes) [40], and T4 outcomes (cost reduction) [40].

The Northwestern thoracentesis SBML program began in 2006 when we became aware of published research using a national sample of internal medicine residents that demonstrated trainees were uncomfortable performing thoracentesis procedures [43]. This was a real medical education challenge because the American Board of Internal Medicine required thoracentesis procedure competence as a graduation requirement [11]. At Northwestern, a targeted needs assessment including discussions with internal medicine trainees revealed that thoracentesis competence was a local as well as a national concern.

We developed a SBML thoracentesis curriculum for third-year (graduating) residents in January 2006. The objective was that all third-year residents would demonstrate thoracentesis competence. Specifically, all graduating residents would meet or exceed a MPS on a simulated thoracentesis mannequin, graded using a skills checklist, before the end of training.

We selected SBML as our educational strategy because it had been previously shown to be effective and highly regarded by internal medicine residents learning advanced cardiac life support protocols [24]. Deliberate practice (DP) was a core component of the SBML curriculum. We developed multiple-choice written examinations and a thoracentesis skills checklist using strategies described in Chap. 3 including review of relevant literature and techniques described by Stufflebeam [44]. Pre- and post-written examinations were created so that each was equally difficult and covered identical content (Chap. 3). An expert panel provided feedback about the initial written examinations and skills checklist allowing for revisions using the modified Delphi technique. The final thoracentesis skills checklist can be found in Appendix 13.1.

The first step in the SBML curriculum required residents to complete a pretest. The pretest included the multiple-choice written examination and a simulated thoracentesis procedure measured by the skills checklist. The pretest is a key feature of mastery learning education interventions. After the pretest, residents watched a lecture discussing thoracentesis indications, contraindications, and complications. Learners also watched a video demonstrating thoracentesis techniques. Next, learners engaged in DP on a thoracentesis simulator with 1:1 supervision and feedback from a trained faculty instructor. Residents subsequently completed a posttest involving a complete simulated thoracentesis including obtaining informed consent, performing the procedure, and providing post-procedure instructions. Each resident was graded using the skills checklist and was required to meet or exceed the MPS. Each resident also completed a written examination posttest.

An expert panel set the MPS at 80% (20/25 items correct on the thoracentesis skills checklist) using the Angoff and Hofstee standard setting methods before launching the curriculum. The interrater reliability (kappa coefficient) for the skills checklist data was 0.94. Checklists were not shared with trainees, but each skill evaluated by the checklist was included in the video, lecture, and deliberate practice sessions. The reliability coefficients (KR-20) for the pre- and post-written examinations were 0.72 and 0.74, respectively.

Implementation across all residents was feasible because participation in the SBML curriculum was required by the training program director. Earlier success with ACLS also led to resident excitement about thoracentesis mastery training [24]. Core program faculty members served as the instructors for the SBML program. The Department of Medicine purchased a thoracentesis simulator and provided training space and scheduling staff. Forty graduating internal medicine residents were eligible to participate in the initial SBML thoracentesis intervention, and all completed the protocol.

T1 Thoracentesis Outcomes

The thoracentesis SBML program was very effective revealed by several T1 outcomes. Simulated skill performance improved from 51.7% (SD = 15.1) items correct at pretest to 88.3% (SD = 8.1) items correct at posttest, $p < 0.001$. Written examination performance improved from 57.6% to 89.8% items correct $p < 0.001$ [11]. A small number of learners (7%) who did not originally meet the MPS returned for additional skills practice and retesting until they achieved the MPS. At the end of training, all learners met or exceeded the MPS on the simulated thoracentesis procedure. Learners also felt the program raised their skills and improved their self-confidence and that the simulation sessions were a valuable addition to their clinical education [11].

Periodic refinement and updating is a critical component of successful SBML programs. We revisited thoracentesis procedure training several years later to update the curriculum and investigate skill retention and downstream patient outcomes as part of our continuous quality improvement process [45]. With new funding from the Agency for Healthcare Research and Quality, we updated the curriculum with a new online interactive lecture and video that learners could review on their own time. Due to new clinical standards, we incorporated ultrasound use into the teaching program and assessment (skills checklist) [40]. We reconvened an expert panel to determine the MPS for the amended checklist which was set at 84.3% (22/26 items correct) [39, 40]. The updated curriculum included all the core features of SBML such as (a) a skills pretest on the simulator; (b) deliberate practice with individualized, actionable feedback; and (c) a simulated skills posttest. We employed a randomized wait-list control design for the study, and 112 internal medicine residents participated. Similar improvements in pre- to posttest performance were observed as internal medicine residents' thoracentesis skills improved from mean 60.3% checklist items correct at pretest (SD = 20.3) to 96.7% checklist items correct at posttest (SD = 3.7) ($p < 0.001$) [40]. Thirty-six residents participated in follow-up testing at 6 months and 1 year to assess skill retention. At 6 months, mean performance was 92.0% items correct (SD = 7.5) and at 1 year 93.9% (SD = 5.0%). Eight residents did not meet or exceed the MPS at the 6-month retest. One resident did not meet the MPS after 1 year. Residents who did not meet the MPS completed additional skill training and were retested until they could meet or exceed the MPS. Of note, skills retention may be considered a T1 or T4 outcome (Chap. 16).

T2 Thoracentesis Outcomes

An important goal of our next thoracentesis SBML study was to evaluate T2 outcomes. We compared clinical referral patterns between traditionally trained residents (who did not receive the SBML intervention) and SMBL-trained residents [39]. We found that traditionally trained residents were more likely to not perform the procedure at the bedside and referred their patients to interventional radiology (IR) instead. Traditionally trained residents cited low self-confidence and perceived competence as the reasons for this clinical decision. Conversely, after completing the education protocol, SBML-trained residents were more likely to perform thoracentesis procedures at the bedside rather than referring them to IR, a more expensive and resource-intensive option [39].

T3 and T4 Thoracentesis Outcomes

The final study in our thoracentesis research program focused on T3 and T4 outcomes and assessed actual procedures performed during clinical care. We compared outcomes of procedures performed by four groups of clinicians: (a) traditionally trained residents, (b) SBML-trained residents, (c) pulmonary medicine specialists, and (d) IR [40]. We found that SBML-trained residents caused fewer clinically meaningful iatrogenic pneumothoraces compared to all other groups ($p = 0.02$; T3 outcome). SBML-trained residents also performed procedures with lower combined clinically meaningful complications compared with other groups ($p = 0.008$; T3 outcome) [40]. SBML-trained residents performed procedures with a trend toward lower combined clinically meaningful complications (iatrogenic pneumothorax, hemothorax, re-expansion pulmonary edema) compared with only traditionally trained residents (0% vs. 7.9%; $p = 0.06$ (Table 13.2)) [40]. Based on our results and data from the University HealthSystem Consortium, we estimated that widespread thoracentesis SBML training could save an estimated $4.9 million and 1194 hospital days in the United States due to a reduction in clinically meaningful iatrogenic pneumothoraces (T4 outcome) [40].

A critical review of the SBML education research agenda shows that thoracentesis SBML is linked to T1 through T4 outcomes. SBML was superior to the traditional apprenticeship model of learning because internal medicine residents were not well prepared to enter into practice and perform thoracentesis procedures in the traditional model (T1 outcome). Additional investigation also yielded sustained and meaningful clinical benefits to patients and the healthcare system (T2–T4 outcomes) from this intervention.

Table 13.2 Thoracentesis procedure complications in patient procedures performed by simulation-based mastery learning (SBML)-trained and traditionally trained residents and procedures referred to pulmonary medicine or interventional radiology (IR)

Clinical outcomes	SBML-trained resident procedures $N = 58$	Traditionally trained resident procedures $N = 63$	Pulmonary medicine procedures $N = 297$	IR procedures $N = 499$	P-value chi-square
Any iatrogenic pneumothorax (n, %)	5 (8.6%)	6 (9.5%)	20 (6.7%)	29 (5.8%)	0.62
Iatrogenic pneumothorax requiring intervention (n, %)	0	3 (4.8%)	1 (0.3%)	3 (0.6%)	0.02
Hemothorax (n, %)	0	2 (3.2%)	1 (0.3%)	1 (0.2%)	0.07
Re-expansion pulmonary edema (n, %)	0	0	1 (0.3%)	2 (0.4%)	1.0
Combined clinically meaningful complications (pneumothorax, hemothorax, and REPE)	0	5 (7.9%)	3 (1%)	6 (1.2%)	0.008

Adapted with permission from Barsuk et al. [40]

CVC Insertion and Maintenance Skills

CVCs are intravenous catheters that are inserted into the large veins of the neck, chest, or groin. They are used in critically ill patients to monitor vital signs and deliver medications. Insertion and maintenance of a CVC is a complex procedure usually done to care for very sick patients. Only healthcare providers who understand CVC indications, contraindications, and complications and have documented competency should insert a CVC. After a CVC is inserted, it can be used to infuse medications and draw blood. Nurses who access CVCs must also be trained to ensure that sterile technique is continuously maintained during access and dressing changes. Training for CVC insertion is necessary because complications during CVC insertion such as iatrogenic pneumothorax and arterial puncture can be life-threatening [15]. Furthermore, central line-associated bloodstream infection (CLABSI) is another life-threatening complication that can occur during CVC insertion and/or maintenance [15].

In 2008, hospitals in the United States began intense efforts to reduce hospital-acquired complications such as CLABSI because the Centers for Medicare and Medicaid Services announced these publically reported conditions would no longer be reimbursed [46]. This national pressure also affected academic institutions where CVC insertion is done by resident and subspecialty fellow physicians whose skills are often untested. We developed a CVC insertion SBML curriculum to address this education need. Consistent with our other curricula, CVC insertion SBML provided standardized learning objectives and feedback as well as the requirement that all learners meet or exceed a predetermined MPS before completion of training (Chap. 3). Residents at our institution are not allowed to perform CVC insertions on patients until this requirement is met. In addition to curriculum development and assessment of education outcomes, our research group designed studies to measure the impact of the curriculum on CVC insertion clinical care.

Our teaching strategy included the key instructional components of SBML interventions described in Chap. 4 including a strong dose of DP. Trainees first completed a simulated CVC insertion and written examination pretest. Next, they watched a digital video lecture that included a step-by-step demonstration of how to perform an ultrasound-guided CVC insertion at either the internal jugular (IJ) or subclavian (SC) site. After this didactic content, each learner participated in DP of CVC insertion with individualized feedback from a trained instructor. Finally, trainees completed a simulated skills and written examination posttest and were required to meet or exceed a predetermined MPS on the clinical skills examination. Trainees who did not meet the MPS at initial posttest were referred back to the simulation center for additional skills practice and retesting until the MPS was reached.

We used the techniques described in Chap. 3 to develop the written examinations and CVC insertion skills checklist. After initial 27-item IJ and SC checklists were developed, an expert panel refined the checklist using the modified Delphi technique. The MPS was set at 79.1% items correct using the average of the Angoff and Hofstee techniques for both the IJ and SC checklists (requiring 22/27 items correct). After setting the MPS for CVC insertion skills, the expert judges determined that two checklist items (cannulation of vein and use of two or fewer needle passes through the skin to complete the procedure) could not be missed. This meant that if a learner used more than two needle passes through the skin or cannulated the artery, a passing score could not be achieved and additional skills practice was necessary. The checklists were later revised as part of our curriculum quality improvement process and now include 29 items each. The final 29-item checklists for IJ and SC CVC insertion can be found in Appendix 13.2. A panel of clinical experts used the Angoff and Hofstee standard setting techniques to set new MPSs for the 29-item checklists. This MPS was set at 88% items correct for the IJ CVC insertion checklist and 87% items correct for the SC CVC insertion checklist (requiring 26/29 items correct on each checklist). There was high interrater reliability for the IJ and SC checklists ranging from Cohen's kappa of 0.83–0.94 [6–8].

Implementation of a SBML intervention is never easy, and support from the Department of Medicine and Northwestern Memorial Hospital (NMH) leadership was critical to the success of this project. Key faculty members with dedicated academic time and clinical expertise served as faculty trainers. Faculty members purchased an ultrasound device and a CVC insertion simulator with funding from NMH. The Department of Medicine also provided administrative oversight to help schedule residents for training sessions. We used "just in time training" for all internal medicine and emergency medicine residents who were about to rotate through the medical intensive care unit (MICU) at our institution. Residents completed CVC insertion SBML the month before their MICU rotation and were required to meet or exceed the MPS before attempting any supervised CVC insertions on MICU patients. The program director of the internal medicine residency program and the medical director of the MICU were critical partners to ensure this occurred.

The curriculum was launched in 2006, and we began an iterative process to evaluate and refine it over the next decade. Modifications and improvements were based on learner and instructor feedback, review of educational and clinical outcomes, and changes in clinical practice standards. We cover translational science outcomes in the next sections.

T1 CVC Insertion Outcomes

We studied the education outcomes of 41 internal medicine resident physicians who completed CVC insertion SBML prior to their MICU rotations [7]. At pretest, none of the residents about to rotate in the MICU met the MPS for CVC insertion at the IJ or the SC sites (mean 48.4% (SD = 23.1) items correct and mean 45.2% (SD = 26.3) items correct, respectively). Although a small fraction of residents required additional DP and retesting, all residents reached or exceeded the MPS at final posttest (mean IJ score 94.8% (SD = 10.0) items correct, mean SC score 91.1% (SD = 17.8) checklist items correct, both $p < 0.001$) as required by the 4 hour SBML protocol [7]. Residents who participated in SBML also reported higher levels of self-confidence inserting CVCs in MICU patients than residents who did not participate in SBML training ($p = 0.02$) [7].

We performed a follow-up study on a new cohort of 76 internal medicine and emergency residents who were about to rotate in the NMH MICU [8]. At pretest, only 12 residents (16%) met the MPS for IJ CVC insertion skills, and 11 (14%) met the MPS for SC CVC insertion skills. Despite meeting or exceeding the MPS, these residents all voluntarily completed SBML training because they believed they would benefit from participation. The mean IJ skills checklist score at pretest was 50.6% (SD = 23.4) items correct and 48.4% (SD = 26.8) items correct for SC. After training, mean posttest scores improved to 93.9% (SD = 10.2) items correct for IJ and 91.5% (SD = 17.1) items correct for SC (both $p < 0.0005$). Written exam scores improved from a pretest mean of 70.3% (SD = 7.7) items correct to 84.8% (SD = 4.8) items correct, $p < 0.0005$ [8].

We implemented our curriculum at a local academic community hospital to compare results across institutions and assess the potential for dissemination of our CVC insertion SBML model [31]. At this site, fifty-one residents completed the SBML protocol. Yet only three (6%) met the MPS at pretest for the IJ CVC insertion and four (8%) for the SC CVC insertion. Mean IJ pretest scores were 35.5% (SD = 8.3) items correct and 23.0% (SD = 9.6) items correct for simulated SC CVC insertion. At posttest, residents at this second institution performed very similar to residents in the original NMH cohorts. Mean posttest scores were 93.0% (SD = 1.5) items correct for IJ CVC insertion and 96.1% (SD = 1.4) items correct for SC CVC insertion, both $p < 0.001$ compared to pretests.

In a final study demonstrating T1 outcomes, we implemented our CVC insertion SBML curriculum at 58 Veterans Affairs Medical Centers (VAMC) across the United States [6]. We developed a train-the-trainer curriculum to teach attending physicians to deliver the SBML CVC insertion curriculum to their colleagues. Each participating VAMC selected 1–3 attending physicians who performed CVC insertions independently and supervised insertions by residents and fellows to participate in the train-the-trainer curriculum. One hundred and eight attending physicians participated in the study and averaged 20 years in practice. Each attending physician performed a simulated IJ or SC CVC insertion as part of the train-the-trainer curriculum [6]. This included 67 simulated IJ and 47 simulated subclavian assessments (six attending physicians performed both assessments) [6]. Somewhat surprisingly, these expert attending physicians performed poorly with a mean IJ CVC insertion score of 72.6% (SD = 19.0) checklist items correct and mean subclavian CVC insertion score of 71.4% (SD = 21.6%) checklist items correct. Only 12 of 67 (17.9%) attending physicians met the MPS for IJ CVC insertion, and only 11 of 47 (23.4%) met the MPS for SC CVC insertion. Among physicians who reported inserting at least 500 CVCs during clinical practice, only one of 10 (10%) met the MPS for the IJ clinical skills assessment, and only four of nine (44%) met the MPS for the subclavian CVC clinical skills assessment.

Although we had convincing evidence about the immediate impact of CVC insertion SBML on T1 education outcomes, we did not know if the skills were retained over time. Thus we assessed clinical skill retention after SBML with a sample of 49 internal medicine residents. These residents completed SBML and returned to the simulation laboratory for additional assessments using the CVC insertion skills checklists 6 months and 1 year after initial training [47]. Mean scores during follow-up testing remained high but fell from immediate posttest. The mean immediate posttest score for IJ CVC insertion was 96.5% (SD = 4.7), 84.6% (SD = 18.9) at 6 months, and 87.9% (SD = 16.1) at 1 year ($p < 0.001$). For SC, residents scored 94.6% (SD = 10.6) at posttest, 88.2% (SD = 15.8) at 6 months, and 88.2% (SD = 16.8) at 1 year ($p = 0.002$). For IJ CVC insertion, all participants met the MPS at immediate posttest, 82.4% met the MPS at 6 months, and 87.1% met the MPS at 1 year ($p = 0.013$). For SC CVC insertion, all participants met the MPS at immediate posttest, 85.3% met the MPS at 6 months, and 83.9% met the MPS at 1-year follow-up ($p = 0.016$) [47]. Examinees who did not meet the MPS were different on each follow-up occasion. Demographic and clinical information such as postgraduate year of training, number of CVC insertions performed in clinical practice, or self-confidence did not predict the residents who did not meet the MPS at follow-up testing. Based on these results, we concluded that CVC reassessment should be performed every 6 months [47].

Our research findings, including a national sample of practicing physicians, make a strong argument that traditional training is inadequate to ensure that physicians are competent to insert CVCs. However, SBML is a proven strategy that produces a high level of competence among physicians who insert CVCs. Based on our findings, we recommend that all healthcare providers who insert CVCs undergo rigorous training and assessment similar to the SBML curriculum. The following sections address the downstream patient impact of CVC insertion SBML.

T2 CVC Insertion Outcomes

Two studies from Northwestern University (NMH) evaluated the impact of CVC insertion SBML on patient care practices. In a pilot study [7], the outcomes of CVC insertions by 13 internal medicine residents rotating in the MICU before the SBML training intervention began were compared to the outcomes of CVC insertions performed by 28 internal medicine residents who completed CVC insertion SBML. Forty-six CVCs were inserted during the study period. SBML-trained residents required fewer needle passes than non-SBML-trained residents ($p = 0.04$) to successfully insert CVCs into actual MICU patients [7]. This was an important finding because the number of needle passes during insertion is directly linked to serious complications such as pneumothorax. In a larger follow-up study, CVC insertion patient care practices were compared between 76 SBML-trained internal medicine and emergency medicine residents and 27 non-SBML-trained (traditionally trained) residents rotating in the MICU [8]. In a pre- and post-intervention comparison (4 months pre-intervention and 8 months post intervention), SBML-trained residents reported fewer needle passes ($p < 0.0005$), arterial punctures ($p < 0.0005$), need for catheter adjustments ($p = 0.002$), and higher success rates ($p < 0.005$) for CVC insertions in MICU patients than non-SBML-trained residents.

T3 CVC Insertion Outcomes

We next performed a study to evaluate the effect of our SBML insertion curriculum on CLABSI rates, an important patient safety outcome [29]. Ninety-two internal medicine and emergency medicine residents completed SBML training before rotating in the NMH MICU from December 2006 to February 2008. Outcomes of CVC insertions from these residents were compared to a historical control group of residents who did not complete SBML and rotated in the NMH MICU from August 2005 to December 2006 and a concurrent control group of residents who did not complete SBML and rotated in the NMH surgical ICU from August 2005 to February 2008. CLABSI rates were reported per routine guidelines by the NMH infection control team during the entire study period. There were 3.20 CLABSIs per 1000 catheter days in the MICU and 4.86 per 1000 catheter days in the surgical ICU during the pre-SBML intervention period (16 months). CLABSI rates sharply decreased to 0.50 per 1000 catheter days in the MICU after the SBML intervention (16 months), despite a higher severity of illness in patients during the post-intervention period in the MICU ($p = 0.001$). However, the surgical ICU CLABSI rate was 5.26 per 1000 catheter days during this same period. The reduction in infections in the MICU remained significant after including the surgical ICU infections and patient comorbidities as independent variables ($p = 0.001$, Fig. 13.1). Based on these findings, we concluded that SBML was responsible for the 85% (95% CI, 56–95%) reduction in CLABSI rates in the MICU, while rates in the surgical ICU remained elevated.

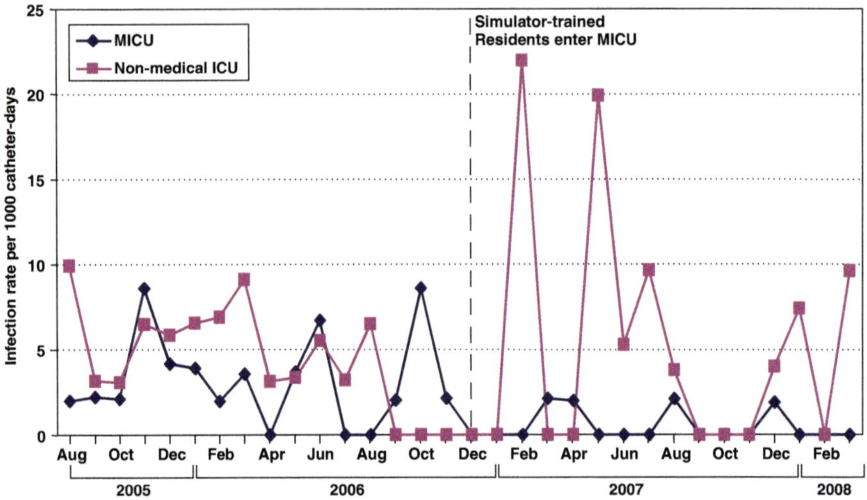

Fig. 13.1 CLABSIs in the medical and surgical ICUs before and after SBML-trained residents rotate in the medical ICU. (Reprinted with permission from Barsuk et al. [29])

To study the impact of SBML on CLABSI rates at another institution, we disseminated our intervention at a local academic community hospital [31]. We compared CLABSI rates in the community hospital MICU from a pre-intervention period of October 2008 to August 2010 to a post-intervention period from September 2010 to May 2012. Fifty-one internal medicine and emergency medicine residents completed the SBML intervention using our protocol and subsequently rotated in the MICU during the post-intervention period. There were 3.82 CLABSIs per 1000 catheter days in the MICU during the pre-intervention period and only 1.29 CLABSIs per 1000 catheter days after the intervention ($p = 0.019$). This translated into a 74% reduction in CLABSI rates (95% CI, 26–91%) during the post-intervention period after controlling for patient severity of illness (Fig. 13.2), thereby reproducing the T3 outcome of CLABSI reduction in a second hospital setting.

T4 CVC Insertion Outcomes

Collateral Effects

The Northwestern CVC SBML training was required for second- and third-year residents 1 month before they rotated through the MICU. Longitudinal pretest data showed that a growing number of residents were meeting or exceeding the MPS without any training. Statistical evaluation confirmed this observation because the passing rate for IJ CVC insertion at baseline was 7% in 2007, 16% in 2008, and 38% in 2009 ($p = 0.004$). Similarly, the pretest passing rate for SC CVC insertion was 11% in 2007, 19% in 2008, and 38% in 2009 ($p = 0.028$) [48]. This increase was also confirmed when assessing mean pretest scores because mean IJ pretest

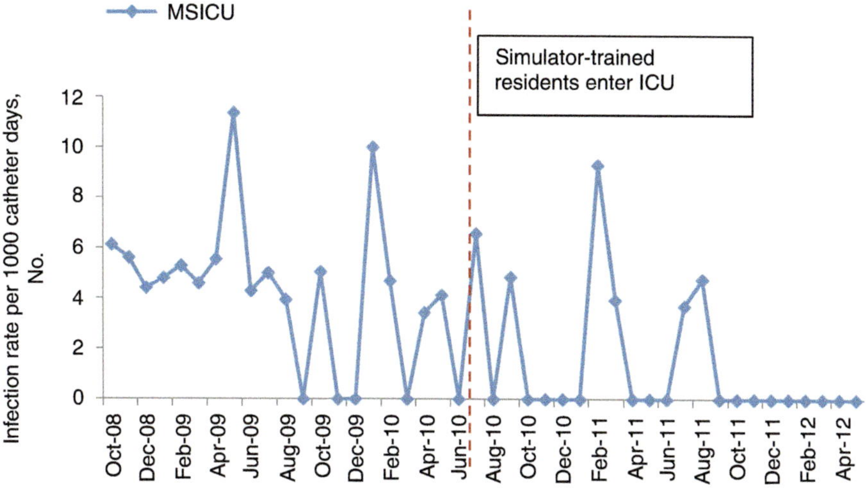

Fig. 13.2 Central line-associated bloodstream infections in the medical intensive care unit before and after SBML-trained residents rotated. (Adapted with permission from Barsuk et al. [40])

scores improved from 46.7% (SD = 20.8%) in 2007 to 55.7% (SD = 22.5%) in 2008 and to 70.8% (SD = 22.4%) in 2009 ($p < 0.001$) [48]. Mean subclavian pretest scores dropped slightly from 48.3% (SD = 25.5%) in 2007 to 45.6% (SD = 31.0%) in 2008 but rose significantly to 63.6% (SD = 27.3%) in 2009 ($p = 0.04$). We believe the improved performance (increased pretest passing rates and mean scores across both CVC insertion approaches) occurred due to changes in the safety culture of the MICU. Second- and third-year residents who completed SBML taught first-year residents (who had not completed the SBML intervention) how to insert CVCs at the bedside. When these residents became second-year residents and were assessed in the simulation lab before their MICU rotation, their CVC insertion skills were significantly better than expected. This unanticipated and collateral effect of SBML contrasts with traditional training approaches in which even highly experienced providers may pass poor techniques and errors down to the next generation of learners.

This unexpected outcome of the SBML intervention led our team to reconsider the original MPS set at 79.1% items correct on the CVC insertion checklist. When an expert panel of judges reassessed the MPS using the Angoff and Hofstee standard setting methods, they set a new more rigorous MPS for both IJ and SC CVC insertion procedures (see Chap. 6) [49]. Trainees were previously allowed to miss up to five items on the IJ and SC checklists and still achieve the MPS. After the more rigorous MPS was imposed, trainees could miss no more than three items on the IJ and SC checklists.

Return on Investment

To further assess T4 outcomes from the CVC SBML project, we measured the return on investment (ROI) produced by the intervention [30] (Chap. 19). In this study, we used NMH quality data to estimate a reduction of 9.95 CLABSIs during the year following implementation of the CVC insertion SBML curriculum. We calculated cost and hospital length of stay attributed to these anticipated CLABSIs to compute cost savings. We calculated the cost of SBML including space charges and staff and faculty salary support. We also calculated supply costs including the simulator, supply cart, vascular ultrasound, sterile personal protective equipment, and CVC insertion kits. The cost for SBML training was $111,916 in the first year of the intervention. However, the total annual estimated savings was $823,164 (141 hospital days and 120 MICU days plus the cost of care related to the 9.95 CLABSIs). This produced a net savings of $711,248 (7 to 1 rate of return on the original investment) during the first year alone. This study was the first to document ROI after simulation training in healthcare and has been widely cited as evidence to support simulation-based education at institutions worldwide.

Dissemination and Implementation

Our first opportunity to disseminate and implement the curriculum was on a smaller scale at a local academic community hospital [31]. This intervention is described in more detail in Chap. 7. We used the implementation science model of Damschroder et al. to ensure success [50]. The attention to these details paid off, and CLABSI reductions were observed at the local community hospital, similar to the results at the academic teaching hospital [29]. However, after 2 years of chief residents delivering the curriculum, a new chief resident stopped training residents using the curriculum. When we discovered this information, we reevaluated CLABSI rates in the MICU and found that they had risen over a 6-month period from 1.29 infections per catheter day to 2.97 [31]. The SBML intervention was reinstated, and CLABSI rates immediately dropped (Fig. 13.3). This emphasized the need to constantly be vigilant and control successful interventions over time.

More recently, we used a train-the-trainer model adapted from our work at the local community hospital to implement the SBML CVC insertion program at 58 Veterans Affairs (VA) hospitals across the United States. During this project, we used qualitative methods (interviews) of physicians, ICU nurses, and trainees to determine how our CVC insertion SBML curriculum was anticipated to effect skills, patient care, and safety [18, 51]. We used the Diffusion of Innovation framework described in Chap. 7. We specifically sought to understand how participants perceived the definition of competence in CVC insertion and their perceptions of the barriers and facilitators to implementation of the CVC SBML curriculum.

We identified varied understanding of how competency in CVC insertion was determined at each site [18]. Some sites used a number-based systems to determine competency, while others had no systems in place, or if they did have a system, participants were not sure what it was or how to access it. Numerous barriers to CVC insertion were identified including lack of familiarity with the CVC insertion kit and ultrasound and lack of standardized training, experience, and provider confidence in CVC insertion [51]. Forces promoting CVC insertion included training on the use of ultrasound and a good patient safety culture. Overall, the SBML

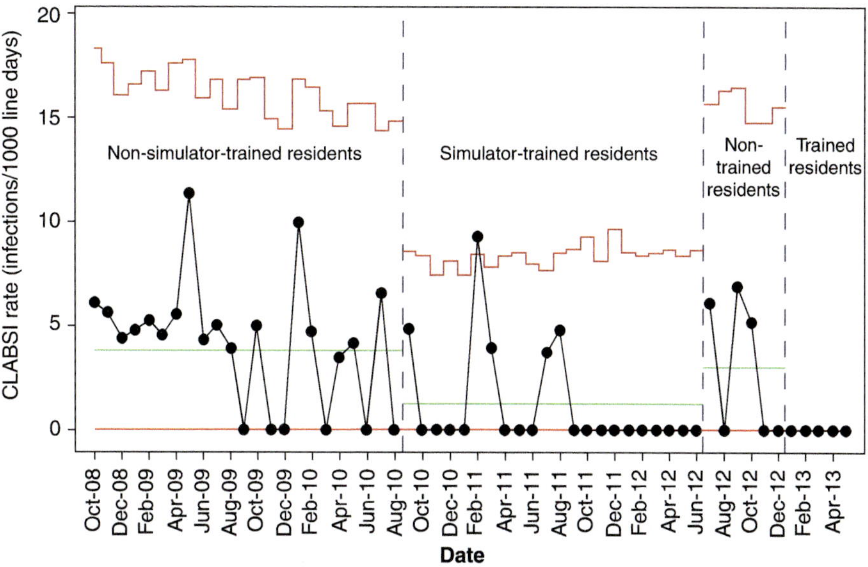

Fig. 13.3 P-chart (control chart) showing monthly central line-associated bloodstream infection rates during time periods where SBML-trained residents were present and absent from the intensive care unit. Dotted blue vertical lines = time transitions. Red lines = upper control limits (three SDs). Green horizontal lines = means. Upper control limits vary because there were a different number of line days each month. (Reprinted with permission from Barsuk et al. [31])

curriculum addressed the issue of defining competency at each of the VA sites. The curriculum also addressed a majority of identified barriers and took advantage of the facilitators. However, one barrier that was identified during our VA interviews was that nurses were not involved in the SBML training curriculum which we addressed by creating new curricula.

T1 and T2 Temporary Hemodialysis Catheter (THDC) Insertion Outcomes

We extended our SBML curriculum to include training for nephrology fellows in THDC insertion due to the success of our program in CVC insertion. When patients require emergent dialysis, clinicians often insert a THDC using the IJ vein insertion approach. THDC insertion is a required procedure for nephrology fellows to master during training [5]. Since the THDC procedure is similar to CVC insertion, we adapted our CVC insertion curriculum to incorporate THDC insertion using the original MPS of 79.1% and the 27-item checklist in 2008. Once the curriculum was adapted, NMH nephrology fellows were required to complete SBML training before performing supervised THDC insertions on actual patients.

We first assessed T1 outcomes from the THDC curriculum. We evaluated graduating third-year nephrology fellows from three institutions in Chicago to compare their THDC insertion skills to those of first-year fellows after SBML [5]. Six graduating and 12 first-year fellows participated in the study. Overall performance was poor, with only one graduating and one first-year fellow meeting the MPS at baseline. The mean overall score for the six graduating fellows was 53.1% (SD = 28.8%) checklist items correct, suggesting that traditional fellowship education did not always prepare graduating nephrologists to insert THDCs competently. However, scores of first-year fellows who completed SBML improved from a pretest mean of 29.5% items correct (SD = 31.5%) to 88.6% (SD = 17.0%; $p = 0.001$) at posttest. The education program for fellows was rated highly. All fellows agreed that the SBML program should be incorporated into nephrology fellowship training.

Two follow-up studies confirmed these T1 outcomes in additional settings. Participants at the 2014 Canadian Society of Nephrology annual meeting in Vancouver, BC, were invited to participate in THDC SBML training as part of a precourse [52]. Twenty-two individuals volunteered to participate and completed the baseline assessment (pretest). No nephrology fellows in their first or second year of training met or exceeded the MPS at baseline because the mean checklist score was 55.4% (SD = 25.7%). Seventeen of 22 participants (77%) completed THDC SBML and improved their scores to a mean of 96.2% (SD = 3.9%; $p < 0.001$), all of whom met the MPS at first attempt [52]. In a follow-up study performed in Toronto, we assessed the baseline THDC insertion performance of 19 experienced nephrologists and compared them to 20 nephrology fellows who completed the SBML intervention [53]. These nephrologists were faculty members from the University of Toronto's training programs and had clinical responsibilities including oversight of fellows during supervised THDC insertions in actual patients. The faculty nephrologists' baseline mean checklist scores were similar to fellows (46.1% items correct, SD = 29.5% and 41.1%, SD = 21.4%, respectively; $p = 0.55$), and only two met or exceeded the MPS. These findings were surprising because these faculty routinely supervised THDC insertions and had a median number of 9 years of faculty experience [53]. These findings were similar to the large VA study of CVC insertion described earlier showing that extensive clinical experience was not a proxy for actual procedural skill [6].

T2 outcomes were assessed by performing direct observations of actual THDC insertions. This study showed that nephrology fellows translated the skills they obtained in the simulated setting to actual patient care. Three fellows who completed THDC insertion SBML were reassessed while performing 15 supervised THDC insertions on patients requiring emergent dialysis [38]. SBML-trained fellows performed similarly at 6 months during actual THDC insertions compared to their original SBML posttest score (mean actual patient insertion score 86.2% (SD = 22.3%) items correct vs. mean SBML posttest score 93.5% (SD = 5.3%) items correct, $p = 0.32$).

Taken together, the THDC studies illustrate that mastery learning yields powerful outcomes in the classroom and at the bedside that cannot be replicated by traditional clinical training and experience.

T1 CVC Maintenance Skills Outcomes

In 2015, NMH infection control personnel noted a rise in the rate of late-onset (more than 4 days after insertion) CLABSIs. We partnered with nursing leadership and extended our CVC insertion program to also include CVC line maintenance to address the late-onset CLABSI problem. The new CVC line maintenance SBML curriculum enabled us to assess the impact of SBML on nursing skills. This partnership was critical because high-quality bedside CVC placements require both safe insertion and maintenance. Including nursing in CVC training was also deemed necessary from our VA interviews [51].

Consistent with other projects, the SBML curriculum included a pretest, didactic content including a video, DP, individualized instructor feedback, and posttest. Learners were required to meet or exceed the MPS on each aspect of CVC line maintenance before completing training. Eight experienced nurse educators developed skills checklists using the modified Delphi technique, incorporating relevant literature and expert nursing and infection control guidelines and opinion. The CVC line maintenance checklists focused on five tasks: (a) medication administration, (b) tubing change, (c) injection cap change, (d) blood draw, and (e) dressing change (total of 72 items; Appendix 13.3) [9]. Rater training was accomplished during a 4-hour train-the-trainer session where checklist scoring of the eight nurse educators was calibrated. An expert panel of clinicians and nursing educators used the Angoff and Hofstee standard setting methods to set the MPS for each skill. The MPSs were set at 91% checklist items correct for medication administration, 92% checklist items correct for tubing change, 88% checklist items correct for injection cap change, 91% checklist items correct for blood draw, and 93% items correct for dressing change. In addition to achieving the MPS on the checklist, several components of the checklist could not be missed. These mandatory items include the following: (a) perform hand hygiene, (b) properly scrub the injection cap, and (c) maintain sterile technique [9].

Implementation of this project was complex because there were over 2000 nurses at NMH who performed CVC line maintenance tasks and were eligible for training. We partnered with nursing leadership to perform a pilot study in the cardiothoracic ICU where the majority of patients have a CVC and short-term effects could be easily determined to assess the impact of the SBML intervention. Beginning in July 2014, all nurses in the cardiothoracic ICU were required to complete SBML training.

Forty-nine ICU nurses participated in the SBML intervention [9]. Baseline performance was uneven. Specifically, only 57% met the MPS for medication administration, 90% met the MPS for tubing change, 67% met the MPS for injection cap change, 57% met the MPS for blood draw, and only 49% met the MPS for dressing change during pretests. Scores improved dramatically after SBML. Medication administration scores improved from a pretest mean score of 38.1% (SD = 19.2) items correct to 97.4% (SD = 11.8) items correct at posttest ($p < 0.001$). Tubing change scores increased from a pretest mean of 25.7% (SD = 38.3) items correct to 80.0% (SD = 44.7%) items correct at posttest ($p < 0.01$). Injection cap change scores improved from a pretest mean of 64.4% (SD = 18.8) items correct to 96.6% (SD = 3.9) items correct at posttest ($p < 0.001$). Blood draw scores improved from a pretest mean of 35.4% (SD = 26.8) items correct to 91.7% (SD = 19.0%) items correct at posttest ($p < 0.001$). Dressing change scores improved from a pretest mean of 53.8% (SD = 25.0) items correct to 96.3% (SD = 16.2) items correct ($p < 0.001$; T1 outcomes). Consistent with findings of our other studies in physicians, total years in nursing had a significant negative correlation with overall baseline (pretest) performance ($r = -0.30$, $p = 0.04$).

As a result of this project, nursing leadership now requires all nurses who interact with CVCs to complete CVC line maintenance SBML assessments annually. Nurse educators also use the checklist during frequent bedside assessments on actual patients (T2 outcomes). In terms of reducing CLABSI rates (T3 outcomes), rates have fallen and remain low hospital-wide. We are unable to fully attribute this reduction to the CVC line maintenance curriculum because multiple interventions occurred at the same time as CVC line maintenance SBML.

Paracentesis Skills

Paracentesis is a bedside procedure performed to remove abnormal fluid from a patient's abdominal cavity. The procedure can be used for both diagnostic and therapeutic purposes in patients with end-stage liver disease or other conditions. First-year internal medicine residents at NMH often perform paracentesis at the bedside under supervision of a senior resident, fellow, or faculty member. The NMH internal medicine residency program requires all residents to complete paracentesis SBML before performing the procedure on patients because paracentesis is performed frequently and serious complications can occur.

We created a paracentesis SBML curriculum incorporating the core principles of mastery learning [23]. Residents performed a simulated skills pretest, completed didactic training including watching a video demonstrating proper procedure techniques, engaged in DP on a paracentesis simulator, and received individualized feedback from a trained instructor. Consistent with the mastery learning model, all residents were required to meet or exceed a predetermined MPS at posttest before training ended. Residents who did not meet the MPS participated in more DP and retesting until the MPS was achieved.

When we created the paracentesis SBML curriculum, an affordable ultrasound-compatible paracentesis simulator was not commercially available. Therefore, in collaboration with a Northwestern University biomedical engineer, we tested various materials and strategies to create an affordable and realistic ultrasound-compatible paracentesis model. A prototype was produced and tested to obtain feedback and suggested modifications. The simulator was pilot tested, and feedback was obtained at a national conference. Improvements were made based on feedback, and a final improved simulator was created. Our final cost for each simulator was $57 [23].

We created the paracentesis SBML curriculum based on best evidence and expert feedback. A 25-item checklist (Appendix 13.4) was developed using standard methods (Chap. 3). Pilot testing was performed, and data were used to inform expert judges during standard setting exercises. The MPS for the paracentesis skills checklist was set at 83% items correct using the mean of the Angoff and Hofstee methods.

Pilot testing revealed that inter-observer agreement for the educational intervention skills checklist was high (kappa = 0.87) [23].

Implementation of the curriculum occurred during a mandatory boot camp program for first-year residents [54]. Each resident completed multiple SBML curricula during the week-long program including paracentesis. The program allowed for any trainee who did not meet or exceed the MPS at initial posttest to complete additional training and retesting until the MPS was reached. After completing SBML, new residents are allowed to perform supervised bedside procedures on actual patients [23, 54]. The entire program, including staff support, simulators, supplies, space rental, and faculty salary coverage, was supported by the Department of Medicine. Salary support for resident physicians was provided by NMH.

T1–T4 Paracentesis Outcomes

Evaluation of the curriculum initially demonstrated that SBML was necessary because no interns met or exceeded the MPS at pretest. Performance on simulated paracentesis skills improved from an average pretest score of 33.0% (SD = 15.2%) checklist items correct to 92.7% (SD = 5.4%) checklist items correct at posttest ($p < 0.001$) [23]. All participants rated the training highly (T1 outcomes).

We next compared patient outcomes among patients who had bedside procedures performed by SBML-trained residents compared to patients whose procedures were performed in IR by a radiologist (T2/T3 outcomes) [35]. After controlling for severity of illness, we found that bedside procedures were as safe as IR procedures and were less costly. Patients who underwent bedside procedures received significantly fewer platelet and fresh frozen plasma transfusions than patients who had IR procedures (both $p < 0.001$, Fig. 13.4; T2 outcomes) [35]. We suspect this is because the SBML didactic curriculum included a review of evidence-based criteria for blood product transfusions before paracentesis procedures. We also found that ICU transfers also occurred less commonly after bedside procedures as compared to IR procedures ($p = 0.02$, Fig. 13.4) [35]. This finding was surprising because Model for End-Stage Liver Disease scores (a severity of illness/mortality marker for patients with end-stage liver disease) were higher in patients who underwent bedside procedures (indicating these patients were more severely ill). After controlling for severity of illness, patients who had paracenteses performed in IR had an additional 1.86 hospital days ($p < 0.003$; T3 outcome) compared to patients who had the procedure performed at the bedside by a SBML-trained resident [35]. Subsequently, we performed a cost analysis using an ROI methodology. Even without including increased costs due to longer hospital length of stay, we showed a 5:1 ROI for procedures performed at the bedside by SBML-trained residents (T4 outcome) [36].

Next Steps and Future Directions

As described in detail in other chapters that describe curriculum development and instructor training, bedside procedure SBML cannot be done "on the cheap" because SBML requires a significant investment of time and effort from both learners and

Variable	Bedside procedure $n = 294$ patients	IR procedure $n = 208$ patients	Odds Ratio	95% CI Lower	95% CI Upper	*P* value
ICU transfer (%), *n*	28 (9.5%)	32 (15.4%)	2.21	1.13	4.31	.02
Red blood cell transfusion (%), *n*	95 (32.3%)	72 (34.6%)	1.11	0.73	1.70	.62
Platelet transfusion (%), *n*	18 (6.1%)	37 (17.8%)	4.56	2.13	9.78	<.001
Fresh frozen plasma transfusion (%), *n*	19 (6.5%)	38 (18.3%)	4.07	2.03	8.18	<.001
Death (%), *n*	14 (4.8%)	13 (6.2%)	1.39	0.58	3.28	.47
30-day readmission (%), *n*[a]	123 (43.9%)	84 (43.1%)	1.00	0.66	1.50	.99
Emergency Department visit within 30 days (%), *n*[a]	10 (3.6%)	8 (4.1%)	0.95	0.32	2.86	.93

CI confidence interval, *ICU* intensive care unit
[a]*n* 475 patients surviving to discharge

Fig. 13.4 Patient outcomes of procedures performed at the bedside by SBML-trained residents vs. those referred to interventional radiology (IR). (Reprinted with permission from Barsuk et al. [35])

instructors. However, we strongly believe that the education and translational science outcomes reviewed in this chapter justify and demand the resources and effort required to support the widespread implementation of SBML for bedside procedure training and assessment. Although the work of Northwestern University investigators is highlighted here because it provides examples of T1–T4 outcomes, we note that other institutions worldwide have instituted SBML curricula for bedside procedural training [32, 34, 55–57]. Furthermore, an attempt to replace time-based health professions education with a competency-based model is gaining traction as well [57].

At Northwestern, we continue to expand the use and scope of SBML with ongoing studies in areas such as transesophageal echocardiography, point-of-care ultrasound, right heart catheterization, arthrocentesis, and ultrasound-guided intravenous catheter insertion. In addition to physicians, physician assistants, and nurses, we continue to expand our learner base to now include patients and caregivers. One project involves SBML for the self-care tasks required of patients with ventricular assist devices (a mechanical pump implanted into the heart for patients with advanced heart failure) and their caregivers. While we know that the mastery learning approach is effective and ensures "excellence for all," we realize that additional dissemination and uptake are necessary to achieve the ultimate goal of a competency-based credentialing and certification process for bedside procedures.

Coda

In this chapter, we presented the education and translational science evidence to support widespread use of SBML to improve the performance and outcomes of bedside procedures. We acknowledge that SBML requires hard work from learners and significant commitment by expert faculty instructors. However, the translational science outcomes reviewed in this chapter provide unequivocal evidence that rigorous education is a powerful quality improvement strategy linked to improved patient outcomes. More work is needed to incorporate actual and simulated performance of bedside procedures (rather than relying on procedure counts or completion of training) into professional society and institutional credentialing and certification pathways.

Appendix 13.1: Thoracentesis Checklist

Thoracentesis

Skill key: A = done correctly B = done incorrectly/not done

Informed consent obtained	A B
Benefits	
Risks	
Permission given	
Call "time-out"	A B
Wash hands	A B

Identify the landmarks based on ultrasound (identify fluid, the lung, and the diaphragm)	A B
Mark the site using ultrasound	A B
Clean area with chlorhexidine solution	A B
Put on sterile gloves	A B
Drape the area	A B
Set up the kit using the catheter/tubing/stop cock system (making sure the flow is from needle to syringe; this is the default position)	A B
Use 1% lidocaine to anesthetize the skin area above the rib (wheal)	A B
Using lidocaine, anesthetize to the bone and pleura with a longer needle	A B
Aspirate pleural fluid with this needle	A B
Using the thoracentesis needle (catheter/needle complex), enter the skin above the rib while aspirating (two hands)	A B
Once the catheter is about to enter the skin, nick the skin with a scalpel at the entry site, and continue to advance the catheter/needle unit	A B
Identify that the catheter and needle have entered the pleural space. White changes to red to white again, and aspirate fluid	A B
Advance the catheter over the needle until it is in the pleural space, and withdraw the needle syringe unit	A B
Turn the stop cock to direct the flow from the catheter in the pleural space to the tubing	A B
Connect the tubing to syringe, and using the "push and pull method," aspirate fluid into the bag	A B
Aspirate no more than 1.5 L of fluid (1 L is acceptable) unless no symptoms (ask how much are you removing?)	
Withdraw catheter/syringe while patient exhales (resident must communicate)	A B
Place dressing	A B
Demonstrate knowledge as to whether to order a chest x-ray	A B
Blood cx inoculated at the bedside (can verbalize)	
Transfer fluid into appropriate vials, and send for appropriate studies: LDH, protein, cell count, gram stain and culture, cytology, and pH	A B
Communicate with the nurse about procedure completion	A B
Maintain sterile technique	A B

Appendix 13.2: Central Line Insertion Checklist for Internal Jugular (IJ) and Subclavian (SC) Veins

Central Line Insertion (IJ)

Skill key: A = done correctly B = done incorrectly/not done

Informed consent obtained Benefits (medicines, fluids) Risks (infection, bleeding, pneumothorax) Consent given	A B
Call "time-out," and site mark if appropriate (must be done before any needles enter the skin)	A B
Wash hands	A B
Place the patient in slight Trendelenburg position	A B
Area is cleaned with chlorhexidine (30 seconds, scrub back forth) If scrubbing back and forth can ask "how long do you need to scrub?"	A B

Don sterile gown, gloves, hat, and mask	A B
Area is draped in usual sterile fashion (must be full-body drape)	A B
The US probe is properly set up and draped, and sonographic gel is used on inside and outside of sheath (more important inside)	A B
Test each port, and flush the lines with sterile saline	A B
Clamp each port (okay to keep distal port open), or use caps (caps must be flushed)	A B
Keep distal port open to accommodate guidewire	A B
The vein is localized using anatomical landmarks with the ultrasound machine	A B
The skin is anesthetized with 1% lidocaine in a small wheal	A B
The deeper structures are anesthetized	A B
Using the large-needle (or catheter) syringe complex, cannulate the vein while aspirating with proper US technique	A B
Remove the syringe from the needle, or advance the catheter into the vein (must be hubbed) removing both the syringe and needle	A B
Advance the guidewire into the vein no more than about 15 cm (range 10–20 cm)	A B
Make sure to nick the skin to advance the dilator (scalpel)	A B
Advance the dilator over the guidewire, and dilate the tissue tract	A B
Advance the triple lumen over the wire, holding the guidewire steady as moving forward with the catheter	A B
Never let go of the guidewire	A B
Once the line is in place, remove the guidewire in its entirety	A B
Advance the line to approx. 14–16 cm for right side and 16–18 cm for left side	A B
Ensure there is blood flow/flush each port (must aspirate before flushing). Place caps here if not done earlier, and flush through	A B
Secure the line in place using the connector correctly (suturing should be verbalized only)	A B
Place sterile dressing	A B
Get a chest x-ray to confirm location	A B
State "the cxr shows no ptx, and you are at the RA SVC junction (if proper depth of insertion)"	
Notify nurse that line is okay to use	A B
Maintain sterile technique	A B

Central Line Placement (Subclavian)

Skill key: A = done correctly B = done incorrectly/not done. **Only one step in italics is used depending on if ultrasound is used

Informed consent obtained Benefits (medicines, fluids) Risks (infection, bleeding, pneumothorax) Consent given	A B
Call "time-out," and site mark if appropriate (must be done before any needles enter the skin)	A B
Wash hands	A B
Place the patient in slight Trendelenburg position	A B
Area is cleaned with chlorhexidine (30 seconds, scrub back forth) If scrubbing back and forth, can ask "how long do you need to scrub?"	A B
Don sterile gown, gloves, hat, and mask	A B

Area is draped in usual sterile fashion (must be full-body drape)	A B
***The US probe is properly set up and draped, and sonographic gel is used on both sides of the sheath (must do if using ultrasound)*	A B
Test each port, and flush the lines with sterile saline	A B
Clamp each port (okay to leave distal port open), or use caps (caps must be flushed)	A B
Keep distal port open to accommodate guidewire	A B
The vein is localized using ultrasound machine or anatomical landmarks verbalized. "I am going 1 cm under the clavicle at 1/3:2/3 the way"	A B
Okay to ask "how did you determine the site of needle entry?"	
The skin is anesthetized with 1% lidocaine in a small wheal	A B
The deeper structures are anesthetized using a larger needle (must numb the periosteum of the clavicle)	A B
Using the large-needle (or catheter) syringe complex, cannulate the vein while aspirating (optional, confirmed by US)	A B
***If US was not used then expected to state or demonstrate they must direct the needle to the sternal notch (must verbalize) (if US was used, may omit)*	A B
Okay to ask "what direction is your needle pointed, toward what anatomic structure?"	
Remove the syringe from the needle, or advance the catheter into the vein (must be hubbed) removing both the syringe and needle	A B
Advance the guidewire into the vein no more than 15 cm (range 10–20 cm)	A B
Make sure to nick the skin to advance the dilator (scalpel)	A B
Advance the dilator over the guidewire, and dilate the tissue tract	A B
Advance the triple lumen over the wire, holding the guidewire steady as moving forward with the catheter	A B
Never let go of the guidewire	A B
Once the line is in place, remove the guidewire in its entirety	A B
Advance the line to approx. 14–16 cm for right side and 16–18 cm for left side	A B
Ensure there is blood flow/flush each port (must aspirate before flushing). Place caps here if not done earlier, and flush through	A B
Secure the line in place using the connector correctly (suturing should be verbalized only)	A B
Place sterile dressing	A B
Get a chest x-ray to confirm location	A B
State "the cxr shows no ptx, and you are at the RA SVC junction (if proper depth of insertion)"	
Notify nurse that line is okay to use	A B
Maintain sterile technique	A B

Appendix 13.3: Central Line Maintenance Checklists

Central Line Maintenance: PICC and CVC

Skill key: 1 = done correctly 0 = done incorrectly/not done

Task	Correct	Incorrect
Medication administration (IV push or piggyback)		
Maintain aseptic technique and standard precautions during the procedure	1	0
Perform hand hygiene	1	0
Don gloves	1	0

Task	Correct	Incorrect
Scrub injection cap with CHG solution for 15 seconds, and allow to dry for at least 15 seconds (or for units using 70% isopropyl alcohol-impregnated port protectors: Remove and discard port protector)	1	0
Attach a pre-filled NS syringe to the injection cap	1	0
If present, open catheter clamp	1	0
Slowly inject 10 mL NS flush solution	1	0
Scrub injection cap with CHG solution for 15 seconds, and allow to dry for at least 15 seconds	1	0
Administer IV push medication (if IV piggyback, luer lock the secondary infusion pump tubing to the cleansed port. Procedure ends here for IV piggyback medications)	1	0
Scrub injection cap with CHG solution for 15 seconds, and allow to dry for at least 15 seconds	1	0
Flush with 10 mL NS (as described above)	1	0
Detach syringe first to activate the positive pressure valve; then clamp catheter	1	0
For units using 70% isopropyl alcohol-impregnated port protectors, apply port protectors to all CVAD access ports that do not have active infusions	1	0
Tubing change: connection to injection cap or hub		
Maintain aseptic technique and standard precautions during the procedure	1	0
Perform hand hygiene	1	0
Don gloves	1	0
Close the catheter clamp	1	0
Disconnect old tubing and discard	1	0
Scrub the CVAD injection cap with CHG solution for 15 seconds, place on sterile 4 × 4 gauze, and allow to dry for at least 15 seconds	1	0
Connect new infusion tubing to CVAD injection cap/hub. If connecting to the hub, don a mask before disconnection	1	0
Open catheter clamp	1	0
Restart infusion pump(s)	1	0
Apply "date to be changed" label to tubing	1	0
For units using 70% isopropyl alcohol-impregnated port protectors, apply port protectors to all CVAD access ports that do not have active infusions	1	0

Injection cap change	Correct	Incorrect
Maintain aseptic technique and standard precautions during the procedure	1	0
Perform hand hygiene	1	0
Don mask and non-sterile gloves	1	0
Mask the patient if the patient is able to tolerate; otherwise instruct the patient to turn his or her head away from the procedure	1	0
Without removing protective covering from the new injection cap, prime the injection cap with normal saline using aseptic technique. The covering is a flush-through covering	1	0
Close the catheter clamp on CVAD	1	0
Remove and dispose of the old injection cap	1	0
Scrub the CVAD hub with CHG solution for 15 seconds, place on sterile 4 × 4 gauze, and allow to dry for at least 15 seconds	1	0
Connect the new injection cap	1	0
Open catheter clamp on CVAD	1	0
Slowly inject NS flush solution	1	0

Injection cap change	Correct	Incorrect
Detach syringe first to activate the positive pressure valve; then close clamp on catheter	1	0
For units using 70% isopropyl alcohol-impregnated port protectors, apply port protectors to all CVAD access ports that do not have active infusions	1	0

Indirect blood draw through injection cap	Correct	Incorrect
Maintain aseptic technique and standard precautions during the procedure	1	0
Perform hand hygiene	1	0
Don non-sterile gloves	1	0
Stop all infusion(s)	1	0
Clamp all CVAD lumens	1	0
Scrub injection cap for 15 seconds with CHG solution, place on sterile 4 x 4 gauze, and allow to dry at least 15 seconds	1	0
Attach the first of two 10 mL NS syringes to the CVAD cap; slowly inject NS	1	0
Remove syringe	1	0
Scrub the injection cap with CHG solution for 15 seconds, and allow to dry for at least 15 seconds	1	0
Attach second of two 10 mL NS syringes to the injection cap; slowly inject NS	1	0
Using the same syringe, aspirate 10 mL of blood for waste	1	0
Remove 10 mL waste syringe and discard	1	0
Scrub the injection cap with CHG solution for 15 seconds, and allow to dry for at least 15 seconds	1	0
Attach 10 or 20 mL syringe	1	0
Aspirate a minimum of 10 mL but no more than 20 mL of blood	1	0
Remove syringe, and place on sterile 4 × 4 gauze	1	0
Scrub the injection cap with CHG solution for 15 seconds, and allow to dry for at least 15 seconds	1	0
Attach the first of 2 mL NS syringes to injection cap of catheter	1	0
Slowly inject NS; detach syringe	1	0
Scrub the injection cap with CHG solution for 15 seconds, and allow to dry for at least 15 seconds	1	0
Attach the second 10 mL NS syringe to the injection cap; slowly inject NS	1	0
Detach syringe first to activate the positive pressure valve; then clamp catheter if not being used for infusion(s)	1	0
Unclamp CVAD lumen(s) being used for infusion(s)	1	0
Restart infusion pump(s)	1	0
For units using 70% isopropyl alcohol-impregnated port protectors, apply port protectors to all CVAD access ports that do not have active infusions	1	0

Dressing change	Correct	Incorrect
Maintain aseptic technique and standard precautions during the procedure	1	0
Perform hand hygiene	1	0
Don non-sterile gloves	1	0
Open the central line dressing kit maintaining sterility at all times. Add additional sterile supplies needed for procedure to sterile field prior to beginning the procedure	1	0
Don mask found in the kit	1	0

Dressing change	Correct	Incorrect
Mask the patient if the patient is able to tolerate a mask; otherwise instruct the patient to turn his or her head away during the procedure	1	0
Remove the entire dressing; loosen the edges without touching the area under the dressing	1	0
Remove non-sterile gloves, and discard	1	0
Perform hand hygiene	1	0
Don sterile gloves	1	0
Remove securing device if present (must be done with sterile gloves)	1	0
Cleanse catheter insertion site using CHG solution. Scrub the skin with a back and forth motion for 30 seconds, covering a 4 inch surface	1	0
Allow the CHG solution to dry for at least 30 seconds	1	0
If applicable, attach a securing device to the PICC line	1	0
If sutures are loose or no longer intact, secure catheter with sterile tape strips to prevent catheter migration	1	0
Optional: *Apply tincture of benzoin to the perimeter of the dressing area – avoid insertion site – to increase adherence of dressing to the skin, if necessary. Allow to dry*	1	0
When site is completely dry, apply the TSM dressing. Ensure occlusiveness (if the dressing is not occlusive, a new dressing must be reapplied. Do *not* attempt to secure TSM dressing with tape)	1	0
Apply date label with date of change to dressing and initial. TSM dressings are changed 24 hours post CVAD insertion and every 6 days (to coincide with IV tubing changes), whenever the dressing is no longer occlusive or there is blood, other drainage, or signs of inflammation present	1	0

Appendix 13.4: Paracentesis Checklist

Paracentesis

Skill key: A = done correctly B = done incorrectly/not done

Informed consent obtained
  Benefits (relief, diagnosis)
  Risks (infection, bleeding)
  Consent given
	A B

Call "time-out," and site mark if appropriate	A B
Wash hands	A B
Identify the landmarks based on percussion or ultrasound	A B
Clean area with sterilizing solution (chlorhexidine)	A B
Put on sterile gloves	A B
Drape the area	A B
Set up the kit	A B
Use lidocaine to anesthetize the skin (wheal)	A B
Using lidocaine, anesthetize deeper	A B
Use Z technique, lift and drop, or angle	A B
Using the Safe-T-Centesis needle (catheter/needle complex), enter the skin while aspirating (one hand holding the needle plush on the chest wall and the other on the syringe)	A B

Once the catheter is about to enter the skin, nick the skin with a scalpel at the entry site, and continue to advance the catheter/needle unit while aspirating	A B
Identify that the catheter and needle have entered the fluid space. White changes to red to white again, and aspirate fluid	A B
Advance the catheter over the needle until it is in the space, and withdraw the needle syringe unit (care not to advance the needle)	A B
Turn the stop cock to direct the flow from the catheter into the tubing	A B
Connect the tubing to a 1 L Vacutainer or the apparatus connected to the aspirating syringe, and inject fluid into the bag	A B
Will you give the patient albumin and how much?	A B
Withdraw catheter/syringe	A B
Place dressing	A B
Position the patient with area up	A B
Blood cx inoculated at the bedside *(can verbalize)*	A B
What studies need to be sent? Must say cell count, gram stain and culture, albumin	A B
Notify the nurse the procedure is done, and give post-procedure orders	A B
Sterile technique is maintained	A B

References

1. How many procedures makes competency? Hosp Peer Rev. 2014;39(11):121–3.
2. Accreditation Council for Graduate Medical Education [Internet]. Chicago: ACGME; 2000–2018 [cited 2018 Oct 8]. Milestones. Available from: http://www.acgme.org/acgmeweb/tabid/430/ProgramandInstitutionalAccreditation/NextAccreditationSystem/Milestones.aspx.
3. Internal Medicine Policies [Internet]. Philadelphia: American Board of Internal Medicine; 2018 [cited 2018 Oct 8]. Available from: http://www.abim.org/certification/policies/imss/im.aspx-procedures.
4. American Board of Surgery Update [Internet]. Philadelphia: ABS; 2015 [cited 2018 Oct 8]. Update. Available from: http://www.absurgery.org/xfer/APDS_2015.pdf.
5. Barsuk JH, Ahya SN, Cohen ER, McGaghie WC, Wayne DB. Mastery learning of temporary hemodialysis catheter insertion by nephrology fellows using simulation technology and deliberate practice. Am J Kidney Dis. 2009;54(1):70–6.
6. Barsuk JH, Cohen ER, Nguyen D, Mitra D, O'Hara K, Okuda Y, et al. Attending physician adherence to a 29-component central venous catheter bundle checklist during simulated procedures. Crit Care Med. 2016;44(10):1871–81.
7. Barsuk JH, McGaghie WC, Cohen ER, Balachandran JS, Wayne DB. Use of simulation-based mastery learning to improve the quality of central venous catheter placement in a medical intensive care unit. J Hosp Med. 2009;4(7):397–403.
8. Barsuk JH, McGaghie WC, Cohen ER, O'Leary KJ, Wayne DB. Simulation-based mastery learning reduces complications during central venous catheter insertion in a medical intensive care unit. Crit Care Med. 2009;37(10):2697–701.
9. Barsuk JH, Cohen ER, Mikolajczak A, Seburn S, Slade M, Wayne DB. Simulation-based mastery learning improves central line maintenance skills of ICU nurses. J Nurs Adm. 2015;45(10):511–7.
10. Barsuk JH, Cohen ER, Caprio T, McGaghie WC, Simuni T, Wayne DB. Simulation-based education with mastery learning improves residents' lumbar puncture skills. Neurology. 2012;79(2):132–7.
11. Wayne DB, Barsuk JH, O'Leary KJ, Fudala MJ, McGaghie WC. Mastery learning of thoracentesis skills by internal medicine residents using simulation technology and deliberate practice. J Hosp Med. 2008;3(1):48–54.

12. Choudhry NK, Fletcher RH, Soumerai SB. Systematic review: the relationship between clinical experience and quality of health care. Ann Intern Med. 2005;142(4):260–73.
13. Duloy AM, Kaltenbach TR, Keswani RN. Assessing colon polypectomy competency and its association with established quality metrics. Gastrointest Endosc. 2018;87(3):635–44.
14. Barsuk JH, Cohen ER, Feinglass J, McGaghie WC, Wayne DB. Residents' procedural experience does not ensure competence: a research synthesis. J Grad Med Educ. 2017;9(2):201–8.
15. McGee DC, Gould MK. Preventing complications of central venous catheterization. N Engl J Med. 2003;348(12):1123–33.
16. Cohen J, Cohen SA, Vora KC, Xue X, Burdick JS, Bank S, et al. Multicenter, randomized, controlled trial of virtual-reality simulator training in acquisition of competency in colonoscopy. Gastrointest Endosc. 2006;64(3):361–8.
17. Birkmeyer JD, Finks JF, O'Reilly A, Oerline M, Carlin AM, Nunn AR, et al. Surgical skill and complication rates after bariatric surgery. N Engl J Med. 2013;369(15):1434–42.
18. Cohen ER, Barsuk JH, Hertz JR, Wayne DB, Okuda Y, Mitra D, et al. Healthcare providers' awareness and perceptions of competency requirements for central venous catheter insertion. AMEE MedEDPublis; 2018. Available at: https://doi.org/10.15694/mep.2018.0000012.1.
19. McGaghie WC, Siddall VJ, Mazmanian PE, Myers J, American College of Chest Physicians Health and Science Policy Committee. Lessons for continuing medical education from simulation research in undergraduate and graduate medical education: effectiveness of continuing medical education: American College of Chest Physicians Evidence-Based Educational Guidelines. Chest. 2009;135(3 Suppl):62S–8S.
20. Cook DA, Brydges R, Zendejas B, Hamstra SJ, Hatala R. Mastery learning for health professionals using technology-enhanced simulation: a systematic review and meta-analysis. Acad Med. 2013;88(8):1178–86.
21. Didwania A, McGaghie WC, Cohen ER, Butter J, Barsuk JH, Wade LD, et al. Progress toward improving the quality of cardiac arrest medical team responses at an academic teaching hospital. J Grad Med Educ. 2011;3(2):211–6.
22. McGaghie WC, Issenberg SB, Cohen ER, Barsuk JH, Wayne DB. Medical education featuring mastery learning with deliberate practice can lead to better health for individuals and populations. Acad Med. 2011;86(11):e8–9.
23. Barsuk JH, Cohen ER, Vozenilek JA, O'Connor LM, McGaghie WC, Wayne DB. Simulation-based education with mastery learning improves paracentesis skills. J Grad Med Educ. 2012;4(1):23–7.
24. Wayne DB, Butter J, Siddall VJ, Fudala MJ, Wade LD, Feinglass J, et al. Mastery learning of advanced cardiac life support skills by internal medicine residents using simulation technology and deliberate practice. J Gen Intern Med. 2006;21(3):251–6.
25. McGaghie WC. Medical education research as translational science. Sci Transl Med. 2010;2(19):19cm8.
26. McGaghie WC, Issenberg SB, Cohen ER, Barsuk JH, Wayne DB. Translational educational research: a necessity for effective health-care improvement. Chest. 2012;142(5):1097–103.
27. Barsuk JH, Szmuilowicz E. Evaluating medical procedures: evaluation and transfer to the bedside. In: Pangaro LN, McGaghie WC, editors. Handbook on medical student evaluation and assessment. North Syracuse: Gegensatz Press; 2015.
28. Butter J, McGaghie WC, Cohen ER, Kaye M, Wayne DB. Simulation-based mastery learning improves cardiac auscultation skills in medical students. J Gen Intern Med. 2010;25(8):780–5.
29. Barsuk JH, Cohen ER, Feinglass J, McGaghie WC, Wayne DB. Use of simulation-based education to reduce catheter-related bloodstream infections. Arch Intern Med. 2009;169(15):1420–3.
30. Cohen ER, Feinglass J, Barsuk JH, Barnard C, O'Donnell A, McGaghie WC, et al. Cost savings from reduced catheter-related bloodstream infection after simulation-based education for residents in a medical intensive care unit. Simul Healthc. 2010;5(2):98–102.
31. Barsuk JH, Cohen ER, Potts S, Demo H, Gupta S, Feinglass J, et al. Dissemination of a simulation-based mastery learning intervention reduces central line-associated bloodstream infections. BMJ Qual Saf. 2014;23(9):749–56.

32. Udani AD, Macario A, Nandagopal K, Tanaka MA, Tanaka PP. Simulation-based mastery learning with deliberate practice improves clinical performance in spinal anesthesia. Anesthesiol Res Pract. 2014;2014:659160.
33. Gossett DR, Gilchrist-Scott D, Wayne DB, Gerber SE. Simulation training for forceps-assisted vaginal delivery and rates of maternal perineal trauma. Obstet Gynecol. 2016;128(3):429–35.
34. Ahn J, Yashar MD, Novack J, Davidson J, Lapin B, Ocampo J, et al. Mastery learning of video laryngoscopy using the glidescope in the emergency department. Simul Healthc. 2016;11(5):309–15.
35. Barsuk JH, Cohen ER, Feinglass J, McGaghie WC, Wayne DB. Clinical outcomes after bedside and interventional radiology paracentesis procedures. Am J Med. 2013;126(4):349–56.
36. Barsuk JH, Cohen ER, Feinglass J, Kozmic SE, McGaghie WC, Ganger D, et al. Cost savings of performing paracentesis procedures at the bedside after simulation-based education. Simul Healthc. 2014;9(5):312–8.
37. Robinson JK, Jain N, Marghoob AA, McGaghie W, MacLean M, Gerami P, et al. A randomized trial on the efficacy of mastery learning for primary care provider melanoma opportunistic screening skills and practice. J Gen Intern Med. 2018;33(6):855–62.
38. Ahya SN, Barsuk JH, Cohen ER, Tuazon J, McGaghie WC, Wayne DB. Clinical performance and skill retention after simulation-based education for nephrology fellows. Semin Dial. 2012;25(4):470–3.
39. Barsuk JH, Cohen ER, Williams MV, Scher J, Feinglass J, McGaghie WC, et al. The effect of simulation-based mastery learning on thoracentesis referral patterns. J Hosp Med. 2016;11(11):792–5.
40. Barsuk JH, Cohen ER, Williams MV, Scher J, Jones SF, Feinglass J, et al. Simulation-based mastery learning for thoracentesis skills improves patient outcomes: a randomized trial. Acad Med. 2018;93(5):729–35.
41. Ericsson KA. Acquisition and maintenance of medical expertise: a perspective from the expert-performance approach with deliberate practice. Acad Med. 2015;90(11):1471–86.
42. Ericsson KA. Peak: secrets from the new science of expertise. Boston: Houghton Mifflin Harcourt; 2016. xxiii, 307 pp.
43. Huang GC, Smith CC, Gordon CE, Feller-Kopman DJ, Davis RB, Phillips RS, et al. Beyond the comfort zone: residents assess their comfort performing inpatient medical procedures. Am J Med. 2006;119(1):71 e17–24.
44. Stufflebeam DL. The checklists development checklist [Internet]. Kalamazoo: Western Michigan University Evaluation Center; 2000 [cited 2018 Oct 8]. Available at: https://www.wmich.edu/sites/default/files/attachments/u350/2014/guidelines_cdc.pdf.
45. Barsuk JH, Cohen ER, Wayne DB, Siddall VJ, McGaghie WC. Developing a simulation-based mastery learning curriculum: lessons from 11 years of advanced cardiac life support. Simul Healthc. 2016;11(1):52–9.
46. Hospital Acquired Conditions [Internet]. Baltimore: Centers for Medicare & Medicaid Services; 2018 [cited 2018 Oct 8]. Available from: https://www.cms.gov/Medicare/Medicare-Fee-for-Service-Payment/HospitalAcqCond/Hospital-Acquired_Conditions.html.
47. Barsuk JH, Cohen ER, McGaghie WC, Wayne DB. Long-term retention of central venous catheter insertion skills after simulation-based mastery learning. Acad Med. 2010;85(10 Suppl):S9–12.
48. Barsuk JH, Cohen ER, Feinglass J, McGaghie WC, Wayne DB. Unexpected collateral effects of simulation-based medical education. Acad Med. 2011;86(12):1513–7.
49. Cohen ER, Barsuk JH, McGaghie WC, Wayne DB. Raising the bar: reassessing standards for procedural competence. Teach Learn Med. 2013;25(1):6–9.
50. Damschroder LJ, Banaszak-Holl J, Kowalski CP, Forman J, Saint S, Krein SL. The role of the champion in infection prevention: results from a multisite qualitative study. Qual Saf Health Care. 2009;18(6):434–40.
51. Cameron KA, Cohen ER, Hertz JR, Wayne DB, Mitra D, Barsuk JH. Barriers and facilitators to central venous catheter insertion: a qualitative study. J of Patient Saf. 2018. https://doi.org/10.1097/PTS.0000000000000477. [Epub ahead of print].

52. Clark E, Paparello JJ, Wayne DB, Edwards C, Hoar S, McQuillian R, et al. Use of a national continuing medical education meeting to provide training in temporary hemodialysis catheter insertion skills for nephrology trainees: a pretest-posttest study. Can J Kidney Health Dis. 2014;1:25.
53. McQuillan RF, Clark E, Zahirieh A, Cohen ER, Paparello JJ, Wayne DB, et al. Performance of temporary hemodialysis catheter insertion by nephrology fellows and attending nephrologists. Clin J Am Soc Nephrol. 2015;10(10):1767–72.
54. Cohen ER, Barsuk JH, Moazed F, Caprio T, Didwania A, McGaghie WC, et al. Making July safer: simulation-based mastery learning during intern boot camp. Acad Med. 2013;88(2):233–9.
55. Zendejas B, Cook DA, Bingener J, Huebner M, Dunn WF, Sarr MG, et al. Simulation-based mastery learning improves patient outcomes in laparoscopic inguinal hernia repair: a randomized controlled trial. Ann Surg. 2011;254(3):502–9; discussion 9–11.
56. Melchiors J, Petersen K, Todsen T, Bohr A, Konge L, von Buchwald C. Procedure-specific assessment tool for flexible pharyngo-laryngoscopy: gathering validity evidence and setting pass-fail standards. Eur Arch Otorhinolaryngol. 2018;275(6):1649–55.
57. Achieving competency-based time-variable health professions education. Recommendations from the Macy Foundation Conference. Macy Foundation Conference; July 14–17; Atlanta, GA. www.macyfoundation.org: Josiah Macy Jr. Foundation; 2017. p. 1–24.

14 Mastery Learning for Clinical Emergencies

Nabil Issa, David H. Salzman, and Mark Adler

Clinicians who practice on the front line of care such as emergency medical service (EMS) responders, trauma surgeons, and emergency department staff recognize that purposeful, well-planned training is required to provide high-quality emergency care [1]. The horrifying events at the Orlando, Florida, Pulse nightclub on June 12, 2016, demonstrate the value of this perspective. An assailant fired 250 bullets from an assault rifle at 300 club patrons in minutes. The Orlando Regional Medical Center (ORMC) and local EMS were prepared for this event because both programs had practiced for 20 years in disaster preparedness [2]. One hundred seven individuals were shot at close range. Forty-eight patients were transported to ORMC, which is Orlando's Level 1 trauma center. Thirty-eight patients arrived in the first 42 minutes. Nine had fatal injuries that could not be treated despite heroic efforts. Another wave of 10 patients arrived at ORMC in the following 2 hours. Each patient had about four gunshot wounds, ranging between 1 and 10. Five trauma surgeons performed 76 operative procedures. *All of the 39 gunshot victims who survived the first hour of trauma resuscitation were discharged from the ORMC* [3–5]. The coordinated and effective response to the Pulse nightclub shooting event can be attributed to a sustained commitment to clinical emergency training.

N. Issa (✉)
Northwestern University Feinberg School of Medicine, Departments of Surgery and Medical Education, Chicago, IL, USA
e-mail: nissa@northwestern.edu

D. H. Salzman
Northwestern University Feinberg School of Medicine, Departments of Emergency Medicine and Medical Education, Chicago, IL, USA

M. Adler
Northwestern University Feinberg School of Medicine, Departments of Pediatrics and Medical Education, Chicago, IL, USA

W. C. McGaghie et al. (eds.), *Comprehensive Healthcare Simulation: Mastery Learning in Health Professions Education*, Comprehensive Healthcare Simulation, https://doi.org/10.1007/978-3-030-34811-3_14

Clinical Emergency Training

High-quality emergency care is a result of effective education together with quality improvement efforts and robust infrastructure. Patient care suffers when gaps occur in these efforts. This performance gap has been shown in clinical emergency care. In a frequently cited journal article, Abella and colleagues demonstrated poor cardiopulmonary resuscitation (CPR) quality by providers in a tertiary care hospital who had fulfilled certificate training [6]. Subsequent work from the same authors demonstrated that substandard life support was associated with failure to timely defibrillate the patient [7]. Hunt and colleagues reported similar findings for advanced life support in a pediatric patient population [8]. Barsuk and the Northwestern Simulation team reported poor baseline performance by experienced US Veterans Administration providers inserting central venous catheters [9].

Large, national resuscitation courses are used routinely to provide education for clinical emergencies. Hospitals and other healthcare entities rely on these programs to provide evidence of workforce readiness. We use these programs as representative cases for clinical emergency education because such programs highlight challenges health professions educators face every day. Barriers and challenges are experienced across the range of programs. Evidence exists about positive outcomes for resuscitation training programs [10], but some data endorse the conclusion that existing curricula may not consistently lead to high-quality care [11]. In the following sections, we review examples of these resuscitation programs. All program durations were found on the authoring entities' websites.

Basic Life Support

Basic Life Support (BLS) [12] is offered by the American Heart Association (AHA) and covers the first steps of field (layperson) or hospital (provider) resuscitation, including initial assessment, cardiopulmonary resuscitation performance, and use of an automated electronic defibrillator (AED). Management of a choking person is included. BLS has the largest target audience(s) of the life support curricula. The course has online pre- and posttests and clinical vignette simulations. An in-person class (4.5 hours for initial, 3 hours for renewal) reviews content and requires learners to demonstrate cardiopulmonary resuscitation and choking management under instructor observation. Renewal is required every 2 years.

Adult Advanced Life Support

Advanced Cardiac Life Support (ACLS) [13] is a long-standing resuscitation course offered by the American Heart Association (AHA) that focuses on adult pulse arrest states, tachy- and bradyarrhythmias, acute stroke, acute myocardial infarction, and post-resuscitation care. ACLS also has content related to teamwork and communication best practices and is targeted at healthcare providers. The current course (2015) has online pre- and posttests and a set of screen-based simulated cases. The cases must be retaken until a passing score is achieved. The in-person class is about 15 hours in duration for initial and 8 hours for renewal classes. Learners participate in groups, and formal individual assessment is limited. Renewal is required every 2 years.

Published research shows that ACLS-based interventions following a mastery learning (ML) model lead to improved education and patient-level outcomes. The evidence is covered in detail in Chap. 3 and is summarized here.

Pediatric Advanced Life Support

Pediatric Advanced Life Support (PALS) [14] targets pediatric healthcare providers and covers the emergent care of infants and children, including acute arrest states, arrhythmias, and septic shock. The course is provided jointly by the AHA and the American Academy of Pediatrics (AAP). The PALS course has an online pre- and posttest, simulated case vignettes, and in-person classroom work involving demonstration of group skills. The ACLS, BLS, and PALS software are all designed by a common software development provider and share user interface and education design approaches. The in-person class is 13.5 hours for initial certification and 6.5–8.5 hours for renewal, with a 2-year renewal cycle. There is strong evidence that PALS, when incorporating simulation-based training, produces improved learning [15].

Neonatal Resuscitation

The Neonatal Resuscitation Program (NRP) [16], offered by the AAP, addresses the immediate postdelivery care of infants transitioning from the uterine environment. The target audience is providers who care for newborns in the delivery room setting. There are online and in-person classroom components. The classroom component is 4 hours for initial and 3 hours for renewal. Renewal is every 2 years.

Trauma (Adult and Pediatric)

Advanced Trauma Life Support (ATLS) [17] is offered by the American College of Surgeons (ACS) and addresses adult and pediatric trauma care, with a target audience of physicians. The course consists of pre-course reading and in-class didactic content followed by simulated cases on management and procedures. The initial course is presented in 2- and 2.5-day formats with renewal offered in ½ day and 1-day formats. The renewal cycle is every 4 years. A Cochrane database systematic review reported no evidence of patient-level benefit [18]. A frequently cited 2014 systematic review claims support for ATLS learner-level outcomes by covering research before 2000 and addressing studies evaluating trainees and students [19].

Each of the resuscitation courses has common approaches, not just a result of sharing a common publisher. The courses have not, to date, satisfactorily captured key education practices that produce strong outcomes. There are several clear flaws in these large-scale curricula:

- Programs are costly at both the system and local levels, requiring:
  - Expenditures to pay for programs/licenses
  - Instructors trained in the course content and educational theory
  - Learners needing time away from work and, in many cases, to be paid for the time
  - Infrastructure including classroom time, administrative support, and equipment (including moderate or high-cost simulators)
- Educationally, these programs:
  - Have long renewal cycles while the events covered are infrequent among adults and very rare in pediatric populations. These factors contribute to observed decay in performance after training [20, 21].
  - Occur in nonclinical environment (e.g., classroom setting).
  - Use classic exemplars of specific conditions that do not reflect clinical variation.
  - Emphasize individual knowledge and performance over teamwork and communication.
  - Are slow to change, given the inherent lag in translation and dissemination of current science into educational content.
  - Create and encourage attendees to adopt pattern recognition exercises or heuristic methods that provide practitioners with rules of thumb to simplify decision-making and allow implementation of appropriate algorithms.
  - Time limited—coursework is fixed and predetermined. Although the courses require learners to meet or exceed a minimum passing standard (MPS) during posttesting, there is not time to permit learners to undergo further practice if standards are not met. Local programs are not resourced to provide additional instruction, and institutions may not be able to support additional learner time away from clinical work.
  - Assessment skews toward knowledge (multiple-choice exam) and individual performance assessed using checklists, while performance level assessment is the desired metric. The assessments now used lack validity data to support judgments about a clinician's ability to practice.

In the next section, we discuss the role of deliberate practice and ML to improve training for clinical emergencies.

Mastery Learning for Clinical Emergencies

In the 2018 *Resuscitation Education Science: Educational Strategies to Improve Outcomes From Cardiac Arrest: A Scientific Statement From the American Heart Association* [1], the authors give a detailed and comprehensive overview about education best practices and proposed a series of future directions about AHA curricula and other programs. The authors begin their recommendations with an endorsement of ML and deliberate practice approaches for life support curricula, stating that "Educators should deliver resuscitation education experiences that allow learners to practice key skills, receive directed feedback, and improve until they attain mastery" [1]. They also recommend education strategies that should form the basis of a well-designed ML program which will focus on spaced and distributed learning, contextual learning, and the use of high-quality faculty development and assessment approaches. In the next section, we discuss the evidence supporting a ML approach and how each AHA recommendation should inform program development and what resources are required to implement these programs.

Mastery Learning, Deliberate Practice, and Rapid-Cycle Deliberate Practice

Mastery learning is a theory-driven education approach that has foundations rooted in the constructivist, behavioral, and social learning theories [22], as discussed in more detail in Chap. 2. ML programs are different from other approaches because the education endpoint is learner-centered. Instruction is complete when the learner meets a MPS, not after a set time has passed. The set time approach is characteristic of the life support programs we have discussed. Mastery learning approaches are particularly important for basic and advanced life support training where the training will be used in high-stakes patient care events.

There is compelling evidence that ML interventions are effective both in general and for emergent care training, which can lead to improved patient outcomes and positive collateral effects [23]. In non-emergent training, Barsuk and colleagues have reported positive education and patient-level and system-level outcomes [24, 25]. In the life support domain, Wayne et al. showed that residents trained using ML with deliberate practice achieved better learning outcomes among the residents and also demonstrated improved patient outcomes [26, 27].

Deliberate practice should form the foundation of emergent care training programs with a ML structure. Deliberate practice, where learners perform skills or activities and receive feedback from individuals with content expertise and educational skills, is a key feature of ML models. The underlying training used to allow learners to reach mastery is best suited to deliberate practice approaches. There is strong evidence favoring use of the deliberate practice model both in general [28] and in healthcare education [29–31].

Rapid-cycle deliberate practice (RCDP) is a specific approach where learners are guided through cycles of practice where individuals or teams receive expert, real-time feedback and then cycle through specific skills or algorithms until mastery is achieved. Hunt and colleagues have shown that RCDP is effective in improving resuscitation performance as have others [8, 10]. Rapid-cycle training approaches can be employed synergistically within a ML model. RCDP is a form of training to a specific endpoint. ML formally sets the target standard.

Spaced (Distributed) Learning

Current life support curricula feature 2–4-year renewal cycles without planned opportunities for practice. This time structure is subject to performance decay and is particularly concerning given the infrequency of some of the targeted training topics [32]. Spaced, short training has been shown to be superior for BLS [33–35] skills retention with more modest evidence for PALS [36–38]. Some models of spaced learning seek to maintain performance skills with a variety of means of learner training and assessment including self-assessment or automated feedback devices to minimize need for faculty involvement. However, one study of 195 practicing healthcare providers failed to show effectiveness of training using an automatic feedback device for long-term retention of chest compression skills. Provider chest compression (rate and/or depth) skills decayed from baseline assessment to three different assessment time periods (1–3 months, 3–6 months, and >6 months) [39].

Within a ML model, spaced training takes the form of a primary session in which mastery is achieved followed by refresher or booster sessions. At all sessions, learners have an opportunity to practice with directed, focused feedback until mastery is achieved. Moazed et al. demonstrated retention of critical care skill performance after a resident boot camp [40]. The frequency of needed spaced learning events is not known in general or in the ML context.

Faculty Development

The role of faculty development within the ML model is addressed in detail in Chap. 9. Skilled educators are required at the design, development, and implementation level for any robust intervention. Mastery learning requires new faculty skills for this specific form of assessment, working with learners to meet mastery standards and to participate in standard setting (Chap. 6). Eppich and colleagues synthesized the findings from several studies and provide insights about the technical aspects of applying ML principles including debriefing strategies [41].

Contextual Learning

Learning and assessment do not occur in vacuum. The location, group composition, and culture impact educational outcomes. In the ML context, resuscitation curricula should try to create team structures consistent with clinical practice such as avoiding single profession teams when not consistent with practice. In situ training offers teams an opportunity to train in the workplace but has not been shown to be superior to classroom instruction. Mannequin or training equipment needs to allow specific skill performance (e.g., CPR, bag-mask ventilation) to be practiced and assessed.

Feedback and Debriefing

Timely, targeted feedback is a key feature of learning programs that produce effective learning among health professionals (Chap. 8) [42]. Actionable feedback fosters development of reflective practice among learners which improves clinical reasoning and contributes to improved practice [43]. Credible instructors help learners to value feedback [44].

Health professions educators must provide clear expectations for learners about the structure and processes used in any curriculum as part of pre-briefing. The prebrief is part of an explicit effort to establish psychological safety [45, 46]. This step is important in general and even more important in ML curricula that include both specific assessment and a variable time to completion. Teachers may share assessment tools with learners and discuss how the mastery standard was set. Others may not share the assessment tools to avoid memorization of steps rather than comprehension of the overall procedure.

Teamwork and task performance are linked in resuscitation and should be taught together. Sources of data can extend beyond the human assessor and include electronic feedback devices such as a defibrillator or haptic simulator [47–49] and peer learners. For example, some haptic simulators give visual electronic feedback of the rate and depth adequacy of chest compressions during CPR [47–49].

Mastery learning curricula often use feedback models that differ from traditional post-event debriefing. RCDP [50], discussed earlier, incorporates a pause-discuss-repeat model where the debriefer provides targeted positive or corrective feedback during breaks that are chosen by the instructor. Eppich and colleagues frame the conceptual basis for this approach, contrasting the reflection-in-action—pause-and-discuss—versus feedback during performance [41]. The ACLS ML program developed by Wayne and colleagues incorporated microdebriefing, a specific model of reflection-in-action in which a trained educator stood nearby to the team leader and gave specific, targeted feedback to the learner in real time [26, 27].

A recent report by Devine and colleagues demonstrated parity between instructor and a "directed self-regulated" ML program teaching ACLS [51]. Self-regulated models have potential for reduced faculty involvement that could affect program scaling to larger audiences, although the data are not yet compelling.

Assessment

The basis of ML is learner achievement to a standard specific to the assessment instrument being used. The MPS is defined in terms of the assessment instrument. When we assert a learner has achieved mastery, we make the decision from scoring data. As discussed in more detail in Chap. 5, this decision must be supported by evidence that the judgment is valid. The argument [52] for the use of a given assessment is supported from a variety of evidence sources. What were the qualifications of the assessment developers? Where raters trained? Did raters agree on scoring when compared quantitatively? Does scoring appear to be biased, for example, do the raters know the learners? Well-designed assessments are informed by curriculum objectives and extensive literature review, require cycles of instrument testing and revision, and must involve rater training and calibration. Chapters 5 and 8 provide more detail about rater training practices.

Existing instruments provided as part of life support courses (BLS, ACLS, PALS, ATLS) do not have published validity evidence to support their use nor is there specific rater training for the use of these instruments. To train and assess rater quality across large-scale life support programs would require substantial investment of time and money. Without this effort, however, it will be difficult to bridge the current resuscitation education model to a ML paradigm. Readers are directed to a table given in the AHA summary statement that offers a list of existing emergency care instruments that have validity evidence to support their use [1].

Coda

This chapter reviews the state of education within national resuscitation programs and makes a case for application of ML approaches for these training programs. These resuscitation education programs are considered exemplars. Many of the same education barriers affect emergency care interventions of any size or scope: limited learner and educator time, no distributed learning plan, limited assessor time, unproven assessment tools, and limited rater training or faculty development. Key issues and future goals provided in the AHA summary statement define a clear and central role for ML in emergency care training programs [1].

References

1. Cheng A, Nadkarni VM, Mancini MB, Hunt EA, Sinz EH, Merchant RM, et al. Resuscitation education science: educational strategies to improve outcomes from cardiac arrest: a scientific statement from the American Heart Association. Circulation. 2018;138(6):e82–122.
2. Cheatham ML, Smith CP, Ibrahim JA, Havron WS, Lube MW, Levy MS, et al. Orlando regional medical center responds to pulse nightclub shooting. Bull Am Coll Surg. 2016;101(11): 12–9.
3. Baker CC, Oppenheimer L, Stephens B, Lewis FR, Trunkey DD. Epidemiology of trauma deaths. Am J Surg. 1980 Jul;140(1):144–50.
4. Pepe PE, Wyatt CH, Bickell WH, Bailey ML, Mattox KL. The relationship between total prehospital time and outcome in hypotensive victims of penetrating injuries. Ann Emerg Med. 1987;16(3):293–7.
5. Petri RW, Dyer A, Lumpkin J. The effect of prehospital transport time on the mortality from traumatic injury. Prehosp Disaster Med. 1995;10(1):24–9.
6. Abella BS, Sandbo N, Vassilatos P, Alvarado JP, O'Hearn N, Wigder HN, et al. Chest compression rates during cardiopulmonary resuscitation are suboptimal: a prospective study during in-hospital cardiac arrest. Circulation. 2005;111(4):428–34.
7. Edelson DP, Abella BS, Kramer-Johansen J, Wik L, Myklebust H, Barry AM, et al. Effects of compression depth and pre-shock pauses predict defibrillation failure during cardiac arrest. Resuscitation. 2006;71(2):137–45.

8. Hunt EA, Vera K, Diener-West M, Haggerty JA, Nelson KL, Shaffner DH, et al. Delays and errors in cardiopulmonary resuscitation and defibrillation by pediatric residents during simulated cardiopulmonary arrests. Resuscitation. 2009;80(7):819–25.
9. Barsuk JH, Cohen ER, Nguyen D, Mitra D, O'Hara K, Okuda Y, et al. Attending physician adherence to a 29-component central venous catheter bundle checklist during simulated procedures. Crit Care Med. 2016;44(10):1871–81.
10. Mosley C, Dewhurst C, Molloy S, Shaw BN. What is the impact of structured resuscitation training on healthcare practitioners, their clients and the wider service? A BEME systematic review: BEME guide no. 20. Med Teach. 2012;34(6):e349–85.
11. Drimousis PG, Theodorou D, Toutouzas K, Stergiopoulos S, Delicha EM, Giannopoulos P, et al. Advanced trauma life support certified physicians in a non trauma system setting: is it enough? Resuscitation. 2011 Feb;82(2):180–4.
12. American Heart Association. Basic life support: provider manual. Dallas: American Heart Association; 2016.
13. American Heart Association. Advanced cardiovascular life support (ACLS) provider manual. Dallas: American Heart Association; 2016.
14. American Heart Association. Pediatric advanced life support (PALS) provider manual. Dallas: American Heart Association; 2016.
15. Donoghue AJ, Durbin DR, Nadel FM, Stryjewski GR, Kost SI, Nadkarni VM. Effect of high-fidelity simulation on pediatric advanced life support training in pediatric house staff: a randomized trial. Pediatr Emerg Care. 2009;25(3):139–44.
16. Weiner GM, Zaichkin J, Kattwinkel J, American Academy of Pediatrics, American Heart Association. Textbook of neonatal resuscitation. 7th ed. Elk Grove Village: American Academy of Pediatrics; 2016.
17. American College of Surgeons. ATLS® student course manual. In: 10th ed. Chicago: American College of Surgeons; 2018.
18. Jayaraman S, Sethi D, Chinnock P, Wong R. Advanced trauma life support training for hospital staff. Cochrane Database Syst Rev. 2014;(8):CD004173.
19. Mohammad A, Branicki F, Abu-Zidan FM. Educational and clinical impact of advanced trauma life support (ATLS) courses: a systematic review. World J Surg. 2014;38(2):322–9.
20. Oermann MH, Kardong-Edgren SE, Odom-Maryon T. Effects of monthly practice on nursing students' CPR psychomotor skill performance. Resuscitation. 2011;82(4):447–53.
21. Arthur W Jr, Bennett W Jr, Stanush PL, McNelly TL. Factors that influence skill decay and retention: a quantitative review and analysis. HHUP. 1998;11(1):57–101.
22. McGaghie WC, Harris IB. Learning theory foundations of simulation-based mastery learning. Simul Healthc. 2018;13(3S Suppl 1):S15–20.
23. McGaghie WC, Issenberg SB, Barsuk JH, Wayne DB. A critical review of simulation-based mastery learning with translational outcomes. Med Educ. 2014;48(4):375–85.
24. Cohen ER, Feinglass J, Barsuk JH, Barnard C, O'Donnell A, McGaghie WC, et al. Cost savings from reduced catheter-related bloodstream infection after simulation-based education for residents in a medical intensive care unit. Simul Healthc. 2010 Apr;5(2):98–102.
25. Barsuk JH, Cohen ER, Feinglass J, McGaghie WC, Wayne DB. Unexpected collateral effects of simulation-based medical education. Acad Med. 2011;86(12):1513–7.
26. Wayne DB, Butter J, Siddall VJ, Fudala MJ, Wade LD, Feinglass J, et al. Mastery learning of advanced cardiac life support skills by internal medicine residents using simulation technology and deliberate practice. J Gen Intern Med. 2006;21(3):251–6.
27. Wayne DB, Didwania A, Feinglass J, Fudala MJ, Barsuk JH, McGaghie WC. Simulation-based education improves quality of care during cardiac arrest team responses at an academic teaching hospital: a case-control study. Chest. 2008;133(1):56–61.
28. Ericsson KA, Krampe RT, Tesch-Römer C. The role of deliberate practice in the acquisition of expert performance. Psychol Rev. 1993;100(3):363–406.
29. Sawyer T, Sierocka-Castaneda A, Chan D, Berg B, Lustik M, Thompson M. Deliberate practice using simulation improves neonatal resuscitation performance. Simul Healthc. 2011 Dec;6(6):327–36.

30. Cordero L, Hart BJ, Hardin R, Mahan JD, Nankervis CA. Deliberate practice improves pediatric residents' skills and team behaviors during simulated neonatal resuscitation. Clin Pediatr (Phila). 2013;52(8):747–52.
31. Burden AR, Pukenas EW, Deal ER, Coursin DB, Dodson GM, Staman GW, et al. Using simulation education with deliberate practice to teach leadership and resource management skills to senior resident code leaders. J Grad Med Educ. 2014;6(3):463–9.
32. Braun L, Sawyer T, Smith K, Hsu A, Behrens M, Chan D, et al. Retention of pediatric resuscitation performance after a simulation-based mastery learning session: a multicenter randomized trial. Pediatr Crit Care Med. 2015;16(2):131–8.
33. Sullivan NJ, Duval-Arnould J, Twilley M, Smith SP, Aksamit D, Boone-Guercio P, et al. Simulation exercise to improve retention of cardiopulmonary resuscitation priorities for in-hospital cardiac arrests: a randomized controlled trial. Resuscitation. 2015;86:6–13.
34. Sutton RM, Niles D, Meaney PA, Aplenc R, French B, Abella BS, et al. Low-dose, high-frequency CPR training improves skill retention of in-hospital pediatric providers. Pediatrics. 2011;128(1):e145–51.
35. Niles D, Sutton RM, Donoghue A, Kalsi MS, Roberts K, Boyle L, et al. "Rolling refreshers": a novel approach to maintain CPR psychomotor skill competence. Resuscitation. 2009;80(8):909–12.
36. Patocka C, Khan F, Dubrovsky AS, Brody D, Bank I, Bhanji F. Pediatric resuscitation training-instruction all at once or spaced over time? Resuscitation. 2015;88:6–11.
37. Bender J, Kennally K, Shields R, Overly F. Does simulation booster impact retention of resuscitation procedural skills and teamwork? J Perinatol. 2014;34(9):664–8.
38. Kurosawa H, Ikeyama T, Achuff P, Perkel M, Watson C, Monachino A, et al. A randomized, controlled trial of in situ pediatric advanced life support recertification ("pediatric advanced life support reconstructed") compared with standard pediatric advanced life support recertification for ICU frontline providers*. Crit Care Med. 2014;42(3):610–8.
39. Garcia-Jorda D, Walker A, Camphaug J, Bissett W, Spence T, Martin D-A, et al. Bedside chest compression skills: performance and skills retention in in-hospital trained pediatric providers. A simulation study. J Crit Care. 2018;50:132–7.
40. Moazed F, Cohen ER, Furiasse N, Singer B, Corbridge TC, McGaghie WC, et al. Retention of critical care skills after simulation-based mastery learning. J Grad Med Educ. 2013;5(3):458–63.
41. Eppich WJ, Hunt EA, Duval-Arnould JM, Siddall VJ, Cheng A. Structuring feedback and debriefing to achieve mastery learning goals. Acad Med. 2015;90(11):1501–8.
42. Issenberg SB, McGaghie WC, Petrusa ER, Lee Gordon D, Scalese RJ. Features and uses of high-fidelity medical simulations that lead to effective learning: a BEME systematic review. Med Teach. 2005;27(1):10–28.
43. Sandars J. The use of reflection in medical education: AMEE guide no. 44. Med Teach. 2009;31(8):685–95.
44. Watling C, Driessen E, van der Vleuten CPM, Lingard L. Learning from clinical work: the roles of learning cues and credibility judgements. Med Educ. 2012;46(2):192–200.
45. Rudolph JW, Simon R, Raemer DB, Eppich WJ. Debriefing as formative assessment: closing performance gaps in medical education. Acad Emerg Med. 2008;15(11):1010–6.
46. Edmondson A. Psychological safety and learning behavior in work teams. Adm Sci Q. 1999;44(2):350.
47. Yeung J, Meeks R, Edelson D, Gao F, Soar J, Perkins GD. The use of CPR feedback/prompt devices during training and CPR performance: a systematic review. Resuscitation. 2009;80(7):743–51.
48. Kirkbright S, Finn J, Tohira H, Bremner A, Jacobs I, Celenza A. Audiovisual feedback device use by health care professionals during CPR: a systematic review and meta-analysis of randomised and non-randomised trials. Resuscitation. 2014;85(4):460–71.
49. Cheng A, Overly F, Kessler D, Nadkarni VM, Lin Y, Doan Q, et al. Perception of CPR quality: influence of CPR feedback, just-in-time CPR training and provider role. Resuscitation. 2015;87:44–50.

50. Hunt EA, Duval-Arnould JM, Nelson-McMillan KL, Bradshaw JH, Diener-West M, Perretta JS, et al. Pediatric resident resuscitation skills improve after "rapid cycle deliberate practice" training. Resuscitation. 2014;85(7):945–51.
51. Devine LA, Donkers J, Brydges R, Perelman V, Cavalcanti RB, Issenberg SB. An equivalence trial comparing instructor-regulated with directed self-regulated mastery learning of advanced cardiac life support skills. Simul Healthc. 2015;10(4):202–9.
52. Kane MT. Validating the interpretations and uses of test scores. J Educ Meas. 2013;50(1): 1–73.

Readiness for Residency

15

David H. Salzman, Heather L. Heiman, Brigid M. Dolan, and Jennifer Trainor

A pager goes off in early July during rounds and an intern runs off to answer the call. The supervising physician wonders, "Will the intern be able to handle this challenge?" More concerns surface. "Does the intern know how to answer a page?" "Is the communication strategy appropriate?" "Does she know the right questions to ask?" "Does she recognize the limits of her knowledge and experience?" As the event unfolds, the attending physician looks over her shoulder wondering, "Do I trust the intern to answer this call unsupervised?" "Can the intern care for the patient?" The intern completes the call, returns to rounds, and presents a brief summary of the situation. The attending physician is relieved knowing that patient care is moving in the right direction. However, uncertainty still remains about the intern's competence across all of the clinical domains required in her new role.

Medical school graduation is an important milestone on the developmental pathway to becoming a competent physician. The transition from medical student to resident is both an invigorating and a frightening time for new physicians. Earning a medical degree indicates that the new doctor has met the expectations

D. H. Salzman (✉)
Northwestern University Feinberg School of Medicine, Departments of Emergency Medicine and Medical Education, Chicago, IL, USA
e-mail: dsalzman005@northwestern.edu

H. L. Heiman · B. M. Dolan
Northwestern University Feinberg School of Medicine, Departments of Medicine and Medical Education, Chicago, IL, USA

J. Trainor
Northwestern University Feinberg School of Medicine, Departments of Pediatrics and Medical Education, Chicago, IL, USA

W. C. McGaghie et al. (eds.), *Comprehensive Healthcare Simulation: Mastery Learning in Health Professions Education*, Comprehensive Healthcare Simulation, https://doi.org/10.1007/978-3-030-34811-3_15

of the degree-granting program. This is an enormous achievement. However, there is evidence that not all medical school graduates are competent across all of the patient care skills needed for graduate medical education (GME). The traditional approach to medical training produces a classic normal distribution of achievement across different parts of the medical school curriculum. In other words, a student may graduate from medical school yet still be below average in several domains.

This chapter addresses the transition from undergraduate medical education (UME) to GME. Although similar issues may be present in other health professions, this chapter focuses on medical students prior to and immediately after graduation from medical school. We focus on the role that mastery learning can have to prepare students for their health professions roles by creating a uniform, tight set of high-level learning outcomes rather than a wide distribution of education results. Health professions schools can do a better job to ensure that graduating students are ready to perform tasks required of interns and other new care providers from day one. Mastery learning is an ideal education approach to meet this need. This chapter addresses the following points:

1. Medical and other health professions graduates are often underprepared to start postgraduate residency education and deliver safe and effective patient care independently.
2. Recent implementation of Core Entrustable Professional Activities (EPAs) by the Association of American Medical Colleges (AAMC) and learning milestones advocated by the Accreditation Council for Graduate Medical Education (ACGME) and other curriculum innovations clarify key learning requirements and help to close this gap (Chap. 17).
3. General and specialty-specific courses at the end of medical school and start of residency are associated with improved confidence, knowledge, and performance.
4. Despite these innovations, simply meeting the minimum expectations is insufficient and we can do better. Mastery learning curricula have proven successful as culminating courses that teach and assess EPA and milestone components.
5. Several other steps are needed to successfully implement mastery learning curricula to ensure readiness for GME and for competent practice in other health professions.

Medical Student Readiness for Residency

At the July start of each academic medical year in the United States, freshly graduated interns assume responsibility for patient care. Startup of a new provider cohort brings concerns of an associated increase in patient morbidity and mortality. This so-called July Effect [1] has been demonstrated in studies examining medication errors [2], patient mortality [3], and undesirable anesthesia events [4]. The increase in patient morbidity and mortality at the start of the academic year seen in these studies is likely due to gaps in clinical skill and inexperience among new doctors. This inability to meet societal expectations is deeply concerning and warrants close attention [5].

A key goal of UME is to ensure that new graduates provide safe and effective patient care as they transition to GME. However, education outcome data and patient safety studies consistently demonstrate that new interns are not adequately prepared to perform all clinical duties. These deficits span the spectrum of competencies and are not isolated to US medical schools. Deficits are found in basic skill performance (e.g., physical exam) [6], clinical procedures [7, 8], handoffs, fluid and medication management, patient admissions, assessment of unstable patients, communication, pain management [9], treatment, and decision-making [10]. Baseline assessments highlight wide skill variability and nonuniform preparation among interns before beginning internal medicine [11] and surgical [12] training programs. Similar findings in Denmark indicate that on average, only 74% of the recently graduated students who completed a self-assessment questionnaire met minimum skill expectations [13].

An additional concern is that the self-confidence and perceived ability of new interns to perform clinical tasks do not match the performance observed by supervisors. One study involving 30 UK junior medical officers in the first postgraduate year of training assessed readiness for patient care responsibilities. New graduates were asked about their confidence and experience in performing seven routine clinical skills. This cohort was also assessed using a competency-based assessment instrument covering the clinical skills. The authors compared self-reported levels of confidence with faculty assessment of actual competence. For many skills, learner self-reported confidence was high, and for all skills, observed performance was much lower than self-confidence scores [14]. Similar findings have been shown in a systematic review demonstrating the limited ability of physicians (including new graduates) to accurately self-assess their competence [15]. Multiple lines of evidence suggest that the performance of recent medical school graduates conforms with the Dunning-Kruger effect, "Unskilled and Unaware of it" [16]. Dunning and Kruger argue, "incompetence not only causes poor performance but the inability to recognize that one's performance is poor" [16]. The impact is likely most significant in the bottom quartile of performers who not only overestimate their own clinical fitness but also perceive that their competence is above average compared to others. As health professions educators, we cannot rely on the self-reported confidence from learners as a reliable index of readiness for residency training. A more thoughtful approach is needed.

Program Director Expectations and New Resident Skills

Residency program directors are challenged when they receive a new class of trainees from different medical schools. Residency program directors have high expectations about the readiness of incoming interns to provide safe patient care. However, there is a gap between residency program directors' expectations and the measured competence of new doctors. The variability in new interns' skills, when measured objectively using Objective Structured Clinical Examinations (OSCEs) in surgery [12] and the general intern year [11, 17], provides evidence for the gap between the baseline competence of interns and the expectations of program directors [11, 18]. This mismatch has also been shown in a survey of family medicine residency program directors [19]. This dichotomy highlights a need to standardize expectations about clinical skills for new doctors entering GME.

Residency programs in the United States now use a competency-based framework to assess performance during GME. The ACGME transitioned to the Next Accreditation System (NAS) with phased implementation beginning in 2013. A principal aim of this new system is to "accelerate the ACGME's movement toward accreditation on the basis of educational outcomes" [20]. Each medical specialty has developed a set of developmental milestones corresponding to sub-competencies within the six core ACGME competencies: (a) patient care and procedural skills, (b) medical knowledge, (c) interpersonal and communication skills, (d) professionalism, (e) practice-based learning and improvement, and (f) systems-based practice. Each sub-competency contains multiple developmental milestones that progress incrementally through more advanced tasks. Level 1, the lowest category, corresponds to performance that is expected of a medical school graduate. Level 5, the highest category, corresponds to the expected level of performance of a senior attending physician.

Given this approach, it is reasonable to expect that all new trainees would be able to meet the Level 1 milestones upon entering GME and be prepared to advance through medical specialty milestones during training. Unfortunately, early studies during NAS implementation revealed that new residents are not meeting this benchmark. In one study, a large group of emergency medicine (EM) residents were surveyed at the beginning of their intern year to find out if they recalled being taught and assessed on the Level 1 EM milestones [21]. The study findings indicated a gap between the material covered in medical school curricula and the Level 1 milestones, including performance and assessment of many of the sub-competencies identified by the ACGME.

Core Entrustable Professional Activities for Graduating Medical Students

Due to the success of competency-based education as a framework in GME, medical schools are currently building their own outcome frameworks based on EPAs. First described in 2005 [22], the EPAs were conceived as a way to translate competency-based medical education objectives into more practical frameworks for learners and faculty. Activities considered EPAs must meet these criteria:

1. Be part of essential professional work in a given context
2. Require adequate knowledge, skills, and attributes, generally acquired through training

3. Lead to recognized output of professional labor
4. Be confined to qualified personnel
5. Be independently executable
6. Be executable within a time frame
7. Be observable and measurable in their process and their outcome, leading to a conclusion ("well done" or "not well done")
8. Reflect one or more of the competencies to be acquired [22]

The AAMC formed an expert task force in 2013 to define the activities that all medical school graduates should perform with limited supervision on the first day of residency. These activities are known as the Core EPAs for Entering Residency [23]. The thirteen EPAs (Table 15.1) apply to all graduating students regardless of specialty choice.

The Core EPA Task Force paid particular attention to the challenge of assessing each of the EPAs [24]. A program of frequent, directly observed, formative assessment of each task has been proposed, and the sum of these assessments should culminate in a final entrustment decision [25].

How Do We Measure Entrustment?

A key benefit of assessing learners using EPAs lies in the intuitive assessment scale. Assessors ask, "Can I entrust this health professional to perform this activity?" [25]. The trust concept is complex, and proponents of EPAs note that clinical supervisors make frequent, implicit entrustment decisions every day when deciding how a learner may engage a patient in the clinical environment. Specific dimensions of trustworthiness that inform these implicit decisions include the following [26]:

Table 15.1 Core entrustable professional activities for entering residency

	Description
EPA 1	Gather a history and perform a physical examination
EPA 2	Prioritize a differential diagnosis following a clinical encounter
EPA 3	Recommend and interpret common diagnostic and screening tests
EPA 4	Enter and discuss orders and prescriptions
EPA 5	Document a clinical encounter in the patient record
EPA 6	Provide an oral presentation of a clinical encounter
EPA 7	Form clinical questions and retrieve evidence to advance patient care
EPA 8	Give or receive a patient handover to transition care responsibility
EPA 9	Collaborate as a member of an interprofessional team
EPA 10	Recognize a patient requiring urgent or emergent care and initiate evaluation and management
EPA 11	Obtain informed consent for tests and/or procedures
EPA 12	Perform general procedures of a physician
EPA 13	Identify system failures and contribute to a culture of safety and improvement

Data from AAMC [23]

1. What is the trainee's fund of knowledge and skill?
2. How aware is the trainee of her own limitations?
3. Is the trainee conscientious? Does he attend to detail, follow through with tasks, and gather and report patient data reliably?
4. Is the learner truthful? Has the learner ever misreported information, e.g., reported an exam that was not performed?

Entrustment may also depend on factors external to the trainee being assessed. Entrustment may stem from the clinical context, the task itself, the supervisor and her experience, and the relationship between the trainee and the supervisor [27]. Issues that underlie entrustment decisions are complex. Many assessment scales have been proposed to simplify these issues and simplify judgement of trainee trustworthiness. These scales focus on the level of supervision that a trainee requires to perform a professional activity. Olle ten Cate originally proposed a five-point scale [25] to determine the degree of learner supervision needed for any EPA (Table 15.2). This work was modified by Chen and colleagues [28] to better capture the assessment of EPAs in the undergraduate medical education setting where full independence typically is not allowed (Table 15.3) (see also Chap.17).

Table 15.2 ten Cate entrustment scale [25, 67]

Scale	Entrustment and supervision scale
1	Not allowed to practice EPA
2	Allowed to practice EPA only under proactive, full supervision
3	Allowed to practice EPA only under reactive/on-demand supervision
4	Allowed to practice EPA unsupervised
5	Allowed to supervise others in the practice of EPA

Data from Ref. [25]

Table 15.3 Chen scale

Scale	Entrustment and supervision scale
1	Not allowed to practice EPA
1a	Inadequate knowledge/skill; not allowed to observe
1b	Allowed to practice EPA—adequate knowledge, some skill; allowed to observe
2	Allowed to practice EPA only under proactive, full supervision
2a	As coactivity with supervisor
2b	With supervisor in room ready to step in as needed
3	Allowed to practice EPA only under reactive/on-demand supervision
3a	With supervisor immediately available, all findings double checked
3b	With supervisor immediately available, key findings double checked
3c	With supervisor distantly available (e.g., by phone), findings reviewed

Adapted from Ref. [28], with permission

Table 15.4 Zwisch scale [29]

Scale	Description	Comments
1	Show and tell	The attending performs the critical portion while explaining each step to the resident
2	Active help	The attending actively guides the resident through the critical portion of the procedure
3	Passive help	The resident performs critical portions of the operation independently, while the attending physician assists only when needed
4	Supervision only	The resident performs the procedure, and the attending does not need to directly assist

Data from Ref. [29]

Table 15.5 Ottawa clinic assessment tool

Scale	Description	Comments
1	I had to do	Requires complete guidance, unprepared to do, or had to do for them
2	I had to walk them through	Able to perform some tasks, but requires repeated directions
3	I had to direct them from time to time	Demonstrates some independence, but requires intermittent prompting
4	I needed to be available just in case	Independent but needs assistance with nuances of certain patients and/or situation, unable to manage all patients, still requires supervision for safe practice
5	I did not need to be there	Complete independence, can safely manage a general clinic in your specialty

Adapted from Ref. [30], with permission

The Zwisch scale (Table 15.4) and the Ottawa clinical assessment tool (Table 15.5) were created and tested to evaluate entrustment in surgical graduate medical education settings, focusing on operating room cases [29] and the outpatient surgery clinic [30], respectively. These instruments differentiate skills between learners with good interrater reliability (see also Chap. 17).

Mastery Learning to Assess EPAs

Given the assessment frameworks for the EPAs, consider the interplay of the seven key steps in the mastery learning model: (a) baseline or diagnostic testing, (b) clear learning objectives, (c) engagement in educational activities and practice with feedback to reach the objectives, (d) a set minimum passing standard, (e) formative assessment with (f) specific feedback, and (g) continued practice until the passing standard is reached [31]. The AAMC Core EPAs should be considered the learning objectives that guide a mastery learning approach to skill achievement (see Chap. 17). The subsequent curriculum (often a clerkship, foundation course, or similar environment) must provide learners with opportunities to practice the skills associated with each EPA. Clinical supervisors provide formative assessment, and the passing standard may be assessed in either a simulated or workplace setting. When merging the EPAs with the mastery learning model, a new approach to standard setting (Chap. 6) may need to be used where judges are asked to consider the student who can reach a higher level of "can perform with indirect clinical supervision," in the case of medical students who are typically not allowed to practice with complete independence.

Although educators have not yet completely merged the Core EPAs with mastery learning, several authors have described assessment tools used to evaluate the EPAs. Aylward and colleagues developed a measure to assess patient handoffs for new interns (Core EPA 8) [32]. Using ten Cate's five levels of entrustment, expert faculty identified the observed behaviors, specific to handoffs, that correspond to each of the five entrustment levels. The measure was used to give learners formative feedback after each observed handoff with the goal that learners would reach the stage of "can perform independently." Checklist-based assessments of other EPAs have been developed including diagnostic reasoning [33]; clinical documentation [34]; oral presentations [35]; and informed consent, admission orders, and discharge prescriptions [36]. To merge these assessment tools with the mastery learning framework, educators can apply mastery standards (i.e., a minimum passing standard) to each of these EPA-based assessments.

Transition to Residency Courses

The EPAs offer a universal minimum expectation of graduates, but their implementation is a work in progress. There continue to be differences between what medical schools teach and what specific residency programs need. Medical school curricula are designed to produce pluripotent physicians, yet US internships are specialized, each with particular cognitive and technical requirements. Although students select their specialties many months before graduation, the final year of medical school is replete with "audition" rotations and interviews. Students have little time to hone the specific skills required for their internship. Internships receive students with a range of abilities from a range of medical schools. Even within a single institution, educators of medical students are not necessarily the same faculty who are responsible for residents.

The gap between residency program expectations and medical school graduates' skill sets can be closed despite these challenges. Published data describe the knowledge and skills that incoming interns need to improve. Over 20,000 internal medicine residents (IM) were surveyed coincident with an IM in-training examination about the key skills they should have acquired before beginning residency. The most frequent responses were (a) knowing when they needed to ask for additional help, (b) managing time and prioritizing work, and (c) discussing care transitions with other healthcare providers [37]. Many of these needs are not unique to specific specialties. Program directors from diverse specialties share similar concerns about their interns according to a recent survey [38]. Program directors would like to see stronger medical knowledge, professionalism, organization, and self-reflection among trainees, and they agree on the clinical rotations during medical school that might best prepare students.

Pre-residency "boot camps" have become common over the past decade. Some occur in the final months of medical school. Others are implemented at the start of internship. There is strong evidence that these experiences improve procedural skills and some evidence that they improve other clinical competencies.

Fourth-year medical school courses for students planning to enter surgical residencies have yielded higher confidence [39–41] and improved surgical skills [42] among participants. A Mayo Medical School study compared interns who had completed a comprehensive 4-week preparatory course in the last year of medical school to interns who had not taken the course. Results showed that course participants outperformed their peers in 32 diverse domains rated by senior residents who were blinded to the participation status of the interns [43]. Preparatory courses for students entering EM, obstetrics-gynecology, and pediatrics have also shown improved confidence [44] and knowledge [45–47].

Capstone courses designed for all students regardless of their planned residency have also been described [48, 49]. A required 4-week course at Duke University School of Medicine focused on nine milestones expected at completion of a transitional internship ranging from planning a quality improvement (QI) project to managing emergencies. Performance varied widely among students by course conclusion. Student clinical performance was much better on skills such as breaking bad news and planning a QI project compared to others such as self-assessment and managing emergencies [49].

Boot camps that take place at the start of internship have focused on discrete technical skills such as central venous catheter insertion and suturing [50, 51] or patient handoffs [52]. However, there are no "best practices" for boot camps. Boot camps for the same specialty differ widely in their objectives, format, duration, and whether or not they are mandatory. Most pre-graduation boot camps do not insist on mastery of knowledge or skills. More standardization would help ensure that best practices are established as outcome evidence grows. Standardization would also reduce duplication of effort between medical school and residency faculty. The American College of Surgeons has called for medical schools to adopt a specific curriculum for students bound for surgical training. In response, national leaders in surgical education are now developing a modular pre-residency curriculum focused on patient care and patient safety [53]. The Society of Neurological Surgeons now requires a "boot camp" in the initial month of internship containing didactics and skills sessions [54]. This neurological surgery boot camp is delivered at six regional centers in the United States. Reports from the inaugural cohort show high satisfaction among participants and improvement in written test scores. In Israel, the health ministry requires a 5-day boot camp focused on basic and advanced life support, manual skills such as suturing and catheter insertion, cognitive skills such a safe prescribing, communication skills, and teamwork [55]. Seven years of data show this national program is highly rated by learners, but performance and knowledge outcomes have not been reported.

How can we move more trainees from sporadic, optional boot camp or capstone experiences to consistent, required training as done by the Society of Neurological Surgeons and the Israeli Ministry of Health? The answer is simple. We must demonstrate that these preparatory courses have consistent learning and patient care outcomes that ensure readiness in the most essential domains for each medical school graduate who is about to assume patient care responsibility. We believe one solution resides in the mastery learning model.

Mastery Learning to Prepare Medical Students for Residency

Boot camps and capstone courses taught with specific mastery learning techniques might improve learning and patient care outcomes at the UME to GME transition. Some educators propose a more uniform method of training at the end of medical school or the beginning of residency to level the playing field. We now explore current evidence about whether such mastery learning curricula and courses can produce consistent outcomes by starting with an intervention designed to measure a single skill and building to discuss larger programs.

Butter and colleagues evaluated cardiac auscultation skills of third-year medical students. These investigators showed that teaching medical students to a minimum passing standard (MPS) (Chap. 6) improved student performance in comparison with a group of fourth-year students not exposed to the mastery learning education intervention. Moreover, the skills in the intervention group exceeded those in the traditional curriculum group both on the cardiac simulator examination and when auscultating findings in actual patients [56]. Skill transfer to the clinical environment to improve patient care outcomes is the ultimate goal of all of these education interventions. However, measurement of clinical skill transfer is difficult, especially when assessing students at the end of medical school (Chap. 16).

The IM residency program at Northwestern University implemented a simulation-based mastery learning (SBML) intern boot camp in 2011 [57]. Educators compared outcomes among interns trained to a mastery MPS with historical controls who started residency in 2009 and 2010 but had not participated the mastery learning boot camp. All interns completed the same clinical skills examination (CSE). Interns in the intervention cohort participated in 3 days of small-group teaching sessions, deliberate practice, and individualized feedback. Measured outcomes included five parts of a clinical skills examination: (a) recognition of physical examination findings (cardiac auscultation) and performance of two clinical procedures, (b) paracentesis, (c) lumbar puncture, (d) management of critically ill patients (intensive care unit skills), and (e) communication with patients (code status discussion). Boot camp participants were required to meet or exceed the MPS on each clinical skill before starting patient care. All interns in the intervention group met or exceeded the MPS and performed significantly better than historical controls on all skills, even after controlling for age, sex, and United States Medical Licensing Examination Step 1 and 2 scores. Downstream improved clinical care was also seen in patients undergoing paracentesis procedures performed by trainees who completed the mastery boot camp program [58].

In an emergency medicine clerkship-based intervention, Reed and colleagues studied whether a mandatory SBML course focusing on six core emergency medicine clinical skills for senior students could produce measurable and consistent performance outcomes [59]. One hundred thirty-five medical students in the intervention were pretested on all six skills: (a) ultrasound-guided peripheral intravenous line insertion, (b) basic skin laceration repair, (c) chest compressions, (d) bag-valve-mask ventilation, (e) using the defibrillator, and (f) leading a patient resuscitation event. Education content was a mix of asynchronous learning via online videos, followed by computer-based skill-related quizzes and one-on-one hands-on skills training. Deliberate practice with feedback was employed until an MPS was achieved for all skills at posttests. All students passed each skill after the education intervention. When unannounced retesting of a convenience sample of students (36% of cohort) was performed from 1 to 9 months later, all students scored at or above the MPS, and there was no significant decrease in mean score between posttest and retention testing for any skill.

To address the Core EPAs, Salzman and colleagues implemented a simulation-based capstone course teaching and assessing individual performance on specific components of several EPAs for a cohort of graduating medical students. They developed two six-station clinical skills examinations (CSEs) to assess performance before and after a simulation-based education intervention with individual checklist performance assessed by trained nurses, standardized patients, and faculty. In this pilot study, the authors demonstrated that graduating medical students could not reliably perform selected EPAs at baseline. However, a focused 3-day simulation-based capstone course produced significant improvement in core clinical skills [36]. The course has subsequently been implemented for the entire graduating class at Northwestern, and at least three components are taught and assessed to a mastery standard. The authors argue that this approach using mastery learning is a feasible strategy to teach and assess components of the EPAs before medical school graduation [60].

The challenge to expand SBML approaches in health professions education is less daunting than critics contend. There are many scales and checklists which have already been created that address EPAs such as handoffs [61], 360° evaluations (receiving feedback from a variety of viewpoints including the learner) [62], and direct mini-clinical evaluation exercise (mini-CEX) observations [63–66]. With the establishment of an MPS and integration into the mastery learning curriculum structure, any of these tools could be used in a mastery learning approach.

Future Directions

Graduating medical students have a wide variety of experiences with uneven clinical knowledge and skills. Within that context, the role of mastery learning may fit best as a teaching tool to improve knowledge and clinical skills in the context of the

EPAs as discussed earlier in this chapter. While no single approach has been agreed on for the determination of entrustment before graduation, current thinking suggests that it could be made by an EPA or entrustment committee which would interpret all of the ad hoc assessments that are collected throughout the curriculum and make a summative entrustment decision [67]. This decision will most likely be based on a series of assessments over time.

Ultimately, in a mastery learning curriculum, the goal is to ensure a uniform, high level of performance from all learners. Through standard setting, expert evaluators can reach consensus about the MPS to provide optimal care and mitigate future harm. Any student not achieving the MPS for a procedure would participate in required education sessions with deliberate practice until mastery is achieved. The EPA or entrustment committee would have multiple assessments leading to mastery of a component of the EPA which would then be used to reach the final entrustment decision.

One of the key hurdles to mastery learning in undergraduate medical education involves the variable time required to achieve uniform outcomes. The goal of uniform outcomes will be critical in closing the gap between program director expectations and the ability of an incoming intern to perform specific tasks. The challenge for all medical school curriculum leaders will be to identify strategies for implementation which allow for and encourage additional time for practice and achievement of mastery in the setting of a traditionally fixed time approach to medical education. The fourth year of medical school has long been identified as a period that lacks clarity of educational purpose, dominated by elective experiences. Restructuring the fourth year to better serve in the transition to residency has been discussed for many years and represents an opportunity to initiate a non-time-bound approach featuring opportunities for mastery learning [68]. Identifying strategic approaches to use different assessments and opportunities for practice within a redesigned fourth year could meet the simultaneous need to improve the fourth year and provide sufficient information for entrustment committees to make summative mastery decisions.

One of the first examples of a program addressing a time variable progression from UME through GME is the Education in Pediatrics Across the Continuum (EPAC) study [69]. This project involves a collaboration among five medical schools with two goals:

1. Establish a model for true competency-based medical education through a variable-time, meaningfully assessed demonstration of competence.
2. Develop a continuous educational pathway linking the continuum of UME, GME, and independent practice using pediatrics as a model.

Students explore the specialty of pediatrics early in medical school in this innovative program. Then they receive an opportunity to match into the program and focus their UME education in pediatrics. These students are guaranteed a position in the school's affiliated pediatrics residency after achievement of competency in the EPAs and satisfaction of the medical school's graduation requirements. During their education, students are assessed across the Core EPAs, progress is monitored by entrustment committees, and the decision to promote to residency training is made when students have achieved the ability perform each of the 13 EPAs with indirect supervision. Students advance to residency training on a timeline that ranges from 6 to 9 months before their peers begin residency training in the traditional pathway. Although the number of students involved in this pilot program is small, it highlights the ability of a competency-based program to allow for a time-variable approach to medical education, one of the key principles of mastery learning.

Coda

Mastery learning curricula for UME meet several specific needs. The first need is the recognition that student performance at the end of UME often does not meet the expectations of residency program directors. The second need driving mastery learning curricula is the need to develop assessments to ensure that graduating students can independently perform the 13 EPA activities identified by the AAMC (Chap. 5). Such needs provide a framework for building curricula using mastery learning and are critical steps in final entrustment or mastery decisions. Thus we endorse a key conclusion of this chapter that a mastery decision can be equivalent to an entrustment decision.

References

1. Young JQ, Ranji SR, Wachter RM, Lee CM, Niehaus B, Auerbach AD. "July effect": impact of the academic year-end changeover on patient outcomes: a systematic review. Ann Intern Med. 2011;155(5):309–15.
2. Phillips DP, Barker GE. A July spike in fatal medication errors: a possible effect of new medical residents. J Gen Intern Med. 2010;25(8):774–9.
3. Jen MH, Bottle A, Majeed A, Bell D, Aylin P. Early in-hospital mortality following trainee doctors' first day at work. PLoS One. 2009;4(9):e7103.
4. Haller G, Myles PS, Taffé P, Perneger TV, Wu CL. Rate of undesirable events at beginning of academic year: retrospective cohort study. BMJ. 2009;339:b3974.
5. Barach P, Philibert I. The July effect: fertile ground for systems improvement. Ann Intern Med. 2011;155(5):331–2.
6. Remmen R, Scherpbier A, Derese A, Denekens J, Hermann I, van der Vleuten C, van Royen P, Bossaert L. Unsatisfactory basic skills performance by students in traditional medical curricula. Med Teach. 1998;20(6):579–82.
7. Board P, Mercer M. A survey of the basic practical skills of final-year medical students in one UK medical school. Med Teach. 1998;20(2):104–8.
8. Promes SB, Chudgar SM, O'Connor Grochowski C, Shayne P, Isenhour J, Glickman SW, Cairns CB. Gaps in procedural experience and competency in medical school graduates. Acad Emerg Med. 2009;16(Suppl 2):S58–62.
9. Kelly C, Noonan CLF, Monagle JP. Preparedness for internship: a survey of new interns in a large Victorian health service. Aust Health Rev. 2011;35(2):146–51.
10. Wall D, Bolshaw A, Carolan J. From undergraduate medical education to pre-registration house officer year: how prepared are students? Med Teach. 2006;28(5):435–9.

11. Lypson ML, Frohna JG, Gruppen LD, Woolliscroft JO. Assessing residents' competencies at baseline: identifying the gaps. Acad Med. 2004;79(6):564–70.
12. Sachdeva AK, Loiacono LA, Amiel GE, Blair PG, Friedman M, Roslyn JJ. Variability in the clinical skills of residents entering training programs in surgery. Surgery. 1995;118(2):300–8.
13. Moercke AM, Eika B. What are the clinical skills levels of newly graduated physicians? Self-assessment study of an intended curriculum identified by a Delphi process. Med Educ. 2002 May;36(5):472–8.
14. Barnsley L, Lyon PM, Ralston SJ, Hibbert EJ, Cunningham I, Gordon FC, Field MJ. Clinical skills in junior medical officers: a comparison of self-reported confidence and observed competence. Med Educ. 2004;38(4):358–67.
15. Davis DA, Mazmanian PE, Fordis M, Van Harrison R, Thorpe KE, Perrier L. Accuracy of physician self-assessment compared with observed measures of competence: a systematic review. JAMA. 2006;296(9):1094–102.
16. Kruger J, Dunning D. Unskilled and unaware of it: how difficulties in recognizing one's own incompetence lead to inflated self-assessments. J Pers Soc Psychol. 1999 Dec;77(6):1121–34.
17. Burch VC, Nash RC, Zabow T, Gibbs T, Aubin L, Jacobs B, Hift RJ. A structured assessment of newly qualified medical graduates. Med Educ. 2005;39(7):723–31.
18. Lindeman BM, Sacks BC, Lipsett PA. Graduating Students' and surgery program directors' views of the Association of American Medical Colleges core entrustable professional activities for entering residency: where are the gaps? J Surg Educ. 2015;72(6):e184–92.
19. Dickson GM, Chesser AK, Woods NK, Krug NR, Kellerman RD. Family medicine residency program director expectations of procedural skills of medical school graduates. Fam Med. 2013;45(6):392–9.
20. Nasca TJ, Philibert I, Brigham T, Flynn TC. The next GME accreditation system--rationale and benefits. N Engl J Med. 2012;366(11):1051–6. https://doi.org/10.1056/NEJMsr1200117. Epub 2012 Feb 22.
21. Santen SA, Rademacher N, Heron SL, Khandelwal S, Hauff S, Hopson L. How competent are emergency medicine interns for level 1 milestones: who is responsible? Acad Emerg Med. 2013;20(7):736–9.
22. ten Cate O. Entrustability of professional activities and competency-based training. Med Educ. 2005;39(12):1176–7.
23. Association of American Medical Colleges. Core entrustable professional activities for entering residency. 2013. https://www.mededportal.org/icollaborative/resource/887. Accessed 7/1/19.
24. Core Entrustable Professional Activities for Entering Residency – Curriculum Developers Guide. https://store.aamc.org/core-entrustable-professional-activities-for-entering-residency.html. Accessed 7/1/19.
25. Ten Cate O. Trusting graduates to enter residency: what does it take? J Grad Med Educ. 2014;6(1):7–10.
26. Kennedy TJ, Regehr G, Baker GR, Lingard L. Point-of-care assessment of medical trainee competence for independent clinical work. Acad Med. 2008;83(10 Suppl):S89–92.
27. Hauer KE, Ten Cate O, Boscardin C, Irby DM, Iobst W, O'Sullivan PS. Understanding trust as an essential element of trainee supervision and learning in the workplace. Adv Health Sci Educ Theory Pract. 2014;19(3):435–56.
28. Chen HC, van den Broek WE, ten Cate O. The case for use of entrustable professional activities in undergraduate medical education. Acad Med. 2015;90:431–6.
29. George BC, Teitelbaum EN, Meyerson SL, Schuller MC, DaRosa DA, Petrusa ER, Petito LC, Fryer JP. Reliability, validity, and feasibility of the Zwisch scale for the assessment of intraoperative performance. J Surg Educ. 2014;71(6):e90–6.
30. Rekman J, Gofton W, Dudek N, Gofton T, Hamstra SJ. Entrustability scales: outlining their usefulness for competency-based clinical assessment. Acad Med. 2016;91(2):186–90.
31. McGaghie WC. Mastery learning: it is time for medical education to join the 21st century. Acad Med. 2015;90(11):1438–41.

32. Aylward M, Nixon J, Gladding S. An entrustable professional activity (EPA) for handoffs as a model for EPA assessment development. Acad Med. 2014;89(10):1335–40.
33. Baker EA, Ledford CH, Fogg L, Way DP, Park YS. The IDEA assessment tool: assessing the reporting, diagnostic reasoning, and decision-making skills demonstrated in medical students' hospital admission notes. Teach Learn Med. 2015;27(2):163–73.
34. Bierman JA, Hufmeyer KK, Liss DT, Weaver AC, Heiman HL. Promoting responsible electronic documentation: validity evidence for a checklist to assess progress notes in the electronic health record. Teach Learn Med. 2017;29(4):420–32.
35. Heiman HL, Uchida T, Adams C, Butter J, Cohen E, Persell SD, Pribaz P, McGaghie WC, Martin GJ. E-learning and deliberate practice for oral case presentation skills: a randomized trial. Med Teach. 2012;34(12):e820–6.
36. Salzman DH, McGaghie WC, Caprio T, Even EA, Hufmeyer K, Issa N, Schaefer E, Trainor J, Wayne DB. Use of a simulation-based capstone course to teach and assess Entrustable professional activities to graduating medical students. Med Sci Educ. 2016;26:453–6.
37. Pereira AG, Harrell HE, Weissman A, Smith CD, Dupras D, Kane GC. Important skills for internship and the fourth-year medical school courses to acquire them: a national survey of internal medicine residents. Acad Med. 2016;91(6):821–6.
38. Lyss-Lerman P, Teherani A, Aagaard E, Loeser H, Cooke M, Harper GM. What training is needed in the fourth year of medical school? Views of residency program directors. Acad Med. 2009;84(7):823–9.
39. Esterl RM, Henzi DL, Cohn SM. Senior medical student "Boot Camp": can result in increased self-confidence before starting surgery internships. Curr Surg. 2006;63(4):264–8.
40. Peyre SE, Peyre CG, Sullivan ME, Towfigh S. A surgical skills elective can improve student confidence prior to internship. J Surg Res. 2006;133(1):11–5.
41. Okusanya OT, Kornfield ZN, Reinke CE, Morris JB, Sarani B, Williams NN, Kelz RR. The effect and durability of a pregraduation boot cAMP on the confidence of senior medical student entering surgical residencies. J Surg Educ. 2012;69(4):536–43.
42. Naylor RA, Hollett LA, Castellvi A, Valentine RJ, Scott DJ. Preparing medical students to enter surgery residencies. Am J Surg. 2010;199(1):105–9.
43. Antonoff MB, Swanson JA, Green CA, Mann BD, Maddaus MA, D'Cunha J. The significant impact of a competency-based preparatory course for senior medical students entering surgical residency. Acad Med. 2012;87(3):308–19.
44. Lamba S, Wilson B, Natal B, Nagurka R, Anana M, Sule H. A suggested emergency medicine boot camp curriculum for medical students based on the mapping of Core Entrustable Professional Activities to Emergency Medicine Level 1 milestones. Adv Med Educ Pract. 2016;7:115–24.
45. Morgan H, Marzano D, Lanham M, Stein T, Curran D, Hammoud M. Preparing medical students for obstetrics and gynecology milestone level one: a description of a pilot curriculum. Med Educ Online. 2014;19:25746.
46. Morgan H, Skinner B, Marzano D, Fitzgerald J, Curran D, Hammoud M. Improving the medical school-residency transition. Clin Teach. 2017;14(5):340–3.
47. Burns R, Adler M, Mangold K, Trainor J. A brief boot camp for 4th-year medical students entering into pediatric and family medicine residencies. Cureus. 2016;8(2):e488. https://doi.org/10.7759/cureus.488.
48. Bontempo LJ, Frayha N, Dittmar PC. The internship preparation camp at the University of Maryland. Postgrad Med J. 2017 Jan;93(1095):8–14.
49. Clay AS, Andolsek K, Grochowski CO, Engle DL, Chudgar SM. Using transitional year milestones to assess graduating medical students' skills during a capstone course. J Grad Med Educ. 2015;7(4):658–62.
50. Parent RJ, Plerhoples TA, Long EE, Zimmer DM, Teshome M, Mohr CJ, Ly DP, Hernandez-Boussard T, Curet MJ, Dutta S. Early, intermediate, and late effects of a surgical skills "boot camp" on an objective structured assessment of technical skills: a randomized controlled study. J Am Coll Surg. 2010;210(6):984–9.

51. Fernandez GL, Page DW, Coe NP, Lee PC, Patterson LA, Skylizard L, St Louis M, Amaral MH, Wait RB, Seymour NE. Boot cAMP: educational outcomes after 4 successive years of preparatory simulation-based training at onset of internship. J Surg Educ. 2012;69(2):242–8.
52. Aylward M, Vawter L, Roth C. An interactive handoff workshop to improve intern readiness in patient care transitions. J Grad Med Educ. 2012;4(1):68–71.
53. American Board of Surgery; American College of Surgeons; Association of Program Directors in Surgery; Association for Surgical Education. Statement on surgical preresidency preparatory courses. J Surg Educ. 2014;71(6):777–8.
54. Selden NR, Origitano TC, Burchiel KJ, Getch CC, Anderson VC, McCartney S, Abdulrauf SI, Barrow DL, Ehni BL, Grady MS, Hadjipanayis CG, Heilman CB, Popp AJ, Sawaya R, Schuster JM, Wu JK, Barbaro NM. A national fundamentals curriculum for neurosurgery PGY1 residents: the 2010 Society of Neurological Surgeons boot camp courses. Neurosurgery. 2012;70(4):971–81.
55. Minha S, Shefet D, Sagi D, Berkenstadt H, Ziv A. "See one, sim one, do one"- a national pre-internship boot-camp to ensure a safer "student to doctor" transition. PLoS One. 2016;11(3):e0150122.
56. Butter J, McGaghie WC, Cohen ER, Kaye M, Wayne DB. Simulation-based mastery learning improves cardiac auscultation skills in medical students. J Gen Intern Med. 2010;25(8):780–5.
57. Cohen ER, Barsuk JH, Moazed F, Caprio T, Didwania A, McGaghie WC, Wayne DB. Making July safer: simulation-based mastery learning during intern boot camp. Acad Med. 2013;88(2):233–9.
58. Barsuk JH, Cohen ER, Feinglass J, McGaghie WC, Wayne DB. Clinical outcomes after bedside and interventional radiology paracentesis procedures. Am J Med. 2013;126(4):349–56.
59. Reed T, Pirotte M, McHugh M, Oh L, Lovett S, Hoyt AE, Quinones D, Adams W, Gruener G, McGaghie WC. Simulation-based mastery learning improves medical student performance and retention of core clinical skills. Sim Healthc. 2016;11(3):173–80.
60. Salzman DH, McGaghie WC, Caprio T, Hufmeyer K, Issa N, Trainor J, Cohen E, Wayne DB. A mastery learning capstone course to teach and assess components of three entrustable professional activities to graduating medical students. Teach Learn Med. 2019;31(2):186–94.
61. Arora VM, Berhie S, Horwitz LI, Saathoff M, Staisiunas P, Farnan JM. Using standardized videos to validate a measure of handoff quality: the handoff mini-clinical examination exercise. J Hosp Med. 2014;9(7):441–6.
62. Massagli TL, Carline JD. Reliability of a 360-degree evaluation to assess resident competence. Am J Phys Med Rehabil. 2007;86(10):845–52.
63. Norcini JJ, Blank LL, Arnold GK, Kimball HR. The mini-CEX (clinical evaluation exercise): a preliminary investigation. Ann Intern Med. 1995;123(10):795–9.
64. Norcini JJ, Blank LL, Duffy FD, Fortna GS. The mini-CEX: a method for assessing clinical skills. Ann Intern Med. 2003;138(6):476–81.
65. Kogan JR, Bellini LM, Shea JA. Implementation of the mini-CEX to evaluate medical students' clinical skills. Acad Med. 2002;77(11):1156–1157.4.
66. Weller JM, Jolly B, Misur MP, Merry AF, Jones A, Crossley JG, Pedersen K, Smith K. Mini-clinical evaluation exercise in anaesthesia training. Br J Anaesth. 2009;102(5):633–41.
67. Ten Cate O, Chen HC, Hoff RG, Peters H, Bok H, van der Schaaf M. Curriculum development for the workplace using entrustable professional activities (EPAs): AMEE guide no. 99. Med Teach. 2015;37(11):983–1002.
68. Walling A, Merando A. The fourth year of medical education: a literature review. Acad Med. 2010;85(11):1698–704.
69. Andrews JS, Bale JF, Soep JB, Long M, Carraccio C, Englander R, Powell D, EPAC Study Group. Education in pediatrics across the continuum (EPAC): first steps toward realizing the dream of competency-based education. Acad Med. 2018;93(3):414–20.

Part IV

Transfer of Training from Mastery Learning

Translational Science and Healthcare Quality and Safety Improvement from Mastery Learning

16

William C. McGaghie, Diane B. Wayne, and Jeffrey H. Barsuk

Previous chapters in this book have set a foundation that demonstrates the power and utility of mastery learning in health professions education. The earlier chapters covered an array of topics such as how to develop mastery learning curricula; evaluate mastery learning outcomes; set mastery learning standards; implement and manage mastery learning programs; and use reliable evaluation data for learner feedback, debriefing, and improvement. Other chapters provide concrete examples that show how mastery learning is used to help health professionals acquire foundation knowledge and skills including clinical communication, surgical dexterity, bedside procedures, and managing clinical emergencies. These chapters are essential, sturdy, and practical building blocks about mastery learning in the health professions. The anatomy and physiology of mastery learning are embodied in such bedrock writings.

This chapter extends basic principles of mastery learning into two new and related domains: (a) mastery learning contributions to translational science and (b) mastery learning as a vehicle for healthcare quality improvement. We address three key questions: First, how can we stretch the mastery learning outcome measurement endpoint from proximal educational settings like a medical simulation laboratory to more distal measurement objectives, i.e., "downstream" educational outcomes? Second, how can we translate powerful, mastery learning educational interventions to patient care practices and patient outcomes that really matter? Third, how can we show that powerful health professions education grounded in mastery learning can improve healthcare quality and safety delivered at the bedside, in the clinic, and in the community?

W. C. McGaghie (✉)
Northwestern University Feinberg School of Medicine, Departments of Medical Education and Preventive Medicine, Chicago, IL, USA
e-mail: wcmc@northwestern.edu

D. B. Wayne · J. H. Barsuk
Northwestern University Feinberg School of Medicine, Departments of Medicine and Medical Education, Chicago, IL, USA
e-mail: dwayne@northwestern.edu

W. C. McGaghie et al. (eds.), *Comprehensive Healthcare Simulation: Mastery Learning in Health Professions Education*, Comprehensive Healthcare Simulation, https://doi.org/10.1007/978-3-030-34811-3_16

These questions reveal an unstated and paradoxical situation. For at least the past century, health professions educators have assumed incorrectly that the "see one, do one, teach one" apprenticeship model of clinical education produces physicians, nurses, and others who can deliver effective and safe patient care that yields good patient outcomes as discussed in Chap. 1. Conventional wisdom holds there is no doubt that traditional clinical education "works" because the training method has been used for decades. Years of experience, but little reliable evidence, underscores a belief that today's approach to clinical education produces health professionals who are competent, caring, skillful, and ethical. Thus the clinical education status quo is rarely challenged. Educational innovators, advocates of change, are the only ones who are expected to present hard data to support rival approaches to "business as usual," as pointed out in the preface to this book. Mastery learning interventions that demonstrate translational outcomes are essential to gain support from healthcare CEOs and other stakeholders who often believe that education is a weak means to improve patient care quality and safety.

This chapter presents and consolidates data that demonstrate the superiority of mastery learning—frequently using simulation technology—for clinical skill acquisition, clinical skill application in patient care, and effective patient outcomes from skillful care, all compared to conventional clinical education.

Mastery Learning Contributions to Translational Science

A 2010 report states that translational science in medical (health professions) education is achieved when "… rigorous studies on trainee clinical skill and knowledge acquisition address key healthcare problems and measure outcomes in controlled laboratory settings (T1 translational research); when these outcomes transfer to clinics, wards, and offices where better healthcare is delivered (T2); and when patient or public health improves as a result of educational practices (T3)" [1]. A fourth outcome category (T4) was added in 2015 to include collateral educational results that produce improved education and healthcare outcomes beyond those intended from the original intervention, e.g., skill and knowledge retention; cost savings or return on investment (ROI) to health systems; and unplanned, systemic effects on healthcare education or delivery [2].

A simple conceptual model shown in Fig. 16.1, derived from the two earlier installments [1, 2], provides a framework to picture health professions education as translational science.

The graphic presentation in Fig. 16.1 suggests that powerful mastery learning educational interventions can produce tangible short- and long-run education and healthcare benefits. The benefits are captured by measurements that are increasingly distal from a proximal mastery learning educational program situated in a classroom, healthcare clinic, or simulation laboratory. What follows is a story about a health professions education mastery learning program that has produced reliably measured outcomes in each of the T1 to T4 translational science categories. The

Medical Education Research as Translational Science

Contributions of *powerful medical education interventions* to T1–T4 outcomes

	Level of Translation			
Focus	**T1**	**T2**	**T3**	**T4**
Increased or Improved	Knowledge, skill, attitudes, professionalism	Patient care practices	Patient outcomes	Collateral effects, e.g., skill retention, ROI, indirect outcomes
Target Groups	Individuals and teams	Individuals and teams	Individuals and public health	Individuals, teams, public health
Setting	Education setting, e.g., simulation lab	Clinic and bedside	Clinic, bedside, and community	Clinic, bedside, and community

Fig. 16.1 From T1 to T4 downstream translational science outcomes

story is about educating internal medicine (IM) and emergency medicine (EM) residents to insert central venous catheters (CVCs) to a very high mastery learning standard and the translational effects of this learning on patient care practices, patient health outcomes, and several collateral results. A key point is that demonstration of "downstream" outcomes stems from careful education and patient outcome measurement, planning, and execution. Demonstration of translational outcomes in health professions education does not stem from single, isolated studies. Instead, translational science educational outcomes derive from rigorously designed education and health services evaluation research *programs* that are thematic, sustained, and cumulative.

T1: Does a Mastery Learning Curriculum Work?

CVCs are often inserted into patients' internal jugular (IJ) vein in the neck or the subclavian (SC) vein just below the clavicle and are needed for patient care and survival. CVCs are used to deliver medication and fluids that cannot be given in a smaller, noncentral vein. They may also be used to monitor different types of blood pressure or laboratory data in patients who are critically ill. CVCs are ubiquitous in medical and surgical intensive care units (ICUs) and are usually inserted by physicians, physician assistants, or nurse practitioners and maintained by nurses. Unskilled CVC insertion can produce adverse patient complications including pneumothorax, arterial injury, and central line-associated bloodstream infections (CLABSIs). Poor CVC maintenance can also cause CLABSIs. These complications produce patient discomfort, increase morbidity and mortality, and are very costly to the healthcare system.

A Northwestern University Feinberg School of Medicine (NUFSM) medical and education team led by hospitalist physician Jeffrey Barsuk developed a simulation-based mastery learning (SBML) curriculum designed to prepare IM resident doctors to insert CVCs [3]. The SBML curriculum for CVC insertion was grounded in the seven cardinal features of the mastery learning bundle described in Chap. 3 of this volume: baseline or diagnostic testing (pretest); focus on clear learning objectives; engagement in educational activities, especially deliberate skills practice; attention to a minimum passing (*mastery*) standard (MPS); formative testing with actionable feedback; advancement if learner performance is ≥ MPS; and continued practice or study if needed until the MPS is reached.

The CVC SBML curriculum was delivered in the Northwestern Simulation Laboratory under controlled, clinically realistic conditions. Figure 16.2 provides a portrait of the CVC training "in action." Note that the learner and the teacher/coach are fully gowned and gloved, observe sterile technique, work together, and communicate directly throughout the education session. The intent is to create a SBML space that is a close approximation to the real clinical setting.

A skill-based pretest, the first step of the mastery learning education bundle, was administered to each of 28 IM resident physicians under controlled conditions with IJ and SC outcomes evaluated using a 27-item checklist. As expected, the pretest results showed the residents performed poorly on the simulated CVC insertions. These results were used as an educational tool, not as a weapon, to give each resident physician specific, actionable feedback about how to improve. The pretest data were matched with SBML learning objectives to give each learner a roadmap for improvement. Learners then engaged in focused, intense, CVC skills deliberate practice that was supervised closely by a teacher/coach. Repetitive formative testing and more feedback were used to help each doctor acquire the CVC insertion skills needed to reach the preset MPS for both the IJ and SC insertion sites. Figure 16.3

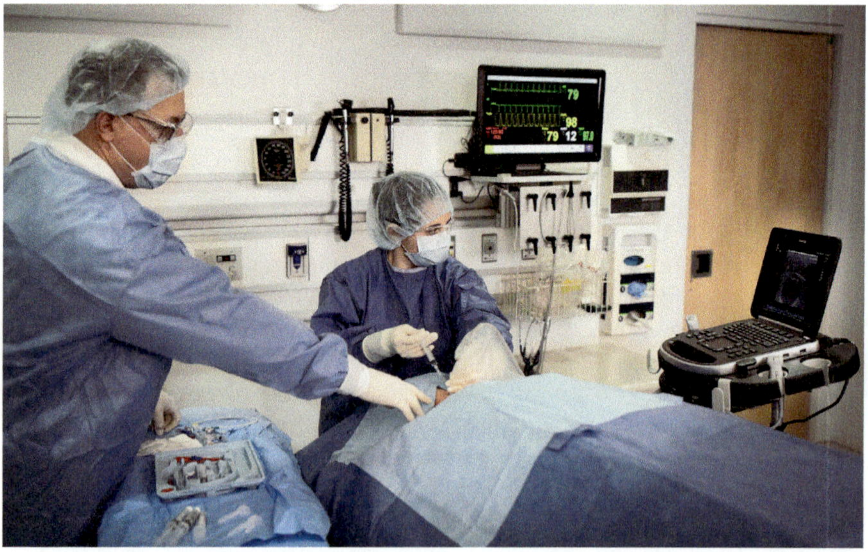

Fig. 16.2 Resident training on the CVC simulator

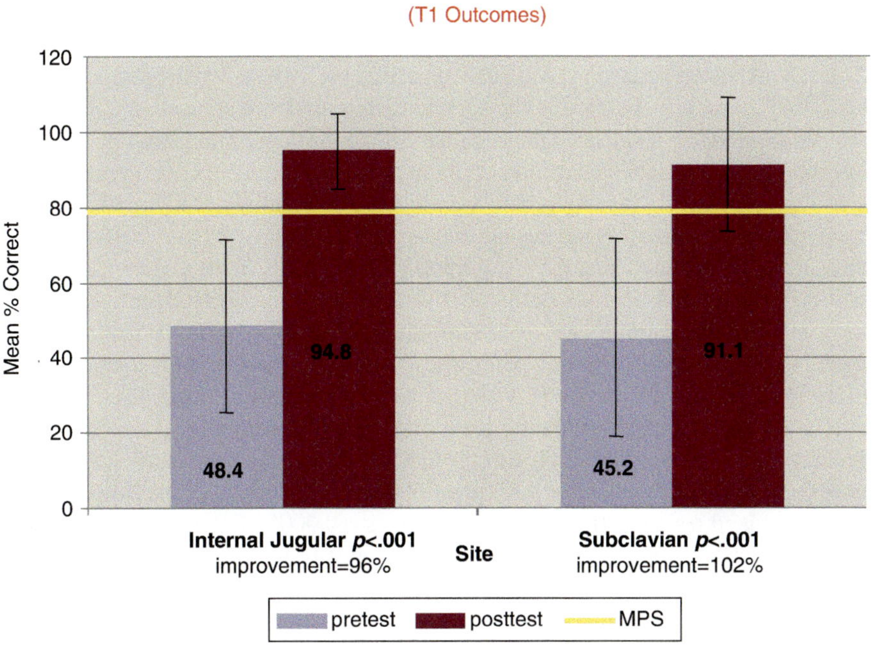

Fig. 16.3 Mean scores and standard deviations on the simulator-based skills exam before and after the educational intervention. MPS = 79.1%. (Adapted from Barsuk et al. [3]. Reprinted with permission from the Society of Hospital Medicine [3])

presents the pretest and posttest mastery learning data for the CVC SBML curriculum for the resident physicians (T1 outcomes). The MPS, set earlier by an expert physician panel, is also indicated [4].

Most of the 28 IM resident physician learners achieved CVC insertion mastery within a uniform 4-hour curriculum in the simulation education laboratory. A handful of the learners, 3 of 28 residents (11%), needed up to an additional hour of deliberate practice, assessment, feedback, and improvement before retesting to achieve the MPS. However, the final result was that all of the resident physicians achieved all of the CVC SBML educational objectives with very little variation in measured outcomes. The residents also expressed genuine self-confidence in their newly acquired clinical skill, confidence verified by outcome data measured objectively and reliably [3].

T2: Does Mastery Learning Improve Patient Care Practices?

The evidence is clear that SBML is a powerful approach to help resident physicians acquire CVC clinical skills in the controlled simulation education laboratory. But a key question is "Do clinical skills acquired in the medical simulation laboratory extend to improved patient care practices in outpatient clinics, hospital floors, ICUs, and other patient care settings?" Do clinical skills learned in an educational environment generalize to better and safer patient care?

The Northwestern team, led by Dr. Barsuk, addressed these questions by conducting a cohort study involving two groups of IM and EM residents [5]. The first group of 27 residents learned to insert IJ and SC central lines via the traditional "see one, do one, teach one" approach common to the apprenticeship model of clinical education. The second group of 76 residents completed the SBML curriculum in IJ and SC catheter insertion in the simulation education laboratory. Patients receiving CVC insertions and care from residents in the two groups were monitored carefully. Daily measurements were taken from patients receiving clinical care from both resident groups. The patient measurements captured four CVC insertion variables: (a) needle passes (associated with an increased risk of pneumothorax), (b) arterial puncture, (c) need for CVC adjustment after initial insertion, and (d) insertion failure rate. All of the patient measurements were recorded by research personnel who were not aware of the training status of the residents who inserted the CVCs (i.e., the recorders were "blinded").

The results of this T2 study are plain and significant on clinical and statistical grounds. Patients receiving CVC care from SBML residents had significantly fewer needle passes (M = 1.32, sd = 0.85) than patients receiving CVC care from traditionally trained residents (M = 1.74, sd = 0.83) ($p < 0.0005$). Patients receiving CVC care from SBML-trained residents also experienced much lower rates of arterial puncture, CVC adjustment, and insertion failure than patients receiving CVC care from traditionally trained resident doctors. This is strong evidence that SBML of CVC insertion skills produces better patient care practices, i.e., T2 outcomes, than traditional clinical medical education (Fig. 16.4) [5].

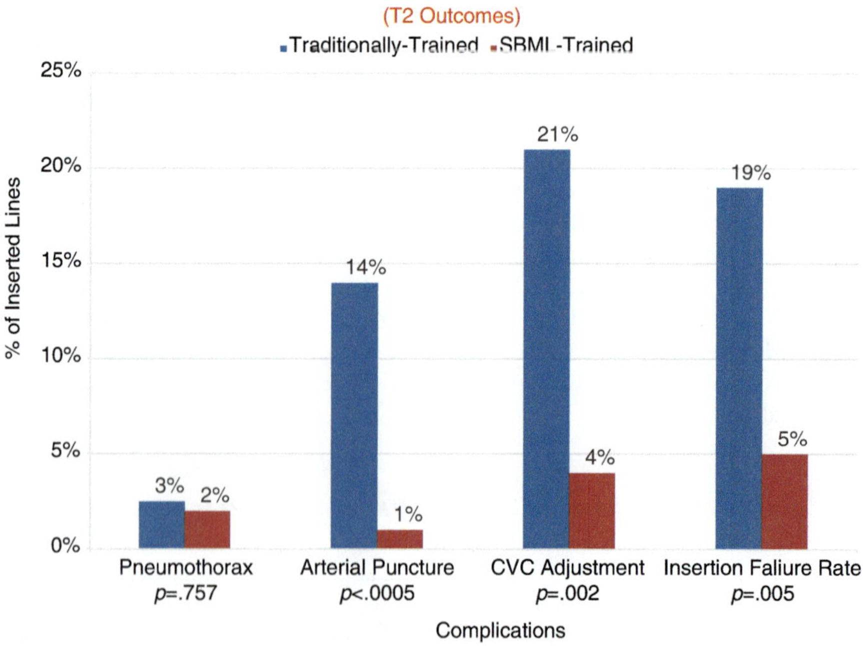

Fig. 16.4 Central venous catheter complications among patients receiving care from traditionally trained residents versus simulation-based mastery learning (SBML)-trained residents. (Data from Ref. [5])

T3: Does Mastery Learning Improve Patient Outcomes?

A subsequent study by the Northwestern group sought to evaluate the impact of the SBML CVC insertion curriculum on patient outcomes (T3) which is another step downstream from (T2) patient care practices [6]. The research question in this project was "Do patients receiving CVC care from medical residents who have mastered the simulation-based curriculum experience lower CLABSI rates than patients receiving CVC care from traditionally trained medical residents?" In short, does SBML of CVC insertion skills lead to better and safer patient outcomes?

The mastery learning curriculum on CVC insertion skills was evaluated using a longitudinal pre-post cohort (incidence) study design that looked at CLABSI rates among two groups of ICU patients who had CVCs inserted across 32 months. The first CVC patient group received care in the medical intensive care unit (MICU) at Northwestern Memorial Hospital (NMH) in Chicago from August 2005 to March 2008. The second CVC patient group received care in the NMH surgical intensive care unit (SICU) during the same time period. During the first 16 months of the education and health services evaluation research study, all CVC patients, in both groups, received care from traditionally trained residents. By contrast, in the second 16 months of the study, all MICU CVC patients received care from residents who were CVC trained to rigorous mastery learning standards, while SICU patients still received CVC care from traditionally trained residents who had not participated in the mastery learning intervention [6].

The results of this T3 evaluation research study are also presented in Fig. 16.5. The figure shows that patients receiving CVC care from medical

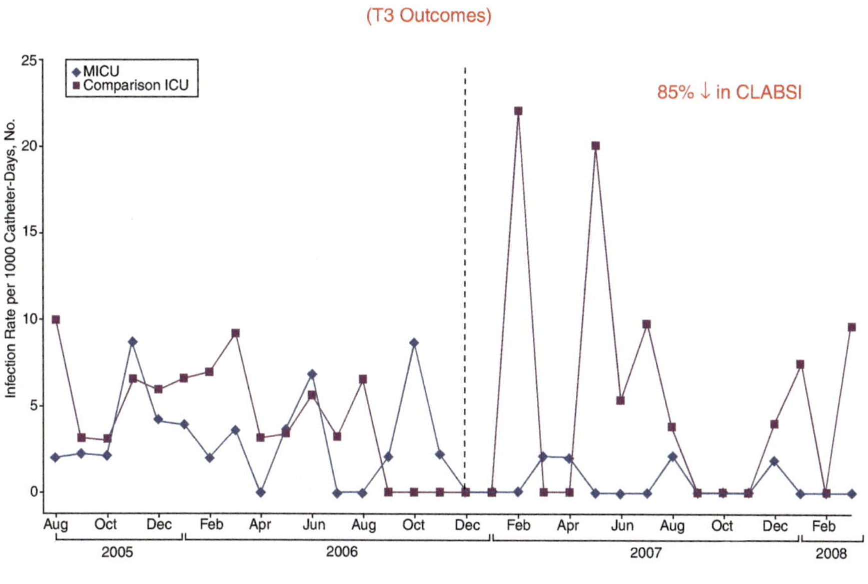

Fig. 16.5 Monthly catheter-related bloodstream infection rates (cental line-associated bloodstream infections) in a medical intensive care unit (MICU) and a comparison intensive care unit (ICU) before and after a simulation-based educational intervention in the MICU. The vertical line at December 2006 indicates the time that simulator-trained residents entered the MICU. (From: Barsuk et al. [6]. Reprinted with permission from the American Medical Association [6])

residents who had mastered the clinical skill from rigorous, simulation-based education experienced an 85% reduction in CLABSI rates both in comparison with the MICU baseline measurement and also in comparison with the SICU CLABSI rate. These results are highly significant on clinical and statistical grounds, where the statistical analysis is controlled for comorbid conditions. These profound patient outcome results are all directly linked to the powerful SBML CVC educational intervention that relies on deliberate practice of clinical skills [6].

T4: Does Mastery Learning Produce Collateral Effects?

The SBML CVC insertion curriculum which was developed, implemented, and evaluated at NUFSM and NMH has produced a variety of collateral effects. Collateral effects in health professions education involve unexpected, yet welcome, accessory results derived from rigorous curriculum interventions. These accessory results are important because they show that new and powerful curricula, once introduced into status quo educational environments, frequently have "ripple effects," i.e., unintended consequences that can affect clinical skill maintenance, healthcare costs, educational and healthcare practices, and other systemic conditions.

Six collateral effects derived from the SBML CVC insertion education program have been reported and are expanded here. The six collateral (T4) education outcomes are (a) CVC skill retention, (b) cost savings and return on investment, (c) systemic effects on healthcare education, (d) increased MPS due to unexpected skill improvement among medical residents, (e) improvement of CVC line maintenance skills among ICU nurses, and (f) questions about attending physician competence doing CVC insertion, especially after longitudinal clinical experience.

CVC Skill Retention

Are clinical skills acquired to a mastery standard in a medical simulation laboratory retained over time? Can we predict clinical skill decay among highly educated physicians?

These questions prompted the Northwestern education and research team to design a follow-up study to evaluate CVC skill decay among doctors who had previously mastered the clinical skill in the simulation laboratory (T1) [3, 5]. The investigators identified 61 Northwestern physicians who had successfully completed the SBML CVC curriculum and were available for follow-up assessment. Forty-nine of the 61 doctors (80.3%) consented to participate in the study. The CVC insertion skills of these doctors were evaluated 6 months and 12 months after skill mastery using the same simulation technology and reliable measurement procedures that were used in the SBML curriculum. The same MPS (79.1% of the skill checklist items needed to be correct on a simulated CVC skills assessment) set by a multidisciplinary expert panel for the SBML curriculum [4] was employed for the follow-up evaluations [7].

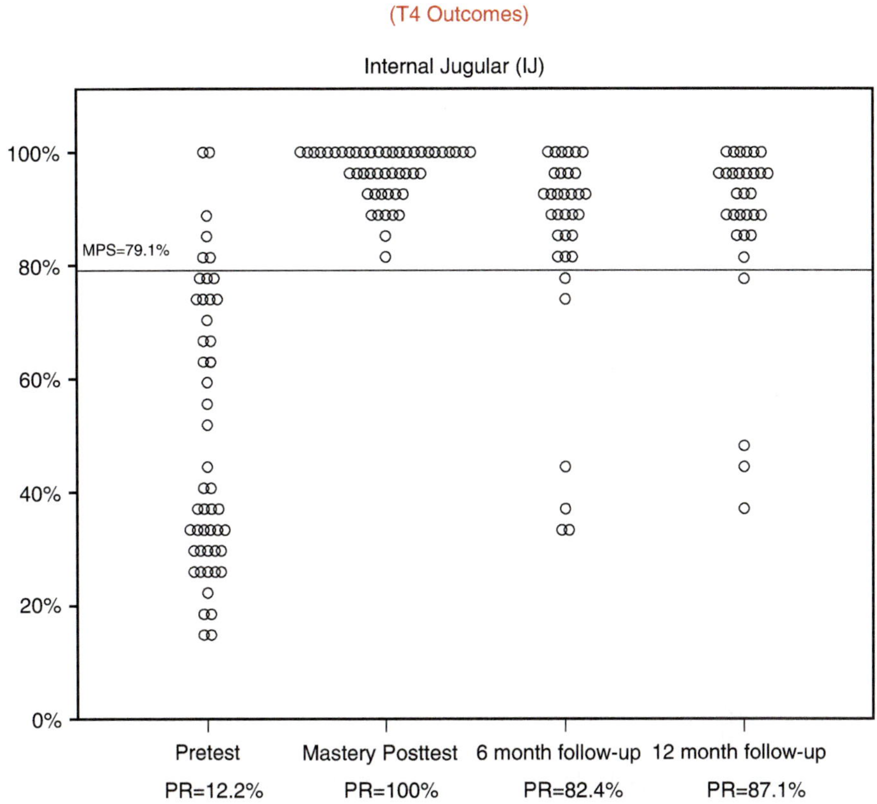

Fig. 16.6 Individual residents' internal jugular (IJ) checklist scores at pretest, posttest, six-month, and one-year follow-up. Pass rate (PR) is reported for each interval, and minimum passing score (MPS) is indicated for the checklist. (Reprinted with permission from: Barsuk et al. [7])

The study results for IJ CVC insertions are presented in Fig. 16.6. (Results for SC CVC insertions are nearly identical.) The IJ pass rates for the four measurement occasions are clear and informative: pretest = 12.2%, mastery posttest = 100%, 6-month follow-up = 82.4%, and 12-month follow-up = 87.1%. The research team discovered that physicians who fell below the MPS at the 6-month follow-up assessment were not the same as those who fell below the MPS at the 12-month follow-up evaluation. The doctors' demographic data and clinical experience did not predict CVC skill decay after mastery was achieved. The Northwestern education scientists conclude, "Procedural skills should be documented through rigorous assessment rather than reliance on clinical experience or reported self-confidence because we cannot reliably predict who will pass or fail follow-up examinations" [7]. The Northwestern team found that it is not enough to train healthcare providers to mastery only once. Providers need follow-up assessment and retraining. Programs must be sustained and ongoing.

Cost Savings and Return on Investment

The expense of SBML of CVC insertion clinical skills can be balanced in comparison with healthcare cost savings expressed as prevented CLABSIs, patient MICU days, pharmacotherapies, and other hospital charges. One report calculated a ratio of per patient cost savings versus expenses from the SBML CVC curriculum [8]. Such calculations allow educational and health services researchers to pinpoint the financial return on investment (ROI) from SBML of CVC clinical skills. This is important because it shows stakeholders that an initial investment in education not only saves lives but also results in cost savings.

A study led by research associate Elaine Cohen with other Northwestern investigators sought to assess the cost savings and ROI of the SBML CVC educational curriculum [8]. The research report states, "After residents completed a simulation-based mastery learning program in CVC insertion, CRBSI [CLABSI] rates declined sharply. … methods were used to estimate savings by comparing CRBSI [CLABSI] rates in the year before and after the intervention. Annual savings from reduced CRBSIs [CLABSIs] were compared with the annual cost of simulation training" [8]. The research report continues, "Approximately 9.95 CRBSI [CLABSIs] were prevented among MICU patients with CVCs in the year after the intervention. Incremental costs attributed to each CRBSI [CLABSI] were approximately $82,000 in 2008 dollars and 14 additional hospital days (including 12 MICU days). The annual cost of the simulation-based education was approximately $112,000. Net annual savings were thus greater than $700,000, a 7 to 1 rate of return on the simulation training intervention" [8].

This is strong evidence from one SBML CVC insertion program that the educational intervention was highly cost-effective. Such data reinforce the view that SBML can produce significant medical care cost savings and ROI.

Systemic Effects on Healthcare Education

The SBML CVC training program has produced consistent, positive T1 results for each consecutive academic year it has been in place. Beginning in 2007–2008, the CVC curriculum has successfully educated successive cohorts of IM residents to be masters of this clinical procedure and, research evidence shows, to provide effective and safe patient care [5, 6].

The SBML CVC curriculum at NMH is embedded strategically in the internal medicine residency education program. The SBML CVC curriculum has been implemented in two annual stages. In stage one, PGY-1 internal medicine residents experience a 1-month MICU rotation where they observe, but do not often perform, CVC insertions. Later, in stage two, PGY-2 internal medicine residents successfully complete the SBML CVC curriculum as a "ticket of admission" to a 1-month MICU rotation. CVC insertion mastery in the medical simulation laboratory certifies that the residents are fit to provide safe venous cannulation to MICU patients. (This is an entrustment decision, to use the language of Chap. 17.) Passing the SBML CVC curriculum is required for the residents to perform this invasive clinical procedure on real, very sick, patients.

The SBML CVC program matured and became more efficient with several years' experience. Another effect was that the annual addition of new SBML-trained cohorts of CVC-educated residents increased the saturation of highly skilled residents in the MICU. Over three consecutive academic years—2007–2008, 2008–2009, and 2009–2010—the density of SBML CVC-educated residents in the NMH MICU increased to nearly 100%. The healthcare microsystem of the NMH MICU became populated with residents who had mastered the invasive CVC clinical procedure.

Plotting and inspection of the SBML CVC education evaluation records produced a startling finding [9]. For each consecutive year of the educational intervention, the *pretest pass rate*, i.e., the rate of residents who passed the mastery learning pretest before experiencing the educational program, climbed every year. Figure 16.7 shows the SBML pretest pass rates for simulated IJ and SC CVC insertions rose from about 10% in 2007, to roughly 18% in 2008, to nearly 40% in 2009 [9]! The Northwestern University education and research team concluded that "... SBE (simulation-based education) for senior residents had an effect on junior trainees, as evidenced by pre-training CVC insertion skill improvement across three consecutive years" [9].

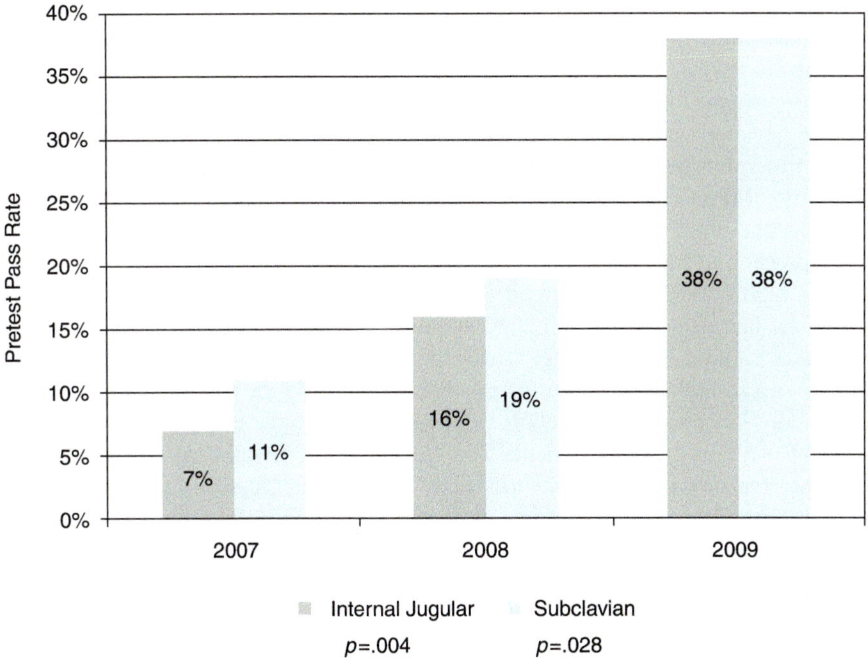

Fig. 16.7 Passing rates for three cohorts (2007–2008, 2008–2009, 2009–2010) of internal medicine residents at Northwestern Memorial Hospital (Chicago, Illinois) in central venous catheter insertion. The increasing passing rates demonstrate improvement over time (internal jugular, $P = 0.004$; subclavian, $P = 0.028$). Pass rate indicates number of residents meeting or exceeding the minimum passing score. (Reprinted with permission from: Barsuk et al. [9])

These unexpected results endorse psychologist Albert Bandura's theory of observational learning [10–12]. People, especially bright and hardworking people like medical residents, acquire skill and knowledge by watching others engage in expert performance. Bandura [11, 12] teaches that observational learning engages four interacting mental processes that likely happen in the NMH MICU for new residents: (a) *attention*, perceiving skilled clinical behavior and judging its utility; (b) *memory*, encoding observations in a form that can be used later; (c) *motor control*, use of observed data to guide one's own actions; and (d) *motivation*, the desire to improve one's clinical skills.

Observational learning is no substitute for sustained, deliberate practice [13, 14] to reach goals of clinical skill acquisition and maintenance among health professions learners. However, we agree with American baseball icon Yogi Berra who said, "You can observe a lot by watching!" You can also learn a lot by watching skillful experts perform invasive clinical procedures. The issue is that skillful experts must be created by participating in SBML with deliberate practice. Before SBML was used to train residents about CVC, junior residents were learning improper techniques from supervising residents. Clinical skills like CVC cannot be mastered without deliberate practice with feedback from an expert instructor.

Increased Minimum Passing Standard

The steady rise in pretest passing rates within the Northwestern SBML CVC curriculum presented an unexpected yet welcome problem. The problem is expressed as two questions by the Northwestern education and research team. First, if the CVC pretest has become so easy for the IM residents to pass before instruction, is the current MPS (79.1%) set in 2006 by a multidisciplinary expert panel [4] now too low? Second, shall we "raise the bar," i.e., reassess and likely increase standards for CVC procedural competence?

The Northwestern team agreed that the steadily rising CVC pretest pass rate called for a revisit to the original 2006 MPS. Thus, a new group of CVC clinical experts was empaneled in 2010 to study the history of IM resident performance and engage in a second standard-setting exercise informed by the historical performance data [15]. The new expert panel provided revised standard-setting judgments about the CVC skill examination. Results from the second CVC standard-setting exercise are that "The new passing standard was 88% for internal jugular and 87% for subclavian central venous catheter insertion compared to 79% for both sites in 2006." The education and research team, in this case led by Elaine Cohen, concluded, "Cumulative performance data influenced experts to set a more stringent minimum passing standard. Standards should be regularly reviewed to ensure they are fair and appropriately rigorous" [15].

Improvement of Central Line Maintenance Skills among ICU Nurses

Effective and safe CVC patient care in the ICU does not reside exclusively with medical staff. Nurses also have a central role in CVC patient care, especially regarding central line maintenance and helping to ensure medical staff perform aseptic insertions. Nurses are the front line of defense to prevent CLABSIs among ICU patients. Nurses' skills at observing ICU patients' conditions, administration of usual and extraordinary catheter care, adjusting patient care as conditions change, and judging patient care outcomes are now commonplace. These nursing skills involve complicated care that requires rigorous clinical education and evaluation to ensure that ICU nurses are fit to care for very sick patients.

The Northwestern SBML CVC learner group was expanded to include ICU nursing staff due to the clinical importance and complexity of CVC line maintenance. A curriculum was created, and an educational program was implemented to educate ICU nurses to mastery learning standards in five CVC maintenance clinical tasks: (a) medication administration, (b) injection cap (needleless connector) changes, (c) tubing changes, (d) blood drawing, and (e) dressing changes. These five clinical nursing tasks all require meticulous attention to sterile technique and are essential for effective and safe nursing care for CVC patient maintenance in the ICU [16].

An initial group of 49 staff nurses working in the NMH Cardiothoracic ICU (CTICU) were enrolled for the first presentation of the SBML curriculum for CVC line maintenance [16]. These continuing professional education trainees were experienced clinical nurses with an average of 10 years of CTICU practice. Results from the report about this innovative SBML curriculum development, implementation, and evaluation study are informative. The research report states, "The number of nurses passing each task at pretest varied from 24 of 49 (49%) for dressing changes to 44 of 49 (90%) for tubing changes. At pretest, scores ranged from a median of 0.0% to 73.1%. At posttest, all scores rose to a median of 100.0%." As an aside, the research report also notes that "Total years in nursing and ICU nursing had significant, negative correlations with medication administration pretest performance" [16]. The report concludes, "ICU nurses displayed large variability in their ability to perform central line maintenance tasks. After SBML, there was significant improvement, and all nurses reached a predetermined level of competency" [16].

This collateral effect of the SBML CVC program on ICU nurses' clinical competence is a short-run (T1) educational outcome achieved in the simulation laboratory [1, 2]. Studies are being planned to evaluate measureable "downstream" results as improved patient care practices (T2) and better patient outcomes (T3) from nursing care in the NMH ICUs.

Questions about Attending Physician Competence at CVC Insertion

Data cited earlier [7] clearly show that CVC skills of residents who have been trained in the simulation laboratory to mastery standards can decay over time (see Fig. 16.6). This research report spawned questions about CVC skill retention among experienced attending physicians who have been performing the clinical procedure for many years and are responsible for training residents in CVC insertion. Do attending physicians maintain their CVC insertion skills over time? How do attending physicians' CVC insertion skills, measured reliably in a medical simulation laboratory, compare with the CVC insertion skills of IM and EM residents measured before and after SBML training?

The Northwestern SBML clinical education and research team, again led by Jeffrey Barsuk, designed and conducted a "prospective cohort study of attending physicians' simulated internal jugular and subclavian central venous catheter insertion skills versus a historical comparison group of residents who participated in simulation training" [17]. This was a train-the-trainer study whose purpose was to use the SBML educational bundle to better prepare attending physicians to teach other healthcare providers to insert CVCs. The SBML education and evaluation program was conducted at 58 Veterans Affairs Medical Centers (VAMCs) across the United States from February to December 2014. The project involved 108 experienced attending physicians, 90% with faculty appointments at academic medical centers, and the historic performance of 143 IM and EM residents from two academic institutions as research participants.

The first step of the mastery learning bundle requires that each SBML trainee must undergo a skills pretest to set a performance baseline for feedback and skill improvement. Pretest scores are also compared with a MPS set previously by an expert panel using systematic methods. All study measurements were obtained under controlled, simulation laboratory conditions, rather than in patient care settings like an ICU, to ensure reliable data.

The study findings show that the attending physicians scored higher on the IJ and SC baseline assessments compared to the residents' baseline assessments. However, the research results also present a concerning outcome because "Overall simulated performance was poor because only 12 of 67 attending physicians (17.9%) met or exceeded the minimum passing score for internal jugular central venous catheter insertion and only 11 of 47 (23.4%) met or exceeded the minimum passing score for subclavian central venous catheter insertion. Resident posttest performance after simulation training was significantly higher than attending physician performance (internal jugular: median, 96% … subclavian: median, 100% … both $p < 0.001$)" [17]. These results are presented graphically in Fig. 16.8.

The attending physician data contained in this research report [17] and from a separate research synthesis that demonstrates residents' procedural experience does not ensure competence [18] clearly indicate that clinical skill acquisition is not a "one time" event for doctors. With or without SBML, clinical experience alone is not a proxy for clinical competence measured objectively and reliably.

Mastery Learning and Healthcare Quality Improvement

Previous sections of this chapter have documented the impact of a powerful SBML CVC curriculum on educational and clinical T1 to T4 outcomes. This is strong evidence that potent health professions education can have robust and lasting effects on patient care practices, patient outcomes, and collateral effects (e.g., observational learning, attention to attending physicians' learning needs) that are frequently overlooked. Rigorous education—the principle that sets mastery learning apart from traditional approaches to health professions education—really matters when the goal is to produce effective and safe clinicians, as discussed in Chaps. 1 and 2 of this book. This observation prompts two questions: Why is health professions education

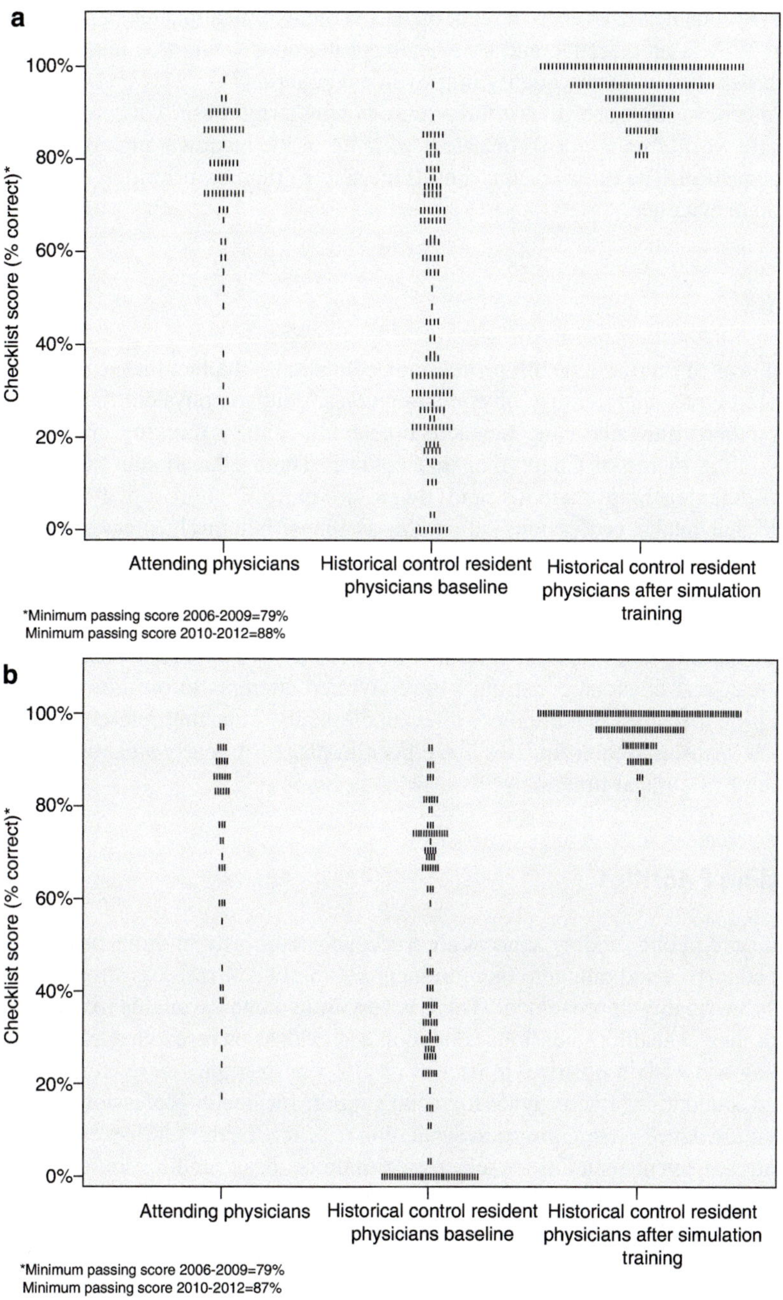

Fig. 16.8 Overall performance of attending physicians (n = 108) and historical control resident physicians (n = 143) on (**a**) internal jugular and (**b**) subclavian central venous catheter (CVC) insertion clinical skill examinations from 2006 to 2012. Attending performance is compared to historical control resident physicians before and after CVC insertion simulation-based mastery learning. Each mark represents one study participant. Residents who elected not to attempt the baseline assessment were given a score of zero checklist items correct. (Source: Barsuk et al. [17]. Reprinted with permission from the Society of Critical Care Medicine and Wolters Kluwer Health, Inc. [17])

so rarely considered, or even thought of, as a vehicle for healthcare quality improvement? Why is an effective and safe health professions workforce not a consistent variable in the healthcare quality improvement equation?

We believe there are at least three reasons why a rigorously educated, effective, and safe workforce is not a consistent variable in the healthcare quality improvement equation. The three reasons are (a) inertia, (b) funding priorities, and (c) inattention to evidence.

Inertia

The power of inertia in health professions education—the fact that we continue to educate twenty-first-century physicians, nurses, dentists, physical therapists, and many other clinicians using obsolete nineteenth-century thinking and technologies—is the theme of Chap. 1 of this volume. These educational habits rely on out-of-date teaching methods and dwell on narrow, short-run T1 outcomes. Traditional health professions education assumes, but rarely measures, that T1 results in the classroom, lecture hall, or simulation laboratory will transfer seamlessly to clinical settings and produce T2 to T4 results. However, in most health professions, there is no accountability mechanism for individuals that counts beyond passing multiple-choice tests of acquired knowledge. Historical, technical, logistical, and financial constraints have stymied attempts to introduce personnel evaluation measures that are more relevant clinically. Thus multiple-choice tests in various forms, and their updates, have been in place for nearly a century as proxy measures of clinical fitness.

Funding Priorities

Private and public funding sources are a second reason why rigorous health professions education and outcome measurement are rarely addressed as strong points of healthcare quality improvement. There is very little money available to support new approaches to health professions education and evaluation research such as mastery learning and sustain positive, impactful results. For example, there are a variety of private foundations that provide financial support for health professions education curriculum development, program evaluation research, health services research, and educational science studies. A selective sample of these funding sources includes the Commonwealth Fund [19], the Robert Wood Johnson Foundation [20], the National Board of Medical Examiners Stemmler Fund [21], and the National League for Nursing [22]. Health professions specialty societies, large and small educational institutions, hospitals, and local family foundations also provide money for innovative educational programs and evaluation research to gauge their effectiveness. However, private financial support in the United States for health professions education program development and rigorous outcome evaluation research is usually in small amounts, for short-run endeavors, and lacks sustainability.

Public funding in the United States for transformative health professions education program and outcome research is equally transient. Translation science scholars [23] argue that the US National Institutes of Health (NIH) and Agency for Healthcare Research and Quality (AHRQ) place high priority on translational science (TS) that seeks "to transform the conduct of biomedical research in the United States by speeding the translation of scientific discoveries into useful therapies and then developing methods to ensure that those therapies reach patients who need them most" [23]. However, the Northwestern mastery learning and evaluation research team has also noted:

> All of these statements about TS policies and priorities focus on biomedical research, the education of biomedical scientists, and conventional treatment options. They do not address the value of a skilled workforce in the clinical medical and health professions and the importance of rigorous clinical education for the delivery of effective health care. We assert that human capital, embodied in competent physicians and other health professionals, is an essential feature of TS even though NIH, Institute of Medicine, and AHRQ policies and priorities are silent about the contribution of clinical medical education to health-care delivery [24].

Medical education research scholars pointed out more than a decade ago that "The majority of published medical education research is not formally funded, and the studies that do receive support are substantially underfunded. ... To improve the quality of medical research, policy reform that increases funding for medical education scholarship will likely be required" [25]. The power of business as usual in health professions education is reinforced by private and public funding agencies that keep educational innovations like mastery learning as a low priority.

Inattention to Evidence

Arguments endorsing the importance of evidence-based medical and, by inference, health professions education have been advanced for nearly two decades [26]. The Best Evidence Medical Education (BEME) Collaboration is an international organization whose mission is (in part) "the implementation by teachers and educational bodies in their practice, of methods and approaches to education based on the best evidence available" [27]. The BEME Collaboration has sponsored medical education scholarship, chiefly in the form of systematic research reviews, to promote evidence-based educational practices.

There is a growing body of empirical evidence, summarized in at least six integrative reviews, that demonstrates the power and utility of simulation-based medical education featuring deliberate practice, often including mastery learning, on measured outcomes ranging from T1 to T4 [28–33]. A groundbreaking international study in nursing education shows a strong association between a highly educated nursing workforce and patient mortality, patient ratings, and quality of care [34]. However, despite compelling data in favor of rigorous, evidence-based medical and health professions education approaches like mastery learning, the educational status quo is steadfast. The authenticity of "reform without change" in health professions education is very real.

Chapter 7 of this book addresses the barriers, whys, and hows of implementing and managing new and different mastery learning education programs in the health professions.

References

1. McGaghie WC. Medical education research as translational science. Sci Trans Med. 2010;2(19):19cm8.
2. Barsuk JH, Szmuilowicz E. Evaluating medical procedures: evaluation and transfer to the bedside. In: Pangaro LN, McGaghie WC, editors. Handbook on medical student evaluation and assessment. North Syracuse, NY: Gegansatz Press; 2015. p. 113–26.
3. Barsuk JH, McGaghie WC, Cohen ER, Balachandran JS, Wayne DB. Use of simulation-based mastery learning to improve the quality of central venous catheter placement in a medical intensive care unit. J Hosp Med. 2009;4(7):397–403.
4. Wayne DB, Barsuk JH, Cohen ER, McGaghie WC. Do baseline data influence standard setting for a clinical skills examination? Acad Med. 2007;82(10, Suppl):S105–8.
5. Barsuk JH, McGaghie WC, Cohen ER, O'Leary KJ, Wayne DB. Simulation-based mastery learning reduces complications during central venous catheter insertion in a medical intensive care unit. Crit Care Med. 2009;37(10):2697–701.
6. Barsuk JH, Cohen ER, Feinglass J, McGaghie WC, Wayne DB. Use of simulation-based education to reduce catheter-related bloodstream infections. Arch Intern Med. 2009;169(15):1420–3.
7. Barsuk JH, Cohen ER, McGaghie WC, Wayne DB. Long term retention of central venous catheter insertion skills after simulation-based mastery learning. Acad Med. 2010;85(10, Suppl):S9–S12.
8. Cohen ER, Feinglass J, Barsuk JH, Barnard C, O'Donnell A, McGaghie WC, Wayne DB. Cost savings from reduced catheter-related bloodstream infection after simulation-based education for residents in a medical intensive care unit. Simul Healthc. 2010;5(2):98–102.
9. Barsuk JH, Cohen ER, Feinglass J, McGaghie WC, Wayne DB. Unexpected collateral effects of simulation-based medical education. Acad Med. 2011;86(12):1513–7.
10. Bandura A. Vicarious processes: a case of no-trial learning. In: Adams JS, Berkowitz L, editors. Advances in experimental social psychology, vol. 2. New York: Academic Press; 1965. p. 1–55.
11. Bandura A. Social learning theory. Englewood Cliffs, NJ: Prentice Hall; 1977.
12. Bandura A. Social foundations of thought and action: a social cognitive theory. Englewood Cliffs, NJ: Prentice Hall; 1986.
13. Ericsson KA. Deliberate practice and the acquisition and maintenance of expert performance in medicine and related domains. Acad Med. 2004;79(10, Suppl):S70–81.
14. Ericsson KA. Acquisition and maintenance of medical expertise: a perspective from the expert performance approach with deliberate practice. Acad Med. 2015;90(11):1471–86.
15. Cohen ER, Barsuk JH, McGaghie WC, Wayne DB. Raising the bar: reassessing standards for procedural competence. Teach Learn Med. 2013;25(1):6–9.
16. Barsuk JH, Seburn S, Cohen ER, Slade M, Mikolajczak A, Wayne DB. Simulation-based mastery learning improves central line maintenance skills of ICU nurses. J Nurs Admin. 2015;45(10):511–7.
17. Barsuk JH, Cohen ER, Nguyen D, Mitra D, O'Hara K, Okuda Y, Feinglass J, Cameron KA, McGaghie WC, Wayne DB. Attending physician adherence to a 29-component central venous catheter bundle checklist during simulated procedures. Crit Care Med. 2016;44(10):1871–81.

18. Barsuk JH, Cohen ER, Feinglass J, McGaghie WC, Wayne DB. Residents' procedural experience does not ensure competence: a research synthesis. J Grad Med Educ. 2017;9(12):201–8.
19. Commonwealth Fund. Commonwealth Fund programs and special initiatives 2017. Retrieved from http://www.commonwealthfund.org/grants-and-fellowships/programs.
20. Robert Wood Johnson Foundation Grants and grant programs 2017. Retrieved from http://www.rwjf.org/en/how-we-work/grants-and-grant programs.html.
21. National Board of Medical Examiners. Stemmler Fund 2017. Retrieved from http://www.nbme.org/research/stemmler.html.
22. National League for Nursing. NLN nursing education research grants 2017. Retrieved from http://www.nln.org/professional-development-programs/grants-and-scholarships/nursing-education.
23. Rubio DM, Schoenbaum EE, Lee LS, Schteingart DE, Marantz PR, Anderson KE, Platt LD, Baez A, Esposito K. Defining translational research: implications for training. Acad Med. 2010;85(3):470–5.
24. McGaghie WC, Issenberg SB, Cohen ER, Barsuk JH, Wayne DB. Translational educational research: a necessity for effective health-care improvement. Chest. 2012;142(5):1097–103.
25. Reed DA, Kern DE, Levine RB, Wright SM. Costs and funding for published medical education research. JAMA. 2005;294(9):1052–7.
26. Petersen S. Time for evidence based medical education. BMJ. 1999;318:1223–4.
27. BEME Collaboration. Best evidence medical and health professions education 2017. Retrieved from https://www.bemecollaboration.org/Publications+Evidence+Based+Medical+Education/.
28. McGaghie WC, Issenberg SB, Cohen ER, Barsuk JH, Wayne DB. Does simulation-based medical education with deliberate practice yield better results than traditional clinical education? A meta-analytic comparative review of the evidence. Acad Med. 2011;86(6):706–11.
29. McGaghie WC, Draycott TJ, Dunn WF, Lopez CM, Stefanidis D. Evaluating the impact of simulation on translational patient outcomes. Simul Healthc. 2011;6(3, Suppl):S42–7.
30. McGaghie WC, Issenberg SB, Cohen ER, Barsuk JH, Wayne DB. Medical education featuring mastery learning and deliberate practice can lead to better health for individuals and populations. Acad Med. 2011;86(11):e8–9.
31. Cook DA, Brydges R, Zendejas B, Hamstra SJ, Hatala R. Mastery learning for health professionals using technology-enhanced simulation: a systematic review and meta-analysis. Acad Med. 2013;88(8):1178–86.
32. McGaghie WC, Issenberg SB, Barsuk JH, Wayne DB. A critical review of simulation-based mastery learning with translational outcomes. Med Educ. 2014;48:375–85.
33. Griswold-Theodorson S, Ponnuru S, Dong C, Szyld D, Reed T, McGaghie WC. Beyond the simulation laboratory: a realist synthesis of clinical outcomes of simulation based mastery learning. Acad Med. 2015;90(11):1553–60.
34. Aiken LH, Sloane D, Griffiths P, Rafferty AM, Bruyneel L, McHugh M, Maier CB, Moreno-Casbos T, Ball JE, Ausserhofer D, Sermeus W, for the RN4CAST Consortium. Nursing skill mix in European hospitals: cross-sectional study of the association with mortality, patient ratings, and quality of care. BMJ Qual Saf. 2017;26:559–68.

Part V

The Road Ahead

Mastery Learning, Milestones, and Entrustable Professional Activities

17

Eric S. Holmboe, David H. Salzman, Joshua L. Goldstein, and William C. McGaghie

A Brief History of Competencies, Milestones, and Entrustable Professional Activities

Competency-based education is not a new concept. In other fields it is often called competency-based education and training (CBET). What is CBET? As Sullivan notes:

> In a traditional educational system, the unit of progression is time and it is teacher-centered. In a CBET system, the unit of progression is mastery of specific knowledge and skills and is learner-centered. [1]

The earliest conception of competency-based training actually arose in the United States during the 1920s as educational reform became linked to industrial and business models of work that centered on clear specification of outcomes and the knowledge and skills needed to achieve the outcome. Chapter 2 provides a

E. S. Holmboe (✉)
Accreditation Council for Graduate Medical Education, Chief Research, Milestone Development, and Evaluation Officer, Department of Milestones, Chicago, IL, USA

Northwestern University Feinberg School of Medicine, Adjunct Professor of Medical Education, Chicago, IL, USA
e-mail: eholmboe@acgme.org

D. H. Salzman
Northwestern University Feinberg School of Medicine, Departments of Emergency Medicine and Medical Education, Chicago, IL, USA

J. L. Goldstein
Northwestern University Feinberg School of Medicine, Departments of Pediatrics, Medical Education, and Neurology, Chicago, IL, USA

W. C. McGaghie
Northwestern University Feinberg School of Medicine, Departments of Medical Education and Preventive Medicine, Chicago, IL, USA

W. C. McGaghie et al. (eds.), *Comprehensive Healthcare Simulation: Mastery Learning in Health Professions Education*, Comprehensive Healthcare Simulation, https://doi.org/10.1007/978-3-030-34811-3_17

Table 17.1 Principles and characteristics of competency-based education

Principles	Characteristics
1. Competencies are role-derived (e.g., physician), specified in behavioral terms, and made public 2. Assessment criteria are competency-based and specify what constitutes mastery level of achievement 3. Assessment requires performance as the prime evidence but also takes knowledge into account 4. Individual learners progress at rates that depend on demonstrated competency 5. The instructional program facilitates development and evaluation of specific competencies	1. Learning is individualized 2. Feedback to the learner is critical 3. Emphasis is more on the exit criteria than on the admission criteria 4. CBET requires a systematic program (approach) 5. Training is modularized 6. Both the learner and the program are held accountable

Data from Ref. [2]

historical overview of mastery learning, highlighting important links between competency-based and mastery education approaches. However, a more recent conception of competency-based education and training (CBET) has its genesis in the teacher education reform movement of the 1960s [2]. Interest in CBET was spawned by a 1968 US Office of Education National Center for Education 10 university research grant program. The program aimed to develop and implement new teacher training models that focused on student achievement (outcomes). Elam laid down a series of principles and characteristics of CBET in 1971 (Table 17.1). Extensions of early CBET thinking and practice generated interest within medical education [3].

Competency-based medical education (CBME) was promoted by McGaghie and colleagues as part of a landmark report to the World Health Organization in 1978 [3]. In that report, the authors state:

> The intended output of a competency-based programme is a health professional who can practise medicine at a defined level of proficiency, in accord with local conditions, to meet local needs. [3]

In a 2002 review, Carraccio and colleagues noted that some sectors in medical education explored competency-based models in the 1970s, but except for one study, no comparisons between competency-based and the traditional structure and process-based curricula were undertaken [4]. In the context of medicine, Carraccio and colleagues compared the elements between the structure and process-based education approach and the competency-based approach in 2002 (Table 17.2) [4].

A group of international educators recently worked to "modernize" the definition of CBME and lay out the theoretical rationale for a CBME system. This group defined CBME as:

> An outcomes-based approach to the design, implementation, assessment and evaluation of a medical education program using an organizing framework of competencies. [5]

A critical principle of CBME is a focus on outcomes, most importantly health and healthcare outcomes for patients and populations [6, 7] (see also Chap. 16). Medical

Table 17.2 Comparison of structure and process-based vs competency-based educational programs

	Educational program approach	
Variable	Structure and process	Competency-based
Driving force for curriculum	Content-knowledge acquisition	Outcome-knowledge application
Driving force for process	Teacher	Learner
Path of learning	Hierarchical (Teacher→student)	Non-hierarchical (Teacher↔student)
Responsibility for content	Teacher	Student and teacher
Goal of education encounter	Knowledge acquisition	Knowledge application
Typical assessment tool	Single subject measure	Multiple objective measures
Assessment tool	Proxy	Authentic (mimics real tasks of profession)
Setting for evaluation	Removed (gestalt)	"In the trenches" (direct observation)
Evaluation	Norm-referenced	Criterion-referenced
Timing of assessment	Emphasis on summative	Emphasis on formative
Program completion	Fixed time	Variable time

Adapted with permission from Carraccio et al. [4]

education can be viewed as a translational science intervention when the measured competencies (i.e., abilities) acquired by learners transfer directly to the care of patients and families. Mastery learning, as highlighted in Chap. 16 and other sources, specifically incorporates this critical philosophy into its design [8–11]. It is simply not enough to know how or show how, health professionals must be able to provide (i.e., "do") care at the highest level of ability. Patients and families deserve no less.

A key distinguishing feature of competency-based education models is that learners can progress through the educational process at *different* rates. Medical education labels this a time-variable approach versus the current time-fixed approach. The most capable and talented individuals should be able to make career transitions *earlier*, while others require more time (up to a point) to attain a sufficient level of knowledge, skills, and professionalism to enter unsupervised practice. Another distinguishing feature lost in current definitions of CBME is the important concept, noted by Sullivan [1], that competency-based education is learner- *and mastery*-centered. If the ultimate goal is better outcomes for patients and populations, it follows that the education goal for learners and training programs is mastery in clinical practice.

The focus on outcomes and mastery heightens the need for robust assessment especially ongoing, longitudinal assessment that enables the faculty to accurately determine the developmental progress of the learner. Robust assessments promote learning via frequent feedback, coaching, and learning plan adjustments [12, 13]. This is consistent with K. Anders Ericsson's work on the acquisition of expertise via deliberate practice that demonstrates the need to tailor education experiences to continually challenge learners with experiences that are neither too easy nor overwhelming (too hard) [14]. As noted in Chapters 2, 4, and 5, mastery-based outcomes and education designs should guide all assessment and curricular experiences.

Competencies provide the framework for defining education outcomes and represent the abilities of an individual or team. As McGaghie and colleagues reported four decades ago and more recently Frank and colleagues noted in 2010, these competencies stem from the health and healthcare needs of patients and populations [3, 5]. Two widely used competency frameworks, the Royal College of Physicians and Surgeons of Canada's CanMEDS roles and the Accreditation Council for Graduate Medical Education (ACGME)/American Board of Medical Specialties (ABMS) General Competencies, were both prompted by public concerns about the effectiveness of medical education to prepare physicians to provide high-quality and safe care [15, 16]. These competency frameworks joined critical domains of essential abilities for effective clinical practice. The ACGME/ABMS General Competencies were officially launched as part of the Outcome Project in 2001 [16].

Operationalizing and implementing competencies proved to be challenging. Residency and fellowship program directors and faculty members worldwide struggled to understand what the competencies meant and, more importantly, what they "look like" in day-to-day clinical practice. This lack of shared understanding (i.e., shared mental models or shared mental representations) slowed curricular changes and the development and evolution of better assessment methods. The challenges to operationalizing the competencies were not restricted to the United States, and over the last 10 years, two notable concepts have emerged in an effort to enable more effective implementation of CBME: milestones, and entrustable professional activities (EPAs) [17].

What Are Milestones?

In general terms, a milestone is simply a significant point in development. The milestones in the United States provide narrative descriptors of the competencies and sub-competencies along a developmental path with varying degrees of granularity. Milestones enable learners and graduate medical education (GME) programs to determine individual trajectories of professional progress using a stage development model. US milestones are heavily influenced by the Dreyfus stage model of development [18, 19]. Milestones describe performance levels residents and fellows are expected to demonstrate for skills, knowledge, and behaviors in six general clinical competency domains. The five stages of the Dreyfus model (Table 17.3) are novice, advanced beginner, competent, proficient, and expert [19]. An application of the Dreyfus model by Carraccio and colleagues can be seen in Table 17.4 of the essential competency of clinical reasoning and judgment [20].

The milestones also help define, in narrative terms, key domains of specialty practice. Domain theory is essential in constructing and using milestones. Messick noted that domain theory is the "the scientific inquiry into the nature of the domain processes and the ways in which they combine to produce effects or outcomes." As Messick points out, "specification of the boundaries of the construct domain to be assessed – that is, determining the knowledge, skills and attitudes, and other

Table 17.3 The stages of learning as proposed by Dreyfus

Stage of learning	Method of instruction (teaching style)	Learning steps	Learner characteristics
1. Novice	Instruction (instructor) Breaks skill into context-free, discrete tasks, concepts, and rules	Recognizes the context-free features Knows rules for determining actions based on these features	Learning occurs in a detached analytic frame of mind
2. Advanced beginner	Practice (coach) Experiences coping with real situations Points out new aspects of material Teaches rules and reasoning techniques for action	Recognizes relevant aspects based on experience that makes sense of the material Learns maxims about actions based on new material	Learning occurs in a detached, analytic frame of mind
3. Competent	Apprenticeship (facilitator) Develops a plan or chooses a perspective that separates "important" from "ignored" elements Demonstrates that rules and reasoning techniques for choosing are difficult to come by Role models are also Emotionally involved in making decisions	Volume of aspects is overwhelming Performance is exhausting Sense of what's important is lacking Stands alone making correct and incorrect choices Coping becomes frightening, discouraging, and elating	Learner is emotionally involved in the task and its outcome Too many subtle differences for rules; student must decide in each case Makes a mistake and then feels remorse Succeeds and then feels elated Emotional learning builds competence
4. Proficient	Apprenticeship (supervisor) Gains more specific experience with outcomes of one's decisions Applies rules and maxims to decide what to do	Rules and principles are replaced by situational discrimination Emotional responses to success or failure build intuitive responses that replace reasoned ones	Learner immediately sees the goal and salient features Learner reasons how to get to the goal by applying rules and principles
5. Expert	Independence (mentor) Experiences multiple, small random variations Observes other experts or experiences nonrandom simulations Working through the cases must emotionally matter	Gains experience with increasingly subtle variations in situations Automatically distinguishes situations requiring one response from those requiring another	Immediately sees the goal and what must be done to achieve it Builds on previous learning experiences

From Dreyfus [58]

attributes to be revealed by the assessment task" is a key issue in validity [21]. Milestones help to define, using the concept of domain theory, both content and performance standards. For medical education and the milestones, the standards should be *mastery learning standards*. Medical education and the milestones are structured in a way that allows for integration of mastery learning principles to become *mastery standards.*

Table 17.4 Example of Dreyfus model stages of development: clinical reasoning and judgment

Stage	Characteristics of stage
1 Novice	Rule driven Uses analytic reasoning and rules to link cause and effect Has little ability to filter or prioritize information, so synthesis is difficult at best to discern the big picture
2 Advanced beginner	Sorts through rules and information to decide what is relevant on the basis of past experience Uses both analytic reasoning and pattern recognition to solve problems Abstracts from concrete and specific information to more general aspects of a problem
3 Competent	Emotional buy-in allows the learner to feel an appropriate level of responsibility Experience tips the balance in clinical reasoning from methodical and analytic to more readily identifiable pattern recognition of common clinical problem presentations Sees the big picture Complex or uncommon problems require reliance on analytic reasoning
4 Proficient	Breadth of past experience allows one to rely on pattern recognition of illness presentation such that clinical problem-solving seems intuitive Relies on methodical and analytic reasoning for managing problems because an exhaustive number of management permutations and responses provide less reasoning experience than illness recognition Comfortable with evolving situations; can extrapolate from a known situation to an unknown situation (capable) Can live with ambiguity
5 Expert	Thought, feeling, and action align into intuitive problem recognition and intuitive situational responses and management Recognizes unexpected events Clever responses Perceptive: discriminates features that do not fit a recognizable pattern

Reproduced with permission from Ref. [20]

In this model achieving a performance "floor," most aligned with the competent stage in the Dreyfus model, is the goal neither of medical education nor of the milestone approach. In addition to the Dreyfus stage model of development, milestones were also influenced by Anders Ericsson's work on purposeful and deliberate practice to achieve expertise [14, 22]. Chapters 2 and 4 in this book provide an overview of purposeful and deliberate practice [22]. Milestones, informed by multiple educational theories and empirical research, were designed to promote mastery as the ultimate goal. In essence, milestone judgments should ultimately be *mastery decisions*. The milestones and entrustable professional activities (EPAs; see below) have the potential to drive learners, with help from their training programs, toward mastery by using an outcomes-based approach (i.e., mastery as outcome) grounded in developmental principles.

The general terminology used within the milestones is included in Fig. 17.1a, b.

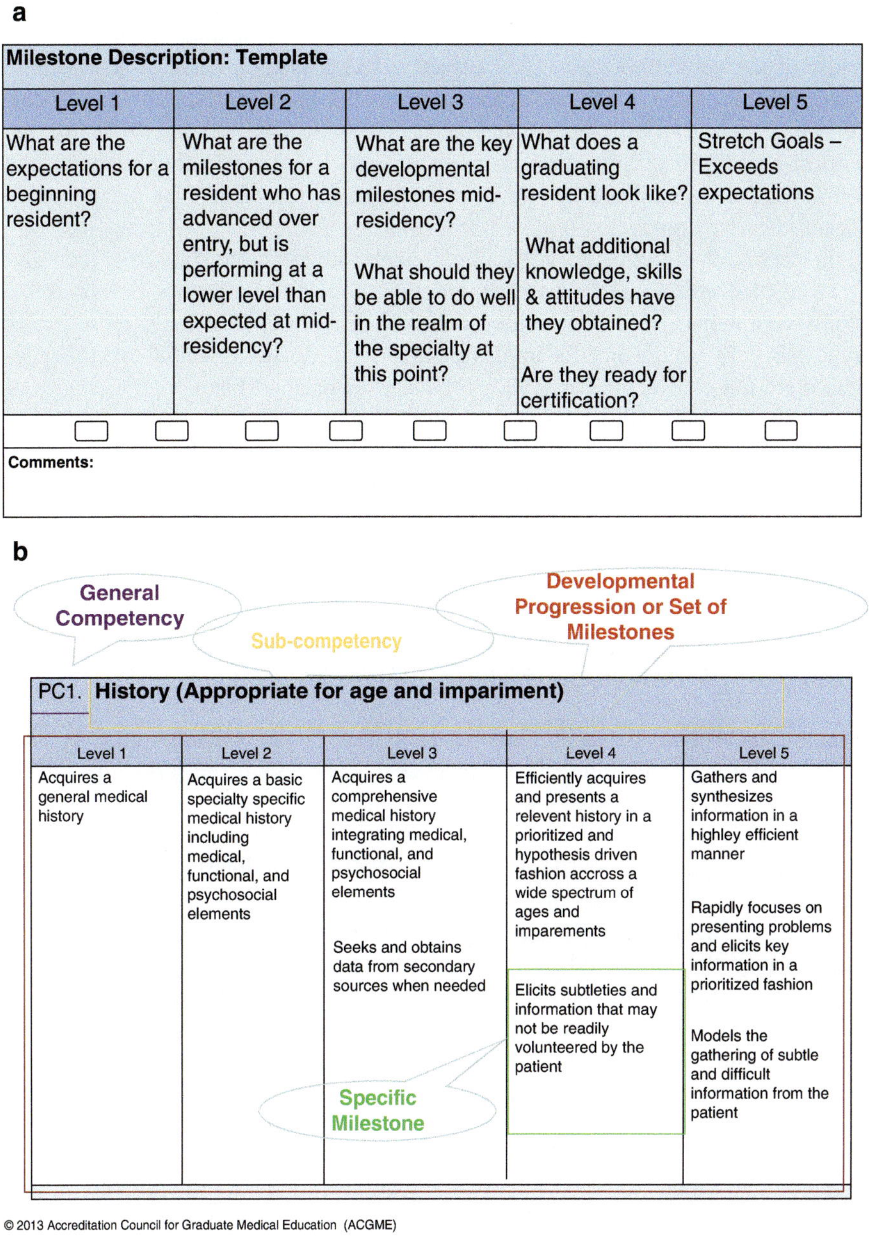

Fig. 17.1 (**a**) General guidance for milestone levels. (**b**) The basic anatomy of a milestone using Patient Care (PC)-1 History Taking as an example. (Adapted from Ref. [18], with permission of ACGME)

Milestones are different from other assessment frameworks. They provide and promote an opportunity for the learner to demonstrate attainment of aspirational levels of the sub-competency (i.e., expertise and mastery). Equally, if not more important, milestones create a mechanism to enable a shared understanding of outcome expectations for the learner and faculty teachers. Milestones provide a framework for all GME programs which grant assurance that graduating residents and fellows across the United States have reached high achievement levels and are ready for unsupervised practice.

In a textbook about mastery learning, it is also important to state what the milestones *do not address*. First and most important, they do not describe or represent a totally comprehensive description of a clinical discipline. Milestones represent an important *core sample* of a discipline (see also Chap. 5). It is essential that the milestones are not considered curricula by themselves or apart from other elements of education. Instead, milestones should guide a thoughtful curriculum analysis to identify strengths and gaps (see Chap. 3). The milestones framework should also guide development and implementation of a robust program of assessment aligned with curricular goals. The mastery learning principles highlighted throughout this book guide integration of curriculum and assessment to achieve desired education outcomes (Chap. 5).

What Are Entrustable Professional Activities?

The concept of entrustable professional activities (EPAs) was introduced in 2005 [23]. An EPA is a unit of professional practice that can be fully entrusted to a trainee as soon as she or he has demonstrated the necessary competence to execute this activity unsupervised. In contrast with competencies, EPAs are not a quality or characteristic of a trainee, but describe the work that must be done [23]. Competencies define the abilities required of a health professional to execute a specific clinical activity (i.e., EPA). Similar to the milestones, EPAs describe a *core sample* of what a graduating student should be fully entrusted to do in an unsupervised setting. Figure 17.2 presents an overview of an EPAs-competencies matrix. The figure shows a typical competency may not be related to a specific task, while an EPA is a concrete clinical task that usually requires several competencies. EPAs represent essential professional work in a given context. EPAs have at least seven features. EPAs (a) account for specific knowledge, skills, and attitudes acquired through training; (b) lead to recognized output of professional labor; (c) are confined to qualified personnel; (d) are done without supervision; (e) are done within a time frame; (f) are observable and measurable in their process and outcome, leading to a conclusion (" well done" or "not well done"); and (g) reflect one or more of the competencies to be acquired [23].

Much of the work in healthcare can be captured by tasks or responsibilities that are entrusted to individuals. EPAs require a practitioner to express and integrate

Entrustable Professional Activities (EPAs)

ACGME/ABMS Competencies	EPA1	EPA2	EPA3	EPA4	EPA5	EPA6
Patient care and procedural skills	☐		☐	☐	☐	
Medical Knowledge		☐	☐	☐		
Interpersonal skills and communication		☐	☐	☐		☐
Professionalism	☐	☐				
Systems-based practice	☐	☐	☐		☐	☐
Practice-based learning and improvement			☐			

Fig. 17.2 Sample matrix of a 6 EPA with the ACGME/ABMS competency framework. (Adapted from Ref. [25], with permission of ACGME)

multiple competencies from several domains simultaneously, such as content expertise; skills in collaboration, communication, and patient management; and many others. Conversely, each competence domain converges on many different activities. Combining competencies (or domains of competence) and EPAs in a matrix reveals which specific competencies a trainee must master before being trusted to perform an EPA [24]. The two-dimensional matrix in Fig. 17.2 provides helpful specifications for assessment, feedback and individual development and to ground entrustment decisions. This makes assessment based on EPAs a more holistic or synthetic approach, rather than evaluating competencies as stand-alone qualities of learners [25]. EPAs are not an alternative for competencies. They constitute a different dimension by grounding competencies in clinical practice.

In the United States, the EPA concept is being pilot tested in undergraduate medical education. Created by the Association of American Medical Colleges (AAMC), the Core Entrustable Professional Activities for Entering Residency (CEPAERs) program describes 13 activities that should be entrusted via indirect supervision to medical students at graduation [25]. For example, conducting an effective, focused history and physical examination is one CEPAER. The entire list of CEPAERs can be found in Box 17.1.

Box 17.1 Core Entrustable Activities for Entering Residency

1. Gather a history and perform a physical examination.
2. Prioritize a differential diagnosis following a clinical encounter.
3. Recommend and interpret common diagnostic and screening tests.
4. Enter and discuss orders and prescriptions.
5. Document a clinical encounter in the patient record.
6. Provide an oral presentation of a clinical encounter.
7. Form clinical questions and retrieve evidence to advance patient care.
8. Give or receive a patient handover to transition care responsibility.
9. Collaborate as a member of an interprofessional team.
10. Recognize a patient requiring urgent or emergent care and initiate evaluation and management.
11. Obtain informed consent for tests and/or procedures.
12. Perform general procedures of a physician.
13. Identify system failures and contribute to a culture of safety and improvement.

Reprinted with permission of [24]

Milestones, EPAs, and Trust

One of the key values of EPAs is the explicit attention they bring to trust and entrustment. To entrust means to invest, to charge, or to give over to another person something for care, protection, or performance [26]. Medical educators frequently make entrustment decisions on a daily basis. A good example is the night float rotation where residents in many specialties provide clinical coverage overnight for hospitalized patients. Faculty are seldom present in the hospital during this overnight activity as residents provide care. In other words, faculty trust residents will provide high-quality care and reach out for help and guidance when needed.

Trust is a critical component of assessment and how faculty make developmental decisions. For example, is this resident ready for a specific activity (or role) such as night float or the next stage of development that coincides with a change in oversight and supervision? What information is the faculty and program using to make such decisions? Ultimately, an entrustment decision must be a mastery decision.

Let's take a deep probe of trust issues before exploring how an entrustment decision should be a mastery decision. Trust can be defined as "the willingness of a party to be vulnerable to the actions of another party based on the expectation that the other will perform a particular action important to the trustor, irrespective of the ability to monitor or control that other party" [26]. As noted by ten Cate et al., trust can be understood by interpreting the dictionary definition to be "the reliance of a supervisor or medical team on a trainee to execute a given professional task correctly and on his or her willingness to ask for help when needed. Trust requires interdependence between truster and trustee, and creates supervisor vulnerability because mistakes made by a trainee may affect the supervisor personally" [26].

Defining Trust

Trust can be defined as presumptive, initial, and grounded. Presumptive trust is based solely on credentials such as graduation from a medical school, performance on licensing examinations, and other credentials. We often use such credentials as proxies for making preemptive "if-then" entrustment decisions. If the new intern graduated from medical school, then she must be able to perform an effective admission history and physical examination. We know from research that this type of presumptive entrustment is often wrong [27, 28].

Initial trust is highly dependent on first impressions and the individual variables that affect trainee behaviors such as wanting to "look good" and perform for the faculty. The faculty's current mood and level of experience also affect initial trust. We know that first impressions, or initial trust, are subject to error and cognitive bias. Finally, grounded trust depends on prolonged interaction with trainees. Prolonged engagement combined with longitudinal, multiple assessments leads to grounded trust. These three main types of trust inform two types of entrustment decisions.

Ad Hoc and Summative Entrustment Decisions

There are two categories of entrustment decisions: (a) ad hoc and (b) summative. Ad hoc *entrustment decisions* happen every day in the moment, usually reached by individual supervisors who must decide whether to grant permission around a series of tasks and clinical decisions. *Summative entrustment decisions* are grounded in more systematic and longitudinal observations, lead to permission to act under a specified level of supervision that formalizes permission to provide care unsupervised from that point onward, but may need to be reviewed at some later point in time [29]. Ad hoc entrustment is usually, but not always, without long-term consequences but will likely stimulate and influence the evaluation of trainee readiness for summative decisions. Conversely, a summative entrustment decision is a general statement that must be documented, explicitly awards a higher level of responsibility for future actions, and should be recognizable by third parties. Both are important in developmental assessments and competency-based educational curricula. The ad hoc decision experiences of a supervisor may be documented in the trainee's portfolio. For example, was this a justified decision? If not, why not? Would the observer recommend a summative entrustment decision soon? These represent an entrustment-type rating scale based on supervision used during a trainee encounter or observation by the faculty.

Summative decisions may be informed by multiple ad hoc decisions supplemented with information gathered through other channels (multisource feedback, knowledge assessment, skills assessment). In the United States and now Canada, group processes through clinical competency committees inform these summative decisions [30]. These summative entrustment decisions should be based on a synthesis of multisource, smaller elements of information. Summative entrustment decisions should be based on *mastery-based criteria and standards*. Mastery-based criteria and standards can inform the appropriate and effective use of milestones and EPAs in competency-based education systems. In the end, a mastery decision is an entrustment decision for the benefit of individual patients and populations.

Milestones and EPAs in Assessment

Competencies represent the abilities, or education outcomes, of an individual, while EPAs define the core activities medical professionals do within their specialties. Milestones at the current time simply describe competencies in developmental narratives. Competencies, and their associated milestones, provide the building blocks or ingredients for EPAs. Competencies are actually essential to constructing EPAs. EPAs that do not attend to the appropriate competency domains lack proper specification of the construct [21] and have no use in reaching mastery-based decisions. Competencies, milestones, and EPAs are currently influencing medical education and assessment in profound ways.

This influence is particularly evident in the United States where all residency and fellowship programs must assess their trainees twice per year using the milestones framework. Each program is required to use a clinical competency committee (CCC) to review and synthesize assessment data to make a judgment about where on the milestones trajectory a trainee is at that point in time [30]. Milestone judgments of the CCC and program director are used as feedback to the learner to support an individualized learning plan.

Figure 17.3 highlights the importance of the quality of the assessment data being considered by the CCC. The CCC judgments, regardless of whether using a milestones or EPA framework, will only be as good and accurate as the data that informs the review discussion. As Edward Deming famously noted in his seminal work in quality improvement, data are not knowledge [31]. Furthermore, most of the assessment data will come from work-based assessments, and a robust body of literature has described the multitude of problems with these types of assessments [12, 32]. From a mastery perspective, it is worth highlighting a few of key limitations in work-based assessment.

The first issue is the "frame-of-reference" problem. Studies have shown that the primary frame-of-reference (i.e., standard) of faculty is often self, or "how I would do it" [33, 34]. Such a standard might be fine under the following two conditions:

1. Self is high competent, i.e., a true expert or, better yet, master in the competency and/or activity (e.g., EPA).
2. Self can describe what mastery actually looks like for the purpose of teaching, feedback, and coaching – key elements in a mastery-based approach.

Unfortunately, a number of studies show condition 1 is not met for many competencies and conditions. For example, Kogan et al., using an objective structured clinical examination (OSCE), found wide variation in basic clinical skills among a

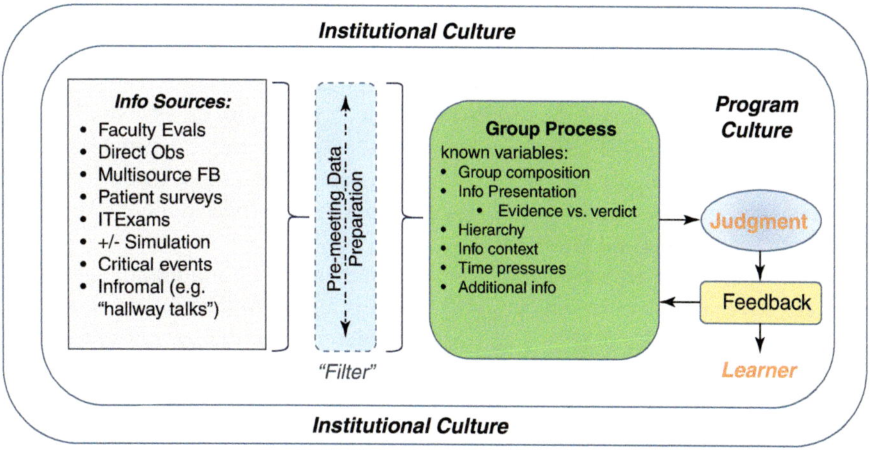

Fig. 17.3 Clinical competency committee process
Info sources: assessment information sources
Faculty Evals: faculty evaluations (e.g., end-of-rotation evaluation forms)
Direct Obs: direct observation-based assessments
Multisource FB: multisource feedback (e.g., 360-degree surveys)
ITExams: in-training medical knowledge examinations
Simulation: includes objective structured clinical examinations; partial and full task trainers; virtual reality
Informal: faculty or others express concern or praise verbally in non-formal settings and/or ad hoc
Group composition: who are the members of the clinical competency committee
Info presentation: how the assessment information is presented to the committee members. Do they start by examining the data (evidence-based approach) or do they start with a decision/judgment (verdict)
Hierarchy: how does the hierarchy of the committee and program affect milestone judgments
Info context: what is the professional and cultural context in which the assessment information is being presented and shared
Adapted from Ref. [30], with permission of ACGME

group of clinician-educators participating in a study of assessment using direct observation [34]. Barsuk and colleagues applied an evidenced-based mastery checklist for central line placement among a group of faculty who perform and teach this skill. They found that only 12 of 67 attending physicians (18%) met or exceeded the minimum passing score for internal jugular central venous catheter insertion. Only 11 of 47 (23%) met or exceeded the minimum passing score for subclavian central venous catheter insertion [35]. Apramian and colleagues in a small study of 11 surgeons found highly variable applications of surgical principles in the operating room, with 1 surgeon notably stating, "when they [trainees] are in my OR, they do it my way" [36].

Thus, while milestones and EPAs have clearly advanced our thinking about professional development, these concepts are still hampered by limitations in work-based assessments and those who complete these assessments. In a word, these and many other studies highlight the lack of shared representations about standards.

Ericsson and Pool in their book *Peak* make the critical point, also articulated in Chaps. 1, 2, and 5, that for most of our work-based assessments, we do not have robust, shared mental representations of clinical practice [22]. The typical response in much of the assessment literature is to treat such variability as a "given" and as useful idiosyncrasy [37–39]. Some argue the best way to handle this variability is to ensure we sample broadly and longitudinally to detect meaningful mean (average) judgment and enhance reliability [37–39]. But does this approach really make sense, especially for patients and families?

From a patient's perspective, the frame-of-reference, at a minimum, should be safe, effective, patient-centered care [40]. There is a limit to the amount of acceptable variability in care delivery. The frame-of-reference for the learner and faculty must always be the patient. In addition, do we really want to place the burden of figuring out what is acceptable and not acceptable practice on the learner, someone very early in her or his own professional development? If the milestones and EPAs address desired educational outcomes and are tightly aligned with high-quality care, should we not also apply mastery-based standards to these educational results? Faculty development using mastery-based, criterion-referenced standards may be one of the best approaches to reduce the unwarranted and harmful variation by promoting shared mental representations of mastery among faculty. In this scenario, everyone "wins" – patients, learners, and faculty.

Mastery Approach to Milestone and EPA Assessment

Milestones and EPAs were developed to define and describe criterion-referenced outcomes developmentally. This is a major shift in thinking and has been a difficult transition. A large part of this difficulty has been the lack of shared mental models around many of the outcomes. The pioneering work of Barsuk and others on the Northwestern Simulation team highlighted in previous chapters clearly demonstrates that a mastery-based approach using simulation can improve performance and patient outcomes in procedural training such as advanced cardiac life support (ACLS) and other skills. The Northwestern group has developed mastery standards in the simulation lab that translate to the clinical care environment. Consistent with Ericsson's notion of the need for clearly defined elements of what expertise looks like, Barsuk and colleagues have achieved this goal for multiple clinical procedures. Since procedural abilities are to be found in many of the milestones, it is fair to ask whether any resident or fellow should be judged on procedural milestones or EPAs without such mastery-based assessments. Stated another way, which of the faculty in the Barsuk central line study cited above [35] would you want to insert a central line in you if such a procedure was indicated?

What about non-procedural competencies and EPAs? Are they simply too messy for a mastery-based approach? Are patients and trainees so highly variable that a mastery-based approach is not warranted or indicated? We believe the answer is no. While indeed clinical skills such as history taking, physical examination, informed decision-making, and breaking bad news, to name a few, might be messier because of the need to interact with diverse patients from different cultural, educational, ethnic, and religious backgrounds, that is not an excuse to ignore high standards of practice. The challenge is not recognizing that a high standard is necessary, but rather in creating approaches to develop assessments that allow for determination of when mastery has been achieved.

For example, we have long known that the quality of history taking is associated with the rate of diagnostic errors. Evidenced-based frameworks, in other words robust mental representations, of medical interviewing already exist [41, 42]. There is a substantial body of literature on effective communication practices for informed (shared) decision-making [43, 44] and breaking bad news [45]. Just like procedures, these are learnable skills judged against a standard. Chapter 10 presents a detailed discussion about mastery learning of clinical communication skills.

One of the biggest barriers to using a mastery-based approach around clinical skills may be the variability among teaching faculty in both their clinical and assessment skills. Given that one significant factor in rater variability is the faculty's own clinical skills as the frame-of-reference, one logical approach would be to improve faculty clinical skills. However, medical education does not need to rely solely on faculty from their own discipline. Trained health professionals from other disciplines can be excellent teachers, assessors, and evaluators. Regardless, faculty would ideally possess mastery in the competency they are teaching and assessing or, at a minimum, would have a deep understanding, or mental representation, of what constitutes mastery [22].

Principles of deliberate practice and mastery-based education could be applied to faculty development, moving beyond the one-time workshop model. Faculty development could start with deliberate practice using standardized patients to improve clinical skills. This activity was included as part of a study on rater training, and one of the authors (ESH) used a formative objective structured clinical examination (OSCE) for faculty as part of the launch of a direct observation initiative [46, 47]. The time has come to incorporate mastery-based learning principles into faculty development around the competencies being applied to medical trainees. Chapter 9 addresses faculty development for mastery learning in detail.

This type of faculty training can serve as a point of departure for purposeful, deliberate practice by faculty in the care of their own patients. Using self-report data, one study found that teaching faculty who applied evidence-based criteria when observing the communication skills of trainees reported these communication skills "spilled over" into their own practice [48].

Stage Models of Development, Mastery-Based Learning, and Context

The milestones and EPAs are grounded in stage models of development such as the Dreyfus model. While the Dreyfus model acknowledges the importance of context, the impact of variable context is not explicitly incorporated in these stage models. The wide variability seen in the clinical contexts where our health professions train and learn is a major issue in reaching mastery. Simulation enables the control, management, and manipulation of multiple contextual factors, but simulation cannot account for all the possible combinations of interactions and interdependences that occur in the clinical work environment.

Evidence is also growing that the performance of clinical microsystems where medical students, residents, and fellows train appears to affect their abilities well beyond training. For example, Asch and colleagues found a strong association between the rate of major obstetrical complications at the institutional level and the rate of complications among its practicing graduates of an obstetrics and gynecology residency program [49]. More concerning is the finding that this association between institutional and individual complication rates appears to last for over 15 years [49–51]. Several articles have reported a relationship between the cost environment where residents train and their subsequent cost patterns when they enter practice [52–54]. Like the Asch study, this effect appears to last for at least 15 years [52].

Since the ultimate goal is to move mastery principles into the clinical training space, what are the implications of the impact of the performance of the clinical microsystems? First, it is hard to imagine that mastery learning can be achieved if the clinical microsystem is performing poorly. Conversely, mastery learning principles could be a mechanism to improve clinical microsystem care. Clinical microsystems depend on effective interactions and interdependences of highly competent health professionals. You cannot insert incompetent providers into interprofessional healthcare teams and expect them to function well. We need high levels of both individual and collective competence.

Onc of the challenges is that we do not as yet have fully developed models of highly effective care delivery in institutions and their multiple microsystems. This lack of understanding of what highly effective care delivery looks like is a challenge for stage models of professional development. Dall'Alba and Sandberg note:

> … an embodied understanding of practice, rather than attributes, forms the basis for professional skill and its development. More specifically, the knowledge and skills that professionals use in performing their work depend upon their embodied understanding of the practice in question. The professionals' way of understanding their practice forms and organizes their knowledge and skills into a particular form of professional skill. When practice is understood in a certain way, knowledge and skills will be developed accordingly. [55]

The key point is that developmental models of professional competence and mastery learning must be embedded into an embodied understanding of highly effective clinical practice. Embodied understanding of practice is analogous to the concepts of shared mental models and shared mental representations. Without this, it is hard to imagine how a training program and its faculty can help a learner achieve mastery.

What we know, however, is that learner and faculty embodied understanding of clinical practice is highly variable which in turn is linked to the highly variable performance of clinical microsystems. Figure 17.4 highlights the point. In this example modified from Dall'Alba and Sandberg, a physician might attain "mastery" in medical interviewing and physical examination yet interact poorly with the interprofessional team and clinical microsystem where (s)he works (curve A).

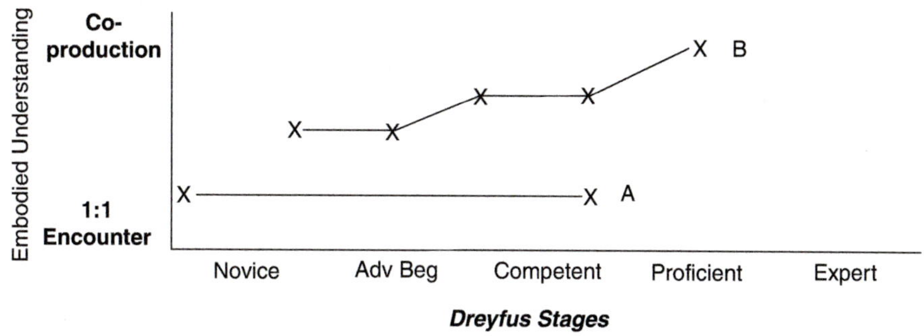

Fig. 17.4 Professional development and embodied understanding of practice. (Adapted from Refs. [55, 58])

However, the ultimate goal is curve B where the physician works within and interacts effective with the clinical microsystem using co-production as an approach to clinical care [56]. Can a physician really attain mastery within a specific skill without an embodied understanding of practice? Furthermore, maintaining mastery is an ongoing process. For example, if the physician moves to another institution or the group that a physician works with changes, there needs to be ongoing deliberate practice to ensure that the highest of standards are met and maintained. Ultimately, mastery is not a one-time destination to achieve a high level of performance, but rather an ongoing journey to maintain and improve that level of high performance.

Coda

Competency-based medical education, with its intense focus on both educational and clinical outcomes, continues to gain traction worldwide. As recently noted by Gruppen and colleagues, CBME requires enhanced requirements for assessment, especially if time-variable training is a goal of the training program [57]. The introduction of developmental assessment and curricular frameworks, using milestones and EPAs, has helped to advance medical education by more explicitly acknowledging the intense professional development trajectories learners experience. These concepts are also signs that medical education is entering a new period of maturity via creation of a common language and shared mental models.

The logical, and necessary, next step is to integrate mastery learning into all developmental models. An entrustment decision should be a mastery decision, and we have a growing body of evidence throughout this book that this is both possible and needed. The next major challenge for mastery learning is to bring these techniques to the patient bedside in day-to-day care. Health professions education is a highly experiential process involving vulnerable patients, families, and communities. A mastery mindset and logic can help accelerate the evolution, if not transformation, now occurring. Further work in refining language and concepts in work-based assessment is still essential to realizing the full promise of CBME using mastery learning methods [57].

References

1. Sullivan RL. The competency-based approach to training. Strategy Paper No 1. Baltimore, MD: JHPIEGO Corporation; 1995.
2. Elam S. Performance-based teacher education: what is the state of the art? Washington, DC: American Association of Colleges for Teacher Education; 1971.
3. McGaghie WC, Miller GE, Sajid AW, Telder TV. Competency-based curriculum development in medical education. Public Health Paper No. 68. Geneva: World Health Organization; 1978.
4. Carraccio C, Wolfstahl SD, Englander R, et al. Shifting paradigms: from Flexner to competencies. Acad Med. 2002;77:361–7.
5. Frank JR, Snell LS, Cate OT, et al. Competency-based medical education: theory to practice. Med Teach. 2010;32(8):638–45.
6. Frank J, Chen L, Bhutta ZA, et al. Health professionals for a new century: transforming education to strengthen health systems in an interdependent world. Lancet. 2010;376:1923–58.
7. McGaghie WC. Medical education research as translational science. Sci Transl Med. 2010;2:19cm8.
8. Schroedl CJ, Corbridge TC, Cohen ER, et al. Use of simulation-based education to improve resident learning and patient care in the medical intensive care unit: a randomized trial. J Crit Care. 2012;27:219.e7–219.e13.
9. McGaghie WC, Issenberg SB, Barsuk JH, Wayne DB. A critical review of simulation-based medical education with translational outcomes. Med Educ. 2014;48(4):375–85.
10. Cook DA, Brydges R, Zendejas B, et al. Mastery learning for health professionals using technology-enhanced simulation: a systematic review and meta-analysis. Acad Med. 2013;88(8):1178–86.
11. Griswold-Theodorson S, Ponnuru S, Dong C, et al. Beyond the simulation laboratory: a realist synthesis of clinical outcomes of simulation-based mastery learning. Acad Med. 2015;90(11):1553–60.
12. Holmboe ES, Sherbino J, Long DM, et al. The role of assessment in competency-based medical education. Med Teach. 2010;32(8):676–82.
13. Kogan JR, Holmboe ES. Realizing the promise and importance of performance-based assessment. Teach Learn Med. 2013;25(Suppl 1):S68–74.
14. Ericsson KA. An expert-performance perspective of research on medical expertise: the study of clinical performance. Med Educ. 2007;41:1124–30.
15. Frank JR, Snell L, Sherbino J, editors. CanMEDS 2015 physician competency framework. Ottawa: Royal College of Physicians and Surgeons of Canada; 2015.
16. Batalden P, Leach D, Swing S, et al. General competencies and accreditation in graduate medical education. Health Aff (Millwood). 2002;21(5):103–11.
17. Holmboe ES, Durning SJ, ten Cate O, Hawkins RE. Assessment challenges in the era of outcomes-based education. In: Holmboe ES, Durning SJ, Hawkins RE, editors. Practical guide to the evaluation of clinical competence. Philadelphia: Elsevier; 2018.
18. Holmboe ES, Edgar RE, Hamstra S. Milestones Guidebook. Available at: http://www.acgme.org.
19. Dreyfus HL, Dreyfus SE. Mind over machine: the power of human intuition and expertise in the era of the computer. New York: Free Press; 1986.
20. Carraccio CL, Benson BJ, Nixon LJ, Derstine PL. From the educational bench to the clinical bedside: translating the Dreyfus developmental model to the learning of clinical skills. Acad Med. 2008;83(8):761–7.
21. Messick S. Standards of validity and the validity of standards in performance assessment. Educ Meas Issues Pract. 1995;14(4):5–8.
22. Ericsson KA, Pool R. Peak: secrets from the new science of expertise. Boston: Houghton Mifflin Harcourt; 2016.
23. ten Cate O. Entrustability of professional activities and competency-based training. Med Educ. 2005;39(12):1176–7.

24. Englander R, Flynn T, Call S, et al. Toward defining the foundation of the MD degree: core entrustable professional activities for entering residency. Acad Med. 2016;91(10):1352–8.
25. Pangaro L, ten Cate O. Frameworks for learner assessment in medicine: AMEE Guide No. 78. Med Teach. 2013;35(6):e1197–210.
26. Ten Cate O, Hart D, Ankel F, et al. for the International Competency-Based Medical Education Collaborators. Entrustment decision making in clinical training. Acad Med. 2016;91(2):191–8.
27. Kogan JR, Holmboe ES. Direct observation. In: Holmboe ES, Durning SJ, Hawkins RE, editors. Practical guide to the evaluation of clinical competence. Philadelphia: Elsevier; 2018.
28. Lypson ML, Frohna JG, Gruppen LD, Woolliscroft JO. Assessing residents' competencies at baseline: identifying the gaps. Acad Med. 2004;79(6):564–70.
29. ten Cate O. Trust, competence, and the supervisor's role in postgraduate training. BMJ. 2006;333(7571):748–51.
30. Andolsek K, Padmore J, Hauer KE, Holmboe ES. Clinical competency guidebook. Available at: www.acgme.org.
31. Deming WE. The new economics for industry, government, education. Cambridge, MA: MIT Center for Advanced Engineering Study; 1993.
32. Lockyer J, Carraccio C, Chan MK, et al. for the ICBME Collaborators. Core principles of assessment in competency-based medical education. Med Teach. 2017;39(6):609–16.
33. Kogan JR, Hatala R, Hauer KE, Holmboe E. Guidelines: the do's, don'ts and don't knows of direct observation of clinical skills in medical education. Perspect Med Educ. 2017;6(5):286–305.
34. Kogan JR, Hess BJ, Conforti LN, Holmboe ES. What drives faculty ratings of residents' clinical skills? The impact of faculty's own clinical skills. Acad Med. 2010;85(10 Suppl):S25–8.
35. Barsuk JH, Cohen ER, Nguyen D, et al. Attending physician adherence to a 29-component central venous catheter bundle checklist during simulated procedures. Crit Care Med. 2016;44(10):1871–81.
36. Apramian T, Cristancho S, Sener A, Lingard L. How do thresholds of principle and preference influence surgeon assessments of learner performance? Ann Surg. 2018;268(2):385–90.
37. Gingerich A, Regehr G, Eva KW. Rater-based assessments as social judgments: rethinking the etiology of rater errors. Acad Med. 2011;86(10 Suppl):S1–7.
38. Gingerich A, van der Vleuten CP, Eva KW, Regehr G. More consensus than idiosyncrasy: categorizing social judgments to examine variability in mini-CEX ratings. Acad Med. 2014;89(11):1510–9.
39. Gingerich A, Kogan J, Yeates P, et al. Seeing the 'black box' differently: assessor cognition from three research perspectives. Med Educ. 2014;48(11):1055–68.
40. Kogan JR, Conforti LN, Iobst WF, Holmboe ES. Reconceptualizing variable rater assessments as both an educational and clinical care problem. Acad Med. 2014;89(5):721–7.
41. Fortin AHVI, Dwamena F, Frankel R, Smith RC. Smith's patient-centered interviewing: an evidence-based method. 3rd ed. New York: McGraw-Hill; 2012.
42. Stein T, Frankel RM, Krupat E. Enhancing clinician communication skills in a large healthcare organization: a longitudinal case study. Pat Educ Couns. 2005;58:4–12.
43. Légaré F, Witteman HO. Shared decision making: examining key elements and barriers to adoption into routine clinical practice. Health Aff (Millwood). 2013;32(2):276–84.
44. Agency for Healthcare Research and Quality. The SHARE Approach. Available at: http://www.ahrq.gov/professionals/education/curriculum-tools/shareddecisionmaking/index.html.
45. Baile WF, Buckman R, Lenzi R, et al. SPIKES-a six-step protocol for delivering bad news: application to the patient with cancer. Oncologist. 2000;5(4):302–11.
46. Kogan JR, Holmboe ES. Preparing residents for practice in new systems of care by preparing their teachers. Acad Med. 2014;89(11):1436–7.
47. Conforti LN, Ross KM, Holmboe ES, Kogan JR. Do faculty benefit from participating in a standardized patient assessment as part of rater training? A qualitative study. Acad Med. 2016;91(2):262–71.
48. Kogan JR, Conforti LN, Bernabeo E, et al. How faculty members experience workplace-based assessment rater training: a qualitative study. Med Educ. 2015;49(7):692–708.

49. Asch DA, Nicholson S, Srinivas S, et al. Evaluating obstetrical residency programs using patient outcomes. JAMA. 2009;302(12):1277–83.
50. Epstein AJ, Srinivas SK, Nicholson S, et al. Association between physicians' experience after training and maternal obstetrical outcomes: cohort study. BMJ. 2013;346:f1596.
51. Asch DA, Nicholson S, Srinivas SK, et al. How do you deliver a good obstetrician? Outcome-based evaluation of medical education. Acad Med. 2014;89(1):24–6.
52. Chen C, Peterson S, Phillips R, et al. Spending patterns in region of residency training and subsequent expenditures for care provided by practicing physicians for Medicare beneficiaries. JAMA. 2014;312(22):2385–93.
53. Sirovich BE, Lipner RS, Johnston M, Holmboe ES. The association between residency training and internists' ability to practice conservatively. JAMA Intern Med. 2014;174(10):1640–8.
54. Phillips RL Jr, Peterson SM, Bazemore AW, al e. The effects of training institution practice costs, quality, and other characteristics on future practice. Ann Fam Med. 2017;15(2):140–8.
55. Dall'Alba G, Sandberg J. Unveiling professional development: a critical review of stage models. Rev Educ Res. 2006;76(3):383–412.
56. Batalden M, Batalden P, Margolis P, et al. Coproduction in healthcare service. BMJ Qual Saf. 2016;25(7):509–17.
57. Gruppen LD, ten Cate O, Lingard LA, et al. Enhanced requirements for assessment in a competency-based, time-variable medical education system. Acad Med. 2018;93:S17–21.
58. Dreyfus HL. On the Internet. Thinking in action series. New York: Routledge; 2001.

18 Mastery Learning, Continuing Professional Education, and Maintenance of Certification

Clara Schroedl, Graham T. McMahon, and William C. McGaghie

Healthcare delivery operates as a purposeful human system. The North American healthcare system seeks to achieve functional and tangible goals including preservation and promotion of individual and public health using means that are just and cost-effective. Human systems are also complicated, dynamic, difficult to manage, and subject to error from many sources as pointed out by the groundbreaking report, *To Err is Human: Building a Safer Health System* [1], published nearly two decades ago. Errors in healthcare come from poor communication; system inefficiencies such as patient handoffs and medication reconciliation; equipment failure; cultural misunderstanding; and imperfect performance by individuals and teams due to aging, indifference, poor basic training, failure to "keep up" with technological advancements, and skill and knowledge decay [2]. In the health professions, continuing professional education (CPE) and maintenance of certification (MOC) programs aim to maintain and improve the quality of healthcare delivered by healthcare individuals and teams.

North American healthcare is often delivered with effectiveness, efficiency, and safety. Millions of patients and their families receive care that improves health and saves lives every day, sometimes with extraordinary results. Yet, there is still much room for improvement, gaps that education programs grounded in adult learning

C. Schroedl (✉)
Northwestern University Feinberg School of Medicine, Departments of Medicine and Medical Education, Chicago, IL, USA
e-mail: c-schroedl@northwestern.edu

G. T. McMahon
Accreditation Council for Continuing Medical Education, President and CEO, Chicago, IL, USA

Northwestern University Feinberg School of Medicine, Adjunct Professor, Departments of Medical Education and Medicine, Chicago, IL, USA

W. C. McGaghie
Northwestern University Feinberg School of Medicine, Departments of Medical Education and Preventive Medicine, Chicago, IL, USA

W. C. McGaghie et al. (eds.), *Comprehensive Healthcare Simulation: Mastery Learning in Health Professions Education*, Comprehensive Healthcare Simulation, https://doi.org/10.1007/978-3-030-34811-3_18

principles aim to close. Many of the gaps are not obvious and are disclosed by research on patient care practices involving licensed and certified health professionals. Several illustrations are telling.

Accurate diagnosis is the cornerstone of healthcare. However, the report, *Improving Diagnosis in Healthcare*, published in 2015 by the National Academies of Science, Engineering, and Medicine states, "5 percent of U.S. adults who seek outpatient care each year experience a diagnostic error; diagnostic errors contribute to approximately 10 percent of patient deaths; diagnostic errors account for 6 to 17 percent of hospital adverse events; and diagnostic errors are the leading type of paid malpractice claims" [3]. These observations are reinforced by new data that show diagnostic decisions made by practicing physicians about common and rare clinical events have much room for improvement [4–6]. Research on the uncertainty of psychiatric diagnoses also shows that the absence of diagnostic "gold standards" contributes to wrong decisions and incorrect patient labelling [7]. Such research findings and a concern for quality standards prompted the National Academies report to assert, "Health care professional certification and accreditation organizations should ensure that health care professionals have and maintain the competencies needed for effective performance of the diagnostic process." In addition, "Educators should ensure that [diagnostic] curricula and training programs [span] the career trajectory" [3].

Scores of studies illustrate that there is much room for improvement in diagnostic accuracy, even when healthcare professionals consider themselves competent [8]. For example, clinical breast examination (CBE) is a diagnostic maneuver commonly performed by primary care physicians, obstetrician gynecologists, surgeons, nurse practitioners, physician assistants, and other professionals engaged in women's healthcare. The CBE involves systematic breast palpation to detect nodules and assess for abnormal nipple discharge. A research team led by surgeon Carla Pugh used four sensor-enabled simulated breast models [9] to assess CBE skills among 533 physicians and surgeons attending three professional meetings [10]. Breast nodule detection rates ranged from 60% to 99.6% depending on nodule size, hardness, and location. Haptic measurements and visual scoring revealed that the physicians displayed wide variation regarding search pattern, search technique, palpation force, and examination time [10]. Findings clearly showed that many physicians who perform the CBE routinely need skill improvement.

The Pugh research team found similar results when they assessed practicing surgeons' laparoscopic ventral hernia (LVH) repair skills in the context of a continuing professional education course [11]. The investigators reported, "... participants scored poorly on the quality and completeness of their hernia repairs." The authors concluded, "... these findings also underscore significant learning needs in the surgical community" [11].

In another example, a multi-institution education research team "sought to determine whether mannequin-based simulation can reliably characterize how board-certified anesthesiologists manage simulated medical emergencies" [12]. The research team evaluated 263 board-certified anesthesiologists participating in MOC courses. The evaluations involved management of high-fidelity crisis scenarios scored by trained, blinded anesthesiologists using standardized measures to yield reliable data. The scores measured the percentage of observed critical performance elements and also used a holistic rating (1 (poor) to 9 (excellent) scale). Results showed that the participants successfully completed 81% of the critical performance elements. However, the average holistic rating of technical and nontechnical performance was just 5/9. Nearly 25% of the anesthesiologists received holistic ratings of three or less. The investigators concluded, "Standardized simulation-based assessment identified performance gaps informing opportunities for improvement. If a substantial proportion of experienced anesthesiologists struggle with managing medical emergencies, continuing medical education activities should be reevaluated" [12].

Central venous catheter (CVC) insertion is an invasive medical procedure that allows doctors to administer drugs, deliver therapies, and evaluate patient health status. Insertion and clinical management of CVCs is associated with preventable adverse events including arterial puncture and central line-associated bloodstream infection. Physicians are usually responsible for CVC insertion, while nurses typically handle indwelling CVC maintenance. Hospitalist physician Jeffrey Barsuk led an education and research team during a mastery learning "train the trainer" program to prepare board-certified attending physicians to educate postgraduate medical residents and subspecialty fellows to insert CVCs via internal jugular (IJ) and subclavian (SC) routes [13]. One hundred eight experienced attending physicians participated in the program. Most of the physicians held faculty appointments at U.S. academic medical centers, reported extensive experience in CVC insertion, and also reported extensive experience teaching the procedure to trainees. Taking a pretest (baseline) measurement is the first step within the mastery learning bundle (Chap. 2). Results from the attending physicians were sobering because only 18% met or exceeded the minimum passing standard (MPS) for IJ insertion and just 23% met or exceeded the MPS for SC insertion [13]. Clinical experience and medical longevity were not predictors of physician competence.

Dr. Barsuk's education and research team also educated experienced (mean = 10 years) intensive care unit (ICU) nurses on central line maintenance skills to a mastery standard [14]. The central line maintenance skills included five tasks: (a) medication administration, (b) injection cap (needleless connector) changes, (c) tubing changes, (d) blood drawing, and (e) dressing changes. Results from the mastery learning education intervention were positive and strong. "The number of nurses passing each task at pretest varied from 24 of 49 (49%) for dressing changes to 44 of 49 (90%) for tubing changes. At pretest, scores ranged from a median of 0.0% to 73.1%. At posttest, all scores rose to a median of 100.0%. Total years in nursing and ICU nursing had significant, negative correlations with medication administration pretest performance" [14]. The brief yet potent mastery learning education program successfully improved central line maintenance skills among the ICU nurses despite many years of inexpert clinical practice most likely due to poor basic training.

Clinical skill deficits have also been recorded from empirical research on experienced, practicing surgeons. Hafford and colleagues presented a fundamentals of laparoscopic surgery (FLS) course to attending surgeons from five state medical schools

[15]. Among the 83 attending surgeons who completed the baseline assessment, 27 (33%) did not meet the competency standard. In another investigation, Birkmeyer and colleagues studied the operative skills of 20 experienced bariatric surgeons in Michigan [16]. Peer surgeons scored (1 to 5 scale; 1 = skill of a general surgery chief resident, 5 = skill of a master bariatric surgeon) video recordings of laparoscopic gastric bypass operations performed by the 20 surgeons in various domains of technical skill. Research results show, "Mean summary ratings of technical skill ranged from 2.6 to 4.8 across the 20 surgeons. The bottom quartile of surgical skill, as compared with the top quartile, was associated with higher complication rates and higher mortality. The lowest quartile of skill was also associated with longer operations, and higher rates of reoperation and readmission" [16]. The authors concluded, "The technical skill of practicing bariatric surgeons varied widely … peer rating of operative skill may be an effective strategy for assessing a surgeon's proficiency" [16].

These few research studies are a small sample of published reports that document professional gaps and education solutions that CPE and MOC programs must address. [Chapter 1 of this volume provides a more extensive discussion about such matters.] There are, however, at least five lessons taken from this work that can frame and channel a productive discussion about mastery learning, CPE, and MOC:

1. Clinical skills acquired, maintained, and used every day by experienced, licensed, and certified health professionals are highly variable. Advanced degrees, certification, and credentials are not reliable or accurate predictors of actual competence.
2. Age and experience are not proxies for competence in the health professions. A recent systematic review about the relationship between clinical experience and quality of healthcare concluded, "Physicians who have been in practice longer may be at risk for providing lower-quality care. Therefore, this subgroup of physicians may need quality improvement interventions" [17].
3. Clinicians are consistently poor assessors of their own skill and cannot be relied on to limit their practice to areas of demonstrable ability.
4. For technical and procedural skills, the research reports underscore the importance of rigorous measurement of skill acquisition and maintenance (see Chap. 5). CPE and MOC programs struggle to create individualized and healthcare team improvement without reliable baseline data. This requires a conceptual shift in the health professions—that assessment data will be used formatively as a tool for improvement [18]. Evaluation apprehension, a widespread barrier to measured improvement in health professions education, must be overcome [19].
5. There needs to be greater recognition that clinical education in the health professions grounded in Osler's clerkship apprenticeship model is increasingly threatened (Chap. 1). Patient safety leader Lucian Leape argued succinctly, "There has always been a strange incongruity between the value placed on technical skill by the specialists who possess them (both surgeons and nonsurgeons) and the casualness with which lesser skills, such as insertion of a chest tube or central venous line, are sometimes taught to those who follow. Much, probably too much, of resident education is still carried out by residents, as embodied in the hallowed, and still oft-repeated, aphorism of 'see one, do one, teach one'" [20].

The chapter sections that follow amplify these opening statements. The next section provides the rationale, evidence of effectiveness, evolution of CPE, CPE requirements, how CPE and MOC differ from undergraduate and postgraduate education, driving self-awareness, and lessons learned about today's CPE and MOC. A subsequent section addresses the relevance, application, and potential of the mastery learning model to CPE and MOC. We conclude with a short section that summarizes the future of mastery learning at work in CPE and MOC programs.

CPE and MOC

Rationale

The importance of continuing professional education should not be underestimated—it is a career-long obligation for practicing health professionals [21]. Based on the well-developed tradition of lifelong learning in the health professions, engagement in CPE reflects everyones' ethical and professional responsibility to be self-aware and to maintain and develop their skills [22]. This engagement is a commitment to patients and their safety. Properly constructed and developed CPE delivers benefits to the individual healthcare provider, our profession, and the public [18].

The medical profession has experimented with a practice-based model of CPE since the 1960s. The succeeding decades have seen an expansive elaboration and extension of this education model [23]. An emphasis on practice has led to research studies that sought to understand the link between medical education, physician performance, and patient health outcomes [24]. These studies, including randomized controlled trials, have been summarized in several reviews which show that education interventions under the right conditions can effectively and efficiently improve physician performance and boost patient health outcomes [25–27]. It is increasingly apparent that education is an essential component of any initiative involving human performance.

CPE refers to expanding medical knowledge, skills, attitudes, and the range of competencies needed to deliver high-quality healthcare, including clinical, managerial, ethical, social, research, and personal skills. The fundamental purpose of CPE is to "facilitate the successful performance of practitioners in the diverse practice characteristic of professional work" [28]. This purpose has been the guiding principle for scholars and leaders across the professions for several decades [29].

Board certification refers to the process of demonstrating sufficient training and knowledge of specialty practice that meets the expectations of a specialty board. Specialty boards create and oversee the standards of specialty and subspecialty practice. MOC is a continuous learning and assessment process that aims to ensure that health professionals keep abreast of the latest knowledge, develop improved practice systems, and, perhaps the most important, show a commitment to lifelong learning through engagement in accredited CPE. Medical MOC requirements were amended recently to include continuous certification, which involves frequent assessment, and inclusion of practice improvement models [30–32]. Over the past several years, and despite widespread modifications to its elements, the value of

MOC and the evidence behind the processes have been the subject of substantial debate within the medical community [33].

In addition to increasing regulatory expectations that health professionals demonstrate their engagement in CPE for MOC, CPE has become increasingly important to a variety of external stakeholders. All health professions have increasingly needed to rely on effective education communities to support better self-awareness and practice improvement due to the rapid pace of change in clinical practice, an explosion of knowledge, problems in patient safety, and changing expectations among patients about their clinicians.

CPE educators have had to rethink the approach to education to provide strategic interventions; address system issues; deliver acceptable, effective, and active learning experiences; and demonstrate meaningful outcomes. Well-designed CPE can be used to create cultural shifts including the elevation of teams and a culture of mutual respect, professionalism, and teamwork [34]. Teams that learn together practice more effectively (Chap. 11). CPE helps clinicians and educators lead, manage, influence, coach, and mentor others—including peers and trainees. CPE can also support and sustain the intellectual growth that attracted many into the health professions, a growth that drives professional satisfaction and prevents burnout. The self-reflection facilitated by CPE helps health professionals develop a greater appreciation about the implications and impact of their work. CPE can lead to increased public confidence in individual professionals and the health professions together.

Evidence of Effectiveness

The question of the overall impact of CPE has been largely settled from 39 systematic reviews published between 1977 and 2014. Major national reports by the Macy Foundation and the National Academy of Medicine in the United States summarize the evidence base showing that CPE is effective and support evidence-based principles for designing effective CPE [35, 36]. Of the 220 articles in the Evidence Library of the American Board of Medical Specialties supporting MOC, 129 demonstrate a positive impact of CPE on physician performance and patient health outcomes. The medical profession has emphasized repeatedly the critical role CPE provides to improve patient outcomes, reduce healthcare costs, improve clinician well-being, and enhance the overall quality and efficiency of the U.S. healthcare system. These results are achieved both in terms of more educated and proficient physicians and by serving as a conduit for medical progress and innovation.

Evolution of CPE

Postgraduate educators emphasize active learning and team-based activities to promote more thorough understanding, assist clinicians in unlearning established though redundant practices, enhance problem-solving skills, and boost self-directed learning among seasoned health professionals. Given their increasingly time-constrained lives, busy clinicians increasingly seek better education opportunities. They are intolerant of passive, weak education and seek activities that are relevant to practice, effective for learning, time-efficient, and that build skills.

Small steps in education design can make a substantial difference in the effectiveness and efficiency of CPE. Grand rounds, conferences, and other live sessions are made more interactive, relevant, and meaningful by limiting the time for formal lecture, incorporating case examples, and allowing substantive time for discussion and for learners to work in pairs or groups to share, reflect on, and solve relevant and challenging problems [21]. Accessible and inexpensive technology facilitates interaction. Comparative performance is especially motivating to clinicians. Creating small groups, discussing, or answering polling questions on smartphones, for example, teaches participants how their attitudes, knowledge, or problem-solving skills compare with peers. Given the opportunity to interact with colleagues, health professionals can measure themselves against professional norms and give each other feedback while building collaborative relationships [37]. Faculty development is needed to support these modest educational innovations and sustain necessary change.

At healthcare institutions, CPE programs and educators can be developed to support strategic objectives and help address important system issues [34]. Hospital and health system leaders worldwide report that investment in CPE has helped them improve provider performance, patient outcomes, and care coordination; drive and manage change, including behavioral and cultural change; improve teamwork and collegiality as well as leadership skills; and reduce burnout and turnover.

CPE Requirements

At its core, CPE is a personal responsibility of health professionals to keep their knowledge and skills current so they can deliver high-quality service that meets the expectations of patients and requirements of their profession and safeguards the public. Nevertheless, there is a long history of using mandates to drive professional engagement in CPE. Such mandates come from professional organizations, licensing authorities, and employers or are required by codes of conduct or codes of ethics.

Mandatory CPE has utility because it increases the number and percentage of clinicians who complete an education activity or program. Mandates communicate the value placed on the skills and competencies being addressed, for example, procedural fitness, communication skill, medication reconciliation, or teamwork. By contrast, many health professions address mandatory CPE, such as programs legislated by U. S. states in different practice realms, with mindless "box-checking behavior." There is little evidence to indicate that mandatory education results in increased knowledge, changes in practice behavior, or improved patient outcomes. If the key measure of success is simply the number of health professionals completing training, then mandatory CPE would be an effective strategy. Regulators who are tempted to impose mandates must understand the conspicuous lack of documented effectiveness of such strategies and the tendency of imposed approaches to create cynicism and backlash among the regulated health professionals.

Voluntary CPE, on the other hand, attracts clinicians who have self-assessed a need for education in their practice settings. This results in motivation not only to complete training but also to increase knowledge and change practice behaviors to improve patient care.

Many organizations present constrained choice as a reasonable and pragmatic alternative that balances mandates with options. We believe a CPE system that presents a range of methods to meet education expectations, even if participation is required, is the best CPE option [38, 39].

Mandates about specific content areas or activities are intrinsically problematic. However, clinicians should be required to engage in professional development. These minimal threshold mandates engage those clinicians who may be least self-aware, most burned out, and most cynical. Minimal threshold mandates can help re-engage clinicians in CPE and performance improvement and connect clinicians with peers and teachers who can support them through that process.

How CPE Differs from Undergraduate and Postgraduate Education

Learners entering health professions schools embark on defined curricula and associated rigorous assessments leading to the award of a professional degree. Health professions educators and their schools are accountable for education quality. Postgraduate programs also present learners with a specific curriculum and competency metrics. Postgraduate learners may receive salaries, largely from government funding. Hospitals and health systems rely on service delivery to fulfill their patient care mission and invest in faculty and educators to comply with accreditation requirements that are necessary for financial support.

CPE differs from medical school and residency training in several ways. There is little need for curricular structure among clinicians who have completed formal education due to wide variation in clinical practice. Practice variation also limits the utility of assessments when the scope of practice is broad. Hospitals and health systems have a vested interest in the professional capacity of their workforce, yet they typically view CPE as a regulatory compliance matter and delegate the responsibility to clinicians themselves. Conflict between the beneficiaries (often the healthcare system) and the funders (often the individual clinician), coupled with the absence of defined curricula, creates unique challenges when working to establish a functional CPE program.

Driving Self-Awareness

Health professionals are typically unaware of their clinical deficits, such as fund of knowledge, procedural skill, reasoning, communication, teamwork, empathy, and others. Clinical defects and professional flaws often hide in the realm of "unknown unknowns" due to a lack of rigorous assessment, feedback, and accountability after health professionals enter practice. This illustrates the well-known "Dunning-Kruger effect" from the behavioral sciences, where even well-trained professionals may be unskilled and unaware of it [40, 41]. Clinical deficits leave doctors and other health professionals with a double burden—not only does their incomplete and misguided knowledge lead them to make mistakes, but the same deficits also prevent them from recognizing when mistakes happen [37].

This recognition problem is particularly troublesome in the health professions because (a) the professions acculturate decisiveness and confidence, (b) stored information becomes dated quickly, (c) practitioners are assessed rarely, (d) bad outcomes can be attributed to sources other than the skill of the clinician, and (e) errors can have very serious consequences. Clinical errors are common, but those errors are linked infrequently to clinical skill deficiencies, and there is minimal feedback to break the cycle that perpetuates inaccurate self-confidence.

Assessment and feedback models that improve self-awareness are key parts of efforts to improve patient safety. Constructive, actionable feedback can be very compelling for individual clinicians who are sustained by a belief that they are performing well. Clinicians who receive formative feedback can be successfully guided to improve. There is ample evidence that health professionals can address competency gaps when they have the humility and motive to improve and engage in effective educational programs.

Lessons Learned: Mistakes of CPE and MOC

1. Compliance Rather Than Learning

Health professionals feel burdened by regulatory and administrative requirements [42]. These requirements prevent clinicians from engaging in activities that deliver professional sustenance and satisfaction (such as spending time with patients or intellectual stimulation) or in balancing home and work lives. Dealing with these administrative burdens is difficult because the needed structures (e.g., electronic health records) are cumbersome and designed to meet reimbursement needs and data management rather than improving clinical efficiency. Health professionals are conflicted. They spend time and energy on activities perceived to deliver value to others but not to themselves or to their patients. Such conflicts produce frustration, cynicism, and burnout. Health professions educators and learning events become contaminated by such cynicism when education opportunities are presented as compliance events.

2. Promoting Credit-Seeking

Education completed to fulfill a mandate is often judged irrelevant and a waste of time. Such CPE is a self-fulfilling prophecy because lack of engagement makes learning and retention impossible and makes participation ineffective and baffling. Learners seek the easiest and cheapest approach to fulfill requirements when CPE is done for regulatory compliance. Health professions educators respond to that need by presenting convenient and simple programs, attributes that promote ineffective learning. Rewarding CPE providers that market programs as easy mechanisms to fulfill regulatory requirements supports negative beliefs about continuing education. When present, mandatory programs and distorted rewards can also imply that the regulatory system and CPE providers are complicit in delivering compliance and obtaining revenue rather than facilitating learning, change, teaming, and professional joy.

3. Reinforcing Redundant Beliefs About Learning

Passive learning is ineffective. Clinicians know when they are learning and value activities that are professionally rewarding, efficient, and effective. Falling grand rounds and clinical conference attendance is a sign of the choices that clinicians make every day about how to spend valuable time. Giving credit for activities that may not be educationally effective risks reinforcing an inappropriate belief among learners that simply "showing up" at education sessions is enough for learning. CPE is effective only if learners engage in active and effortful ways with the material (Chap. 4).

4. Top-Down Approach, Bottom-Up Approach, and the Importance of Relevance

Learning, retention, and consolidation require hard work. Effortful activities will be pursued only if they deliver value to learners. Stressed clinicians want learning experiences that address their specific practice and patients efficiently. Practice patterns are diverse with many specialty areas. Presenting focused CPE activities that are relevant widely to a target population is challenging. "One-size-fits-all" programs are often rejected when a lack of clinical relevance becomes evident. Perceptions of wasted time yield frustration if health professionals believe time is spent on activities that do not generate value.

Relevance is more likely if the top-down learning approach is exchanged for tactics that allow clinicians to choose CPE issues to study. CPE is improved through bottom-up staffing and support, facilitating programs that allow clinicians to identify needs, and then finding activities that help them meet that need. The bottom-up approach makes no a priori decision about what is needed for a clinician and provides a flexible curriculum of diverse activities that maximize choice. Instead, the bottom-up approach uses objective assessment data together with personal aspiration to drive the individual clinician's professional development journey.

Relevance, Application, and Potential of the Mastery Model to CPE and MOC

Case Example

Veno-venous extracorporeal membrane oxygenation (ECMO) is growing in use for patient management of refractory acute hypoxemic respiratory failure. There is much variability in expertise among ICU clinicians about use of ECMO technology. The CPE intent is to design a simulation-based mastery learning curriculum to educate ICU healthcare team members involved in the care of ECMO patients. ECMO educators pose several questions about the most efficient and effective way to prepare clinicians for patient care.

Questions:

1. How shall we assess individual and institutional needs for ECMO training?
2. How shall we develop and pilot test educational interventions that improve learners' clinical skills to assure high-quality care for ECMO patients?
3. What is the best way to assess outcomes for individual learners and the overall ECMO program?
4. How can we maintain a uniformly high level of care for ECMO patients over time?

Principles that describe mastery learning programs have been presented in earlier chapters. Despite the acknowledged differences in the CPE environment compared to those in UME and GME, mastery learning principles can be readily applied to CPE. Much of the prior mastery learning work has focused on health professions trainees rather than practicing clinicians. However, there is great opportunity to advance mastery learning into CPE for health professions individuals and teams. Nurses, physical therapists, physicians, and dentists practice for many decades after their training programs are complete. All are at risk for skill degeneration over time [2]. They all must also learn about new advances including medications, procedures, or technologies. Consistent with the mastery model, evidence supports change in professional practice due to interactive CPE that allows active participation and the opportunity to practice skills [12]. In the next four sections, we discuss the relevance, application, and potential of the mastery model in continuing professional development (CPD) related to (a) needs assessment, (b) developing education interventions, (c) outcome assessment, and (d) skill consolidation and maintenance. More impactful CPE is on the horizon. There is substantial evidence that education interventions that are developed using mastery learning principles will promote both learning efficacy and efficiency.

Needs Assessment

Mastery learning in CPE is not implemented widely. Earlier we provided several published examples to highlight the successful application of simulation-based mastery learning (SBML) in CPE. However, few programs such as the "train the trainer" program of central venous catheter insertion and maintenance for physicians [13] and nurses [14] and programs that are developed to teach surgical or procedural skills have used mastery learning principles.

A 2011 survey by the Association of American Medical Colleges (AAMC) demonstrated that simulation was used at more than 65% of medical schools and teaching hospitals to address a broad range of competencies [43]. The 2018 Harrison Survey, a biennial survey jointly sponsored by the AAMC and the Society for Academic Continuing Medical Education (SACME), found that 92% of responding academic Continuing Medical Education (CME)/CPD programs utilized simulations in their CME/CPD activities >/= 1 time during the last year [44]. Reimagining CPE, away from didactic lectures and toward either cognitive participatory case-based simulation or hands-on, team-based, interactive simulation, is clearly growing with increasing frequency [21]. However, simulation within CPE is not yet routinely designed with the robustness of mastery learning principles or incorporated into a longitudinal curriculum (Chap. 11).

Gaps in knowledge, competence, or performance among core competencies, as determined by a needs assessment, are the foundation for all CPE activities whether designed for individuals or clinical teams. Identifying that gaps exist between what a learner or a clinical team is doing or accomplishing and what is achievable is the key initial step in deciding what to teach. The design of education interventions, of course, must match the desired outcome (Chaps. 3 and 4). Education activities that close these gaps provide value to individuals, teams, health professions institutions, and patients. If proficiency in an invasive procedure such as paracentesis is the desired result, it is incomplete to provide education only in a lecture format. Simulation (cognitive or technical) with deliberate practice and feedback toward a mastery learning goal can achieve the level of proficiency desired in a way that is more educationally effective.

Education needs of health professions learners vary by specialty, practice environment, and experience. Education needs change as the careers of health professionals advance. Healthcare quality improvement or patient safety data used in planning CPE activities can help identify education needs of individual health professionals or teams. However, many CPE units do not use objective data when planning events [45]. Addressing the needs of a group of learners may be insufficient to target the needs of an individual. The core competency of practice-based learning and improvement (PBLI), for example, helps identify the learning needs of a practicing physician. The physicians can review data related to their clinical practice and identify performance gaps. Previous work found that physicians prefer to self-assess their CPD needs [46]. However, the utility of self-assessed educational needs is limited [46]. Physicians may not know what they need to know, a manifestation of

Table 18.1 Example of a robust needs assessment: ECMO case

A robust needs assessment might identify the following practice gaps, based on the education needs of the learners and the system: 1. ECMO team members lack a structured system for evaluating patients who may benefit from ECMO care. Review of indications and contraindications in a time-sensitive manner is necessary to guarantee proper patient selection. 2. Physicians are unaware of equipment selection and lack strategies for ECMO vein cannulation. 3. The physicians, nurses, respiratory therapists, and perfusionists lack clearly identified roles and responsibilities for the care of patients on ECMO. 4. Physicians are ill-equipped to manage ECMO emergencies.

the "Dunning-Kruger effect" [40, 41]. Completion of a pretest, or baseline skills assessment, is another way of identifying learner needs and is a key feature of mastery learning, providing that information is then used to customize the intervention [13]. An example of a robust needs assessment is presented in Table 18.1.

Construction of Education Interventions

Mastery requires deliberate practice and feedback. Unidirectional information sharing, a typical model of didactic programs, is inadequate to build the competencies and skills necessary for mastery. There is great opportunity to design CPE courses that assess participant performance objectively and provide opportunities for deliberate practice and feedback until mastery is reached. Physician learners are not adept at selecting activities based on intentional instructional design and may rather choose activities that are familiar in style and content [46]. Only 23% of physicians who participate in MOC identified simulation-based education as a useful CPD activity. Seventy-two percent of participants felt that traditional knowledge-based CPD or exam preparation courses were most helpful for MOC [46]. There is a disconnect between the education choices of practicing physicians and education events that produce the best outcomes. Mastery learning in CPD should be targeted first to potentially high-impact situations, such as team-training, and content domains that are particularly dangerous or new [13].

The steps involved with the development of mastery curriculum for CPE do not differ from those described in Chap. 3. However, given constraints that exist in CPE settings, educators must attend to:

1. The effectiveness of the education program
2. The efficiency of the learning achieved
3. The relevance of the material to the learners' individual scope of practice
4. Opportunities to leverage peer-, group-, and team-based learning
5. Creating accurate self-awareness of competency
6. Overcoming apprehension about evaluation [19] and new learning modalities
7. Managing conflicts of interest and independence from commercial interests

Experienced health professionals, presumed experts in their field, are often anxious about exposing competency vulnerabilities when flawless performance is expected and presumed. CPE educators must dispel such apprehension to correct knowledge or skill deficits among their learners. Learners are more inclined to seek education voluntarily when a new treatment or procedure is introduced. Attention to the formative value of feedback and sensitivity to evaluation apprehension must be considered [47].

A recent survey of licensed US pharmacists sought to understand their decisions about participation in CPE. The pharmacists reported that time was the most important barrier to their participation [48]. CPE differs from undergraduate or postgraduate professional education because learning time is not part of the health professional's schedule. Research evidence from many sources shows that mastery learning improves outcomes, but it also requires learning time and resources [25–27]. The return on investment from mastery of clinical skills must be weighed against costs regarding time, personnel, price, and lost opportunity to participate in other activities [49] (see also Chap.19), including productive clinical work. In the CPE arena, educators must carefully select the skills for mastery education that ensure learning efficiency from high-value education. Education is an inexpensive solution that improves clinical performance, fosters meaning in work, and reduces burnout among health professionals [34]. Personnel turnover is costly to healthcare institutions. Research shows that education is key to reduce turnover while improving productivity and quality [50]. Institutional investment in CPE that allows time for provider participation without repercussions, such as lost revenue or work backlog, encourages education activities that support individual goals and maximize engagement toward institutional goals.

The earlier example about developing a mastery-based education program for ECMO narrows the scope of a CPE intervention that is feasible for one institution. Evidence about SBML is more robust for procedural training than team training or diagnostic reasoning education. Consequently, health professions educators may decide to start by designing a curriculum for ECMO vein cannulation. A review of the literature showed that a mastery curriculum and skills checklist for this procedure do not exist. Developing an ECMO skills checklist, setting a MPS, and creating a video demonstration of appropriate technique are good points of departure (Table 18.2).

Table 18.2 Education implementation for an ECMO skills program

1. Outline expected competencies to be measured.
2. Align learning and assessment elements with each competency expectation.
3. Recruit learners to the program.
4. Provide a variety of choices for how to complete the mastery curriculum and formative assessment elements incorporating online, live, and simulation.
5. Provide individual feedback and additional deliberate practice and feedback until mastery is achieved.
6. Implement consolidation and reminder approaches to maintain skill over time.

Outcome Assessment

Research evidence clearly demonstrates the effectiveness and value of mastery learning approaches in improving patient care and patient safety [24–27]. This scientific work has focused mainly on medical trainees rather than practicing physicians. However, there is no reason to believe that research results are not transferable to the CPE arena. Outcome assessments are key to evaluate the results of a CPE intervention. The Accreditation Council for Continuing Medical Education (ACCME), one of the bodies responsible for the oversight of U.S. CME programs, values practices that demonstrate the impact of education on healthcare professionals and patients. Educators must measure performance improvement to demonstrate benefits to learners and use a variety of approaches ranging from post-activity self-assessment and tests of knowledge and skill growth to measures of performance, skill, and patient outcomes. Individual improvement relies on tracking relevant data over time. A good mastery-based learning curriculum starts with a skills checklist that can reliably assess baseline performance. Post-intervention data analysis demonstrates the impact of the CPD program [51].

Our example proposes a SBML curriculum for ECMO vein cannulation. Outcomes assessment could evaluate results achieved in the simulated environment (T1), transfer to better patient care practices (T2), or improved patient outcomes (T3) [24]. The potential to impact physician wellness, engagement, and interprofessional collaboration is measured less frequently. Participating in meaningful and high-value education will drive future engagement of the learners (Table 18.3) (see also Chap. 16).

Skill Consolidation and Maintenance

Health professionals are expected to demonstrate and maintain their competence after formal training. Regulatory requirements and public scrutiny expect accountability for professional performance via CPE and engagement with board

Table 18.3 Outcome assessment for the ECMO program [24]

Example outcome	Translational science level
Number of learners who attended and completed the program	N/A
How learners rated their satisfaction with the program	T1 (Attitudes)
How learners performed on a written test of ECMO knowledge	T1 (Knows)
How learners performed on a written test that used a variety of case-based problems about the application of ECMO to different circumstances	T1 (Knows how)
How learners performed when asked to demonstrate the use of the ECMO machine on a simulator	T1 (Shows how)
Number of appropriate patients who were successfully treated with ECMO	T2 (Improved patient care practices)
Mortality rates among patients treated with ECMO at the index facility	T3 (Better patient outcomes)

Data from Ref. [24]

certification requirements. Organizations that regulate maintenance of competence among health professionals must assess the available methods and tools to determine if nurses, doctors, pharmacists, midwives, and other professionals are meeting a predefined standard needed to continue practice and keep patients safe. Medical boards are each examining best strategies to help their diplomates stay current with best practices, maintain skills, and measure competence. There has been demonstrable tension between the acceptability of these education and assessment approaches and their accuracy and precision for individual competency determinations. It is clear that mastery approaches to learning and performance management will become increasingly incorporated into the best practices that certifying boards will accept as meeting their needs and expectations.

Barriers to the mastery learning approach include professional inertia, time and resources, evaluation apprehension, and the absence of professional accountability. It is increasingly clear that health professionals will need to engage in education programs where a rigorous standard is set and participants are given time for deliberate practice until their performance meets a stringent minimum threshold. This strategy includes objective assessment of individual performance in a standardized environment (Chap. 17).

Educators must also evolve. Expertise in education design is needed to create robust curricula (Chap. 3). Health professions educators must also balance time and resources needed to achieve mastery in one skill with the large number of other learner education priorities (Table 18.4).

Coda

After formal training, health professionals spend most of their careers in a CPE phase. Acquired skills are uneven and decay over time. Many clinicians are inappropriately overconfident in their skills, a problem that leads to medical errors. Health professionals rarely undergo rigorous, reliable assessment to identify

Table 18.4 Consolidation and maintenance of ECMO skills

Visual aids placed in conspicuous places to remind clinicians about the key components of ECMO skill that are often forgotten.
Incorporation of checklists and other consolidation approaches that reinforce safe and effective practice in the clinical environment.
Routine and regular feedback to staff about data and lessons learned from the ECMO program over time.
Development of an ECMO core team at the facility with regular meetings to reflect on experience and strategy.
Additional mastery modules could be added as new technology or techniques are introduced. For example, a course on addressing ECMO emergencies could be developed.
Regularly scheduled sessions that serve as reinforcement can be offered to allow skill practice and assessment. Such sessions have value if a physician's participation in ECMO activities has been less than that required to maintain his or her skill or if a new physician is asked to care for ECMO patients without having prior experience.

professional practice gaps and create more accurate self-awareness necessary to stimulate engagement in CPE. Passive CPE education programs can create complacency by reinforcing mistaken beliefs that learning is occurring or has occurred when it has not. Many learners in professional practice are reluctant to engage in education programs that are cognitively demanding and time-consuming, even if this type of program is most likely to produce clinical improvement.

CPE programs also need to account for the remarkable diversity of its learner community. Some health professionals practice with a broad scope, while others narrow their scope of practice to a specialized skill set. Others pursue research, education, or administrative roles that define a professional identity. Acknowledging this diversity and then creating education opportunities to assist health professionals to acquire and maintain skills most pertinent to their practice requires deliberate planning and careful implementation.

The mastery learning model can readily translate to the CPE environment. Competency-based education grounded in mastery learning is becoming the norm in many health professions training programs [52, 53]. Educators will continue to refine assessment methods to guarantee the quality of physicians, nurses, physical therapists, and other professionals entering practice. Mastery learning, a particularly rigorous method of competency-based education, is a key strategy that holds great potential to improve health professions education. Recognizing the limits of the current model of health professions education and assuring mastery learning rigor will boost the quality and value of CPE.

References

1. Kohn LT, Corrigan JM, Donaldson MS, (Institute of Medicine). To err is human: building a safer health system. Washington, DC: National Academy Press; 2000.
2. Arthur W Jr, Bennett W Jr, Stanush PL, McNelly TL. Factors that influence skill decay and retention: a quantitative review and analysis. Hum Perform. 1998;11(1):57–101.
3. National Academies of Sciences, Engineering, and Medicine. Improving diagnosis in health care. Washington, DC: The National Academies Press; 2015.
4. Meyer AND, Payne VL, Meeks DW, et al. Physicians' diagnostic accuracy, confidence, and resource requests: a vignette study. JAMA Intern Med. 2013;173(21):1952–9.
5. Kliegman RM, Bordini BJ, Basel D, Nocton JJ. How doctors think: common diagnostic errors in clinical judgment—lessons from an undiagnosed and rare disease program. Pediatr Clin N Am. 2017;64:1–15.
6. Singh H, Schiff GD, Graber ML, et al. The global burden of diagnostic errors in primary care. BMJ Qual Saf. 2017;26:484–94.
7. Mokros A, Habermeyer E, Küchenhoff H. The uncertainty of psychological and psychiatric diagnoses. Psychol Assess. 2018;30(4):556–60.
8. Davis DA, McMahon GT. Translating evidence into practice: lessons for CPD. Med Teach. 2018;40(9):892–5.
9. Laufer S, Cohen ER, Kwan C, et al. Sensor technology in assessments of clinical skill. N Engl J Med. 2015;372:784–6.
10. Laufer S, D'Angelo A-LD, Kwan C, et al. Rescuing the clinical breast examination: advances in classifying technique and assessing physician competency. Ann Surg. 2017;266:1069–74.

11. Pugh CM, Arafat FO, Kwan C, Cohen ER, Kurashima Y, Vassiliou MC, Fried GM. Development and evaluation of a simulation-based continuing medical education course: beyond lectures and credit hours. Am J Surg. 2015;210:603–9.
12. Weinger MB, Banerjee A, Burden AR, et al. Simulation-based assessment of the management of critical events by board-certified anesthesiologists. Anesthesiology. 2017;127:475–89.
13. Barsuk JH, Cohen ER, Nguyen D, et al. Attending physician adherence to a 29-component central venous catheter bundle checklist during simulated procedures. Crit Care Med. 2016;44:1871–81.
14. Barsuk JH, Seburn S, Cohen ER, et al. Simulation-based mastery learning improves central line maintenance skills of ICU nurses. J Nurs Adm. 2015;45(10):511–7.
15. Hafford ML, Van Sickle KR, Willis RE, et al. Ensuring competency: are fundamentals of laparoscopic surgery training and certification necessary for practicing surgeons and operating room personnel? Surg Endosc. 2013;27:118–26.
16. Birkmeyer JD, Finks JF, O'Reilly A, et al. Surgical skill and complication rates after bariatric surgery. N Engl J Med. 2013;369:1434–42.
17. Choudhry NK, Fletcher RH, Soumerai SB. Systematic review: the relationship between clinical experience and quality of health care. Ann Intern Med. 2005;142:260–73.
18. McMahon GT. Inspiring curiosity and restoring humility: the evolution of competency-based continuing medical education. Acad Med. 2018;93:1757–9.
19. McGaghie WC. Evaluation apprehension and impression management in medical education. Acad Med. 2018;93(5):685–6.
20. Leape LL. The preventability of medical injury. In: Bogner MS, editor. Human error in medicine. Hillsdale: Lawrence Erlbaum Associates; 1994. p. 13–25.
21. McMahon GT. What do I need to learn today? The evolution of CME. N Engl J Med. 2016;374(15):1403–6.
22. McMahon GT. Advancing continuing medical education. JAMA. 2015;314(6):561–2.
23. Cervero RM. Lifespan professional development through practice-based education: implications for the health professions. In: Neimeyer GJ, Taylor JM, editors. Continuing professional development and lifelong learning: issues, impacts, and outcomes. New York: Nova Science Publishers; 2011. p. 265–76.
24. McGaghie WC. Medical education research as translational science. Sci Transl Med. 2010;2:19cm8.
25. McGaghie WC, Draycott TJ, Dunn WF, Lopez CM, Stefanidis D. Evaluating the impact of simulation on translational patient outcomes. Simul Healthc. 2011;6(7, Suppl):S42–7.
26. McGaghie WC, Issenberg SB, Cohen ER, Barsuk JH, Wayne DB. Translational educational research: a necessity for effective health-care improvement. Chest. 2012;142(5):1097–103.
27. McGaghie WC, Issenberg SB, Barsuk JH, Wayne DB. A critical review of simulation-based mastery learning with translational outcomes. Med Educ. 2014;48:373–85.
28. Houle CO. Continuing learning in the professions. San Francisco: Jossey-Bass; 1980.
29. Cervero RM. Effective continuing education for professionals. San Francisco: Jossey-Bass; 1988.
30. American Board of Medical Specialties. Board certification and maintenance of certification. Available at: https://www.abms.org/board-certification/.
31. American Board of Medical Specialties. Steps toward initial certification and MOC. Available at: https://www.abms.org/board-certification/steps-toward-initial-certification-and-moc/.
32. American Board of Medical Specialties. Value of board certification to health care. Available at: https://www.abms.org/board-certification/value-of-board-certification-to-health-care/.
33. Teirstein PS. Boarded to death—why maintenance of certification is bad for doctors and patients. N Engl J Med. 2015;372(2):106–8.
34. McMahon GT. The leadership case for investing in continuing professional development. Acad Med. 2017;92(8):1075–7.
35. Institute of Medicine. Redesigning continuing education in the health professions. Washington, DC: The National Academies Press; 2010.

36. Fletcher SW. Chairman's summary of the conference. In: Hager M, editor. Continuing education in the health professions: improving healthcare throughout lifelong learning. New York: Josiah Macy, Jr. Foundation; 2007.
37. Rifai N, Rose T, McMahon GT, Saxberg B, Christensen UJ. Learning in the 21st century: concepts and tools. Clin Chem. 2018;64(10):1423–9.
38. McMahon GT, Skochelak SE. Evolution of continuing medical education: promoting innovation through regulatory alignment. JAMA. 2018;319(6):545–6.
39. McMahon GT, Aboulsoud S, Gordon J, et al. Evolving alignment in international continuing professional development accreditation. J Contin Educ Health Prof. 2016;36(Suppl. 1):S22–6.
40. Kruger J, Dunning D. Unskilled and unaware of it: how difficulties in recognizing one's own incompetence lead to inflated self-assessments. J Pers Soc Psychol. 1999;77(6):1121–34.
41. Dunning D, Heath C, Suls JM. Flawed self-assessment: implications for health, education, and the workplace. Psychol Sci Public Interest. 2004;5(3):69–106.
42. McMahon GT. Managing the most precious resource in medicine. N Engl J Med. 2018;378(16):1552–4.
43. AAMC. Medical simulation in medical education: results of an AAMC survey. Available at: https://store.aamc.org/medical-simulation-in-medical-education-results-of-an-aamc-survey-pdf.html.
44. SACME. Academic CME/CPD in the United States and Canada: the 2015A AMC/SACME Harrison Survey. Available at: https://store.aamc.org/downloadable/download/sample/sample_id/234/
45. Cook DA, Blachman MJ, Price DW, West CP, Berger RA, Wittich CM. Professional development perceptions and practices among U.S. physicians: a cross-specialty national survey. Acad Med. 2017;92(9):1335–45.
46. Davis DA, Mazmanian PE, Fordis M, Van Harrison R, Thorpe KE, Perrier L. Accuracy of physician self-assessment compared with observed measures of competence: a systematic review. JAMA. 2006;296(9):1094–102.
47. Clark EG, Paparello JJ, Wayne DB, et al. Use of a national continuing medical education meeting to provide simulation-based training in temporary hemodialysis catheter insertion skills: a pre-test post-test study. Can J Kidney Health Dis. 2014;1:25.
48. Tsoi STA, de Boer A, Croiset G, Koster AS, Kusurkar RA. Factors influencing participation in continuing professional development: a focus on motivation among pharmacists. J Contin Educ Health Prof. 2016;36(3):144–50.
49. Cook DA, Brydges R, Zendejas B, Hamstra SJ, Hatala R. Mastery learning for health professionals using technology-enhanced simulation: a systematic review and meta-analysis. Acad Med. 2013;88(8):1178–86.
50. Society for Human Resource Management. Developing and sustaining high performance work teams. Available at: https://www.shrm.org/ResourcesAndTools/tools-and-samples/toolkits/Pages/default.aspx.
51. Prenner SB, Wayne DB, Sweis RN, Cohen ER, Feinglass JM, Schimmel DR. Simulation-based education leads to decreased use of fluoroscopy in diagnostic coronary angiography. Catheter Cardiovasc Interv. 2018;91(6):1054–9.
52. Frank JR, Snell L, Englander R, Holmboe ES, ICBME Collaborators. Implementing competency-based medical education: moving forward. Med Teach. 2017;39(6):568–73.
53. Holmboe ES, Sherbino J, Englander R, Snell L, Frank JR, ICBME Collaborators. A call to action: the controversy and rationale for competency-based medical education. Med Teach. 2017;39(6):574–81.

Return on Investment from Simulation-Based Mastery Learning

19

Jeffrey H. Barsuk, Sidney A. Barsuk, and Diane B. Wayne

Almost 4% of hospitalized patients in the United States experience serious or fatal iatrogenic complications. Medical errors account for more than 1 million injuries and at least 98,000 hospital deaths annually [1]. Invasive medical procedures are the second most common cause of iatrogenic patient complications [2, 3]. These complications lead to increased hospital length of stay (LOS) and higher healthcare costs [4, 5]. The Centers for Medicare and Medicaid Services (CMS) no longer reimburses hospitals for preventable adverse events and instead provides incentives to reduce hospital-acquired conditions (HACs) [6]. CMS-identified preventable adverse events include iatrogenic infections and other hospital or procedure-related complications [7]. Identifying processes, systems, and methods to eliminate preventable adverse events is key to patient safety efforts and to avoid nonreimbursable expenses and penalties.

Chapter 1 of this volume points out that the traditional model of medical education relies heavily on time-based apprenticeship models that do not consistently achieve expected learning outcomes. Another impediment to progress is that healthcare providers are certified using multiple-choice examinations and are not required to demonstrate mastery of clinical skills before completing training. Although the Institute of Medicine identified simulation-based education in its landmark 2000 publication, *To Err is Human: Building a Safer Health System*, as a way to boost patient safety [1], little has changed about how we certify, license, and credential physicians in the last two decades.

J. H. Barsuk (✉) · D. B. Wayne
Northwestern University Feinberg School of Medicine, Departments of Medicine and Medical Education, Chicago, IL, USA
e-mail: jbarsuk@northwestern.edu; dwayne@northwestern.edu

S. A. Barsuk
Northwestern University School of Professional Studies (retired), Chicago, IL, USA

W. C. McGaghie et al. (eds.), *Comprehensive Healthcare Simulation: Mastery Learning in Health Professions Education*, Comprehensive Healthcare Simulation, https://doi.org/10.1007/978-3-030-34811-3_19

Historically, education has been considered a weak strategy to improve healthcare quality and patient safety [8]. This is because traditional methods such as reading, didactic lectures, time-based apprenticeships, expert consultation, and short continuing medical education sessions are largely passive interventions that yield uneven results. However, a growing body of research shows that newer techniques, such as SBML involving deliberate practice, individualized feedback, and rigorous competency assessment, produce robust educational outcomes that yield improved downstream patient care results and reduce healthcare costs [9–15].

SBML interventions have been developed and studied by university-based researchers, yet they are seldom evaluated against quality improvement (QI) metrics endorsed by chief executive officers, chief financial officers, chief medical officers, nursing executives, and other healthcare financial stakeholders. The focus in professional schools is on education, patient care, research, and innovation. Concerns of C-suite executives include improving market share, expense reduction, and reducing clinical variation. Thus, healthcare professional school leaders and healthcare organization executives in the C-suite may have complementary goals but may not speak the same language. This chapter discusses strategies to align academic and commercial stakeholders and provides a business foundation intended to help educators make a business case for SBML educational interventions.

The chapter has four sections exploring how simulation education leaders can approach business-based, return on investment modeling for SBML. The sections are (a) description of the Phillips ROI methodology, (b) an example of use of the ROI model with SBML, (c) additional examples of ROI, and (d) stakeholder engagement: convincing the C-suite.

Phillips ROI Model

Business Alignment, Forecasting, and Needs Assessment

Hospitals and other healthcare institutions are concerned about issues such as patient care quality, market share, reputation, organization morale, and financial returns [16]. Educators can better align with these issues by understanding how to calculate ROI using the Philips ROI model [17]. The first step in the Phillips ROI model is to perform a five-step needs assessment. As shown in Fig. 19.1, the needs include (a) payoff needs, (b) business needs, (c) performance needs, (d) learning needs, and (e) preference needs [17]. The needs assessment helps align the improvement intervention with institutional goals. Steps in the needs assessment can be linked to key outcomes that are of particular interest to healthcare stakeholders (reaction, learning, application/implementation, impact, and ROI) [17].

Payoff Needs

Payoff needs address healthcare problems and evaluate the likelihood of showing positive ROI. The payoff need simultaneously shows that a problem is worth solving and the proposed solution (such as SBML) is acceptable. The payoff needs ask

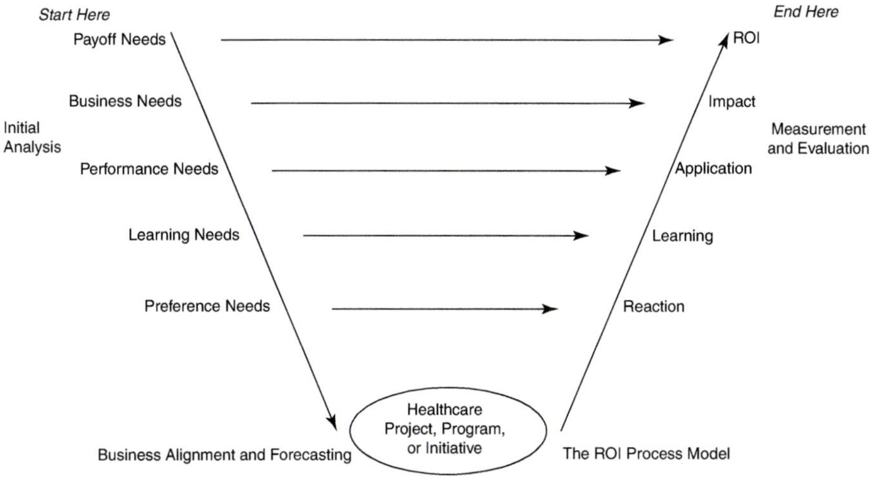

Fig. 19.1 Business alignment model. (Adapted with permission from Buzachero et al. [17]. Copyright © 2013 McGraw-Hill Education)

for an answer to a simple question: Can earning or saving a reasonable amount of money be associated with solving a problem? A payoff can be realized through decreased costs from errors or wasteful spending, higher value from improved clinical outcomes, or expanding population or community health. Avoiding penalties due to the CMS value-based purchasing (VBP) readmission reduction program and incurring costs due to nonreimbursable HACs is also crucial for many hospitals, hospital systems, and clinics to survive [18]. Therefore, many payoff needs lie within these nonpayment programs.

Business Needs

Business needs are addressed by impacts that allow an organization to take advantage of a payoff need. In other words, the business need is the outcome that must be measured to demonstrate the payoff. A business need is a *measurement* of improvements in efficiency, quality, cost, or productivity. These gains involve reductions in overuse, underuse, inefficient, or defective healthcare [16]. For example, if central line-associated bloodstream infections and catheter-associated urinary tract infections are driving HAC nonpayment penalties, measuring reductions of these infections after a SBML intervention reflects a business need.

Performance Needs

Performance needs determine the cause of a payoff need and what applied improvements should be made. There are many ways to determine the source of a problem including surveys, direct observation, simulations, and chart review. Quality improvement methods such as root cause analysis, failure mode effects analysis, or process mapping can also help pinpoint problems [8]. For example, if direct observation of patient care identifies errors in infection prevention techniques, the performance need is the lack of skill shown by personnel performing these tasks.

Learning Needs

Virtually every healthcare quality improvement effort involves education [8, 18]. The learning needs ask about what should be learned to address performance. Examples of learning needs include helping employees become familiar with new equipment, policies, or clinical procedures. Learning needs are discovered from interviews, observations, simulation-based assessments, written tests, or chart reviews.

Preference Needs

Preference needs focus on stakeholder reactions to the project. Preference needs determine if the proposed solution to a healthcare problem is necessary, practical, and useful for patient care. Input from several stakeholders defines preference needs—project scope, timing, resources, and location. This information can be obtained from one-on-one meetings, interviews, or surveys. Once a learning need is identified, the preference need reflects how the hospital employees prefer to receive training, for example, online module vs. simulation-based education.

Measurement and Evaluation: Inputs and Outputs

After the needs of the institution are understood, an intervention can be developed to address them. Calculating the people, time, and costs of the intervention are the inputs, while the outcomes of the intervention are outputs. Both inputs and outputs must be objectively and rigorously evaluated, assessed, and reported to stakeholders during the project span.

Inputs

1. Access: Who needs to be involved, and how much effort or time will it take to participate? Access also accounts for the space and equipment needed to complete the project.
2. Cost: Conservative yet comprehensive cost estimates should be prepared before the ROI project begins. Accurate estimates help build trust with stakeholders for current and future projects. All costs must be calculated prospectively from the start of the project to avoid errors. We recommend keeping a detailed file of all project costs. These costs include salary support for the individuals involved including time spent on planning and preparation, implementation, and assessment of the project. Opportunity costs are included if the team includes healthcare providers who would otherwise be engaged in patient care activities that generate revenue. Other costs include supplies, space, and equipment. Accuracy in cost estimation and actual expenditures is needed to support a reliable ROI calculation.

Outputs

Outputs of the ROI model include reaction, learning, application and implementation, impact, and ROI. Outputs are directly informed by the needs assessment. It is not always necessary to show all five outputs from a project to be successful or obtain continued support:

1. Reaction: Reaction measures the stakeholders' or learners' reaction to the project and relates to the preference needs assessment. Understanding stakeholders' reactions can aid project development by pre-emptively addressing barriers or concerns. Stakeholder meetings, interviews, focus groups, or questionnaires can be used to obtain reactions to a project. There is a strong positive correlation between reaction and successful project application and implementation.
2. Learning: Learning measures show that achievement has occurred and relates to the learning needs assessment. In SBML interventions, learning is measured by comparing pre- and posttest scores. Understanding pretest knowledge gaps and how they have been addressed is an example of a learning outcome.
3. Application and implementation: Application and implementation measures to what extent the new process, skill, or knowledge is being used in actual practice and relates to performance needs assessment. Application and implementation can be measured by medical record review, direct observation, surveys, or interviews. Application and implementation can be reported as a number or percent of the time the new process is being used.
4. Impact: The impact of an ROI project measures and evaluates business needs. An example of a business need is to reduce LOS related to a clinical condition such as pneumonia. A project that reduces LOS for pneumonia admissions by 60% demonstrates meaningful impact related to business needs.
5. ROI. Return on investment measures the value of improvements related to payoff needs. Payoff needs include measurable outcomes such as cost savings, employee engagement, nurse turnover, preventable adverse events, and mortality. For example, cost savings due to reduced LOS from a project can be assigned a monetary value to address the payoff need and demonstrate ROI as a cost/benefit ratio. When calculating costs, always use the most credible sources to obtain trust from stakeholders. This may include the hospital finance department or use of published sources. ROI is calculated using this formula:

$$\mathrm{ROI}(\%) = \frac{\text{Net project benefits}\left(\text{benefits} - \text{costs}\right) \times 100}{\text{Cost}}$$

An ROI of 50% means that after costs were removed, an additional 50% of the costs were made as revenue or savings. Several published SBML studies describe ROI as a benefit/cost ratio [15, 19, 20].

In some cases, value may be hard to measure as cost savings. For example, nurse or other participant satisfaction after an education intervention might be linked to lower nursing turnover and reduced recruitment and onboarding costs for new nurses. Other intangible measures include improved reputation and improved safety culture.

Using the ROI Model with SBML: Central Line Maintenance

We used SBML to train intensive care unit (ICU) nurses at Northwestern Memorial Hospital (NMH) in proper central line maintenance skills [21]. This project received stakeholder support across NMH including physicians, nurses, nurse educators and managers, patients, the patient safety and quality department, chief medical officer, chief nursing officer, and the hospital president. Indirectly CMS (insurers) supported this project through financial incentives to reduce central line-associated bloodstream infections (CLABSIs) and HACs. The plan and details of the project were discussed frequently with stakeholders via monthly meetings. The following section describes the approach we used for this SBML intervention using the Phillips ROI model (Table 19.1).

Business Alignment, Forecasting, and Needs Assessment

NMH hospital epidemiology records revealed that CLABSIs were rising in the ICUs. Consequently, NMH received HAC non-reimbursements from CMS (payoff need) and needed to reduce CLABSI rates and improve hospital reputation (intangible benefit) from this publicly reported measure (business needs).

A chart review and root cause analysis showed that most CLABSIs were occurring 4–5 days after central venous catheter (CVC) insertion. Because most infections were delayed, this suggested that attention should be paid to central line maintenance rather than CVC insertion. An initial review of best practices resulted in changes to policies and equipment, but CLABSI rates did not improve. Therefore, a central line maintenance skills SBML pilot study was performed, training nurses from the cardiothoracic intensive care unit (CTICU), where CLABSI rates were the highest. Pretest results revealed wide variation in skills related to central line maintenance tasks [21]. This performance data identified performance and learning needs and suggested that a major factor contributing to high CLABSI rates was skill variation among nursing staff. Nurses preferred to be trained using simulation (preference need). A central line maintenance SBML curriculum was developed to train and evaluate CTICU nurses in five aspects of central line maintenance: (a) medication administration, (b) injection cap (needleless connector) changes, (c) tubing changes, (d) blood draws, and (e) dressing changes [21]. All participating nurses were expected to demonstrate mastery of the five skills after completion of the SBML education intervention.

Inputs and Outputs

Inputs include space, equipment, and other costs. In this example, we accounted for (a) training costs including classrooms, simulators, and central line supplies; (b) faculty time to develop and pilot test the SBML curriculum and perform training and assessment; and (c) nursing salaries during training.

Table 19.1 Use of the Phillips return on investment (ROI) model to design and evaluate a central line maintenance SBML curriculum for nurses

Phillips model step	What was assessed	What was found
Needs assessment		
Payoff	Hospital-acquired condition (HAC) non-reimbursement penalties	Our hospital wanted to reduce the amount of HAC non-reimbursement penalties it faced every year
Business	Central line-associated bloodstream infections (CLABSIs)	Lowering CLABSI rates would prevent HAC non-reimbursement penalties and improve hospital performance in national surveys
Performance	Root cause analysis and chart review	Timing of infections suggested suboptimal central line maintenance was causing CLABSIs
Learning	Simulation-based training of central line maintenance tasks	Nurses demonstrated high variability in central line maintenance skills and needed further training
Preference	Informal surveys	Nurses preferred to have on-the-job training with simulation as opposed to lectures and online modules
Inputs		
Access	Location for training, number of nurses to be trained, instructors needed to teach the curriculum, sufficient simulators, and supplies	Hospital conference rooms, 2000 nurses, 12 instructors, 6 simulators, and supplies for up to 10,000 simulated skills
Costs	Cost of conference rooms, nursing salary for participants and instructors, simulators, and supplies	Conference rooms were provided by the hospital, nurses and instructors were paid their hourly salary rates, simulators were donated by an industry partner, and supplies were purchased by hospital operations
Outputs		
Reaction	Post-course surveys	Nurses who participated in SBML believed that the educational experience was valuable and prepared them well to perform central line maintenance tasks
Learning	Pre- to posttest comparisons of five central line maintenance tasks using a skills checklist and a simulator	Performance on all five central line maintenance tasks improved significantly from baseline
Application and implementation	Random audits were performed to evaluate if nurses were performing central line maintenance tasks on patients in the ICU the way they were trained in the simulation laboratory	Nurses were almost always performing the tasks as taught during SBML. Nurses received refresher training as needed
Impact	CLABSI rates	CLABSI rates decreased
Return on investment	HAC penalties	HAC non-reimbursement penalties were avoided

Outputs of the ROI model include reaction, learning, application and implementation, impact, and ROI. We used a questionnaire to obtain feedback from learners (reaction) about the SBML intervention. Specifically, participating nurses reported their self-confidence to perform each of the five components of central line maintenance and their satisfaction with the curriculum. Pre- and posttest checklist data about nurse performance for each of the five central line maintenance tasks were collected during the mastery learning education intervention (learning). Random audits of actual ICU patient care were performed to determine how often nurses used the techniques taught during the SBML intervention (application and implementation). NMH records are monitored monthly to document CLABSI rates (impact). The cost of CLABSI non-reimbursed care and any CMS penalties were monitored by our hospital finance and quality departments (ROI).

Since implementation, we reported high nurse satisfaction with SBML (reaction) and significantly improved clinical skills (learning) [21]. Random audits continue to show that nurses are using the skills taught in the simulation laboratory during actual ICU patient care (application). In terms of impact, NMH has also experienced a substantial decline in CLABSI rates since the SBML intervention began leading to elimination of costly HAC penalties (which can range up to millions of dollars annually).

We also discovered several other benefits of our SBML intervention. First, participating CTICU nurses reported on surveys and informally that the investment of time and resources toward their education produced greater engagement and job satisfaction. Additionally, it is likely that the perceived reputation of the institution improved because CLABSI rates are publically reported and factor into quality rankings.

As a result of the outputs reported to hospital leadership, NMH has continued to fund SBML line maintenance training for all nurses who care for patients with CVCs.

Additional Examples Demonstrating ROI from SBML

Currently, three published studies evaluate ROI in terms of cost savings after SBML. All were performed at Northwestern University.

CVC Insertion SBML

The first study to show ROI from SBML evaluated CVC insertion training for physicians [19]. In this report, the cost of CVC insertion SBML was compared to hospital costs for treating a CLABSI. Education intervention costs included purchase of an ultrasound, simulator, CVC kits, sterile equipment, other miscellaneous supplies, facility rental, and faculty and staff salary support. Investigators worked closely with the hospital quality and finance departments to estimate costs for items such as hospital LOS. The estimated cost of the SBML program was $111,916. The estimated cost saving due to CLABSIs that were prevented after training was $823,164 in the first year alone. Therefore, this analysis demonstrated an ROI of 636%, over a 7:1 return (benefit/cost ratio) on investment in 1 year. Important keys to success of this project were partnership with the hospital quality and finance departments and adequate time for training to achieve learning outcomes.

Bedside Paracentesis SBML

The second study to show ROI from SBML addressed bedside paracentesis procedure training for physicians [20]. In this study, the cost of performing bedside paracentesis by SBML-trained internal medicine (IM) residents was compared to the cost of referring the procedure to interventional radiology (IR).

Education intervention costs included the simulator, procedure-related equipment and sterile supplies, and faculty and resident physician time. No costs were incurred for space and ultrasound use in this study. Investigators worked closely with the hospital quality and finance departments to estimate costs for items such blood transfusions, interventional radiology (IR) staffing, and room use. The cost difference for paracentesis procedures performed by SBML-trained internal medicine residents versus procedures performed in IR was considered the net benefit. The estimated cost of a bedside paracentesis procedure was $134.01 compared to $663.42 for each paracentesis procedure referred to IR. Therefore, this analysis demonstrated an ROI of 395%, nearly a 5:1 return (benefit/cost ratio) based on the actual number of procedures performed in 1 year [20].

Laparoscopic Common Bile Duct Exploration

The third study establishing ROI from SBML addressed laparoscopic common bile duct exploration (LCBDE) [15]. Patients often need two invasive procedures to treat cholecystitis (inflammation of the gallbladder) complicated by common bile duct obstruction due to gallstones. The procedures include a laparoscopic cholecystectomy in which the gallbladder is removed by a surgeon, as well as a subsequent endoscopic retrograde cholangiopancreatogram (ERCP) performed by a gastroenterologist to remove gallstones obstructing the common bile duct. LCBDE offers an option to perform both in a single procedure, thus exposing patients to only one anesthesia and potentially shorter LOS and costs.

In this study, surgeons were trained to perform the LCBDE procedure using SBML. Costs were compared between the traditional two-procedure approach (surgery plus ERCP) and the single-procedure approach (LCBDE). SBML intervention costs included creation of the simulator; facility, equipment, and supply rental; and faculty and physician salary. Investigators worked closely with the hospital quality and finance departments to estimate costs for items such as operating and procedure room staffing, supplies, and room use. The cost difference between procedures performed by SBML-trained surgeons (who performed LCBDE) and procedures performed by non-SBML-trained physicians (who never performed LCBDE) was considered the net benefit. The cost of the SBML intervention over a 3-year study period was \$10,254. The average hospital cost of patients cared for by SBML physicians was \$12,987 ± \$3286 versus \$15,022 ± \$4613 for patients cared for by non-SBML-trained surgeons due to patients requiring a second procedure (ERCP) and needing a longer LOS. The intervention provided a 3-year ROI of 277% or 4:1 return (benefit/cost ratio). We anticipate that the cost savings will increase as the operation becomes more common.

As these examples show, using the Phillips ROI model is an effective way to present a data-driven argument for SBML project support. Other strategies including stakeholder engagement and change management (covered in Chap. 7) are also needed to ensure success.

Convincing the C-suite

Stakeholder engagement must occur before, during, and after the needs assessments and the ROI methodology are complete [22–24]. Stakeholders are defined as a group either inside or outside a healthcare organization that are affected or can affect the objectives of an improvement project [22, 23]. Stakeholder engagement includes all stakeholders in the process from start to finish. SBML projects that are linked to improved patient care and are a win-win for all parties (hospital administrators, clinicians, patients, educators) have the best chance of success.

Clear and frequent communication with stakeholders, clinical and operations leaders, and participants is key to any successful quality improvement project. Electronic communication is best for communicating factual information such as project schedules. In-person meetings are needed for high-stakes decisions and to obtain buy-in for projects. Interviews, workshops, focus groups, and surveys are also useful for project development and engagement. Trust will develop from frequent communication, setting agendas, meeting deadlines, and achieving objectives.

We follow at least ten basic rules when developing SBML projects in a clinical environment [22, 23]:

1. Include all stakeholders and obtain buy-in before project implementation.
2. Commit to transparency and meeting shared deadline objectives to build trust.
3. Align with stakeholder objectives and goals. A SBML project that represents a novel research idea for an academic team may fail if key stakeholders do not see the value.
4. Recognize and respect organizational culture. Each institution has a unique culture that affects acceptance and success of new initiatives.
5. Reflect on past experiences and learn from barriers and facilitators of past project failure and success.

6. Foster a long-term commitment.
7. Ensure data are accurate and reliable.
8. Develop credible and conservative ROI calculations.
9. Create clear roles and expectations for team members.
10. Communicate formally and frequently.

Coda

This chapter reviews how to create a business case to support SBML quality improvement projects. Not all projects yield ROI, but understanding business language and strategies helps simulation leaders demonstrate the value of their projects and obtain support for current and future work. SBML is a proven strategy to improve healthcare education and patient outcomes. To maximize its impact, educators must be able to align with the needs and outcomes desired by healthcare organizations.

References

1. Kohn LT, Corrigan JM, Donaldson MS. To err is human: building a safer health system. Washington, DC: National Academy Press; 2000.
2. Brennan TA, Leape LL, Laird NM, Hebert L, Localio AR, Lawthers AG, et al. Incidence of adverse events and negligence in hospitalized patients. Results of the Harvard Medical Practice Study I. N Engl J Med. 1991;324(6):370–6.
3. Duffy FD, Holmboe ES. What procedures should internists do? Ann Intern Med. 2007;146(5):392–3.
4. Giraud T, Dhainaut JF, Vaxelaire JF, Joseph T, Journois D, Bleichner G, et al. Iatrogenic complications in adult intensive care units: a prospective two-center study. Crit Care Med. 1993;21(1):40–51.
5. Rubins HB, Moskowitz MA. Complications of care in a medical intensive care unit. J Gen Intern Med. 1990;5(2):104–9.
6. Rosenthal MB. Nonpayment for performance? Medicare's new reimbursement rule. N Engl J Med. 2007;357(16):1573–5.
7. Leape LL, Brennan TA, Laird N, Lawthers AG, Localio AR, Barnes BA, et al. The nature of adverse events in hospitalized patients. Results of the Harvard Medical Practice Study II. N Engl J Med. 1991;324(6):377–84.
8. Joshi M, Ransom ER, Nash DB, Ransom SB. The healthcare quality book: vision, strategy, and tools. 3rd ed. Chicago: Health Administration Press; 2014.
9. Barsuk JH, Cohen ER, Feinglass J, McGaghie WC, Wayne DB. Use of simulation-based education to reduce catheter-related bloodstream infections. Arch Intern Med. 2009;169(15):1420–3.
10. Barsuk JH, Cohen ER, Potts S, Demo H, Gupta S, Feinglass J, et al. Dissemination of a simulation-based mastery learning intervention reduces central line-associated bloodstream infections. BMJ Qual Saf. 2014;23(9):749–56.
11. Barsuk JH, Cohen ER, Williams MV, Scher J, Jones SF, Feinglass J, et al. Simulation-based mastery learning for thoracentesis skills improves patient outcomes: a randomized trial. Acad Med. 2018;93(5):729–35.
12. Barsuk JH, McGaghie WC, Cohen ER, O'Leary KJ, Wayne DB. Simulation-based mastery learning reduces complications during central venous catheter insertion in a medical intensive care unit. Crit Care Med. 2009;37(10):2697–701.

13. Didwania A, McGaghie WC, Cohen ER, Butter J, Barsuk JH, Wade LD, et al. Progress toward improving the quality of cardiac arrest medical team responses at an academic teaching hospital. J Grad Med Educ. 2011;3(2):211–6.
14. Gossett DR, Gilchrist-Scott D, Wayne DB, Gerber SE. Simulation training for forceps-assisted vaginal delivery and rates of maternal perineal trauma. Obstet Gynecol. 2016;128(3):429–35.
15. Schwab B, Teitelbaum EN, Barsuk JH, Soper NJ, Hungness ES. Single-stage laparoscopic management of choledocholithiasis: an analysis after implementation of a mastery learning resident curriculum. Surgery. 2018;163(3):503–8.
16. Swensen SJ, Dilling JA, Mc Carty PM, Bolton JW, Harper CM Jr. The business case for healthcare quality improvement. J Patient Saf. 2013;9(1):44–52.
17. Buzachero VV, Phillips J, Phillips PP, Phillips ZL. Measuring ROI in healthcare: tools and techniques to measure the impact and ROI in healthcare improvement projects and programs. New York: McGraw-Hill; 2013.
18. CMS's Value Based Programs. Available from: https://www.cms.gov/Medicare/Quality-Initiatives-Patient-Assessment-Instruments/Value-Based-Programs/Value-Based-Programs.html.
19. Cohen ER, Feinglass J, Barsuk JH, Barnard C, O'Donnell A, McGaghie WC, et al. Cost savings from reduced catheter-related bloodstream infection after simulation-based education for residents in a medical intensive care unit. Simul Healthc. 2010;5(2):98–102.
20. Barsuk JH, Cohen ER, Feinglass J, Kozmic SE, McGaghie WC, Ganger D, et al. Cost savings of performing paracentesis procedures at the bedside after simulation-based education. Simul Healthc. 2014;9(5):312–8.
21. Barsuk JH, Cohen ER, Mikolajczak A, Seburn S, Slade M, Wayne DB. Simulation-based mastery learning improves central line maintenance skills of ICU nurses. J Nurs Adm. 2015;45(10):511–7.
22. AHRQ. Engaging stakeholders to improve the quality of children's health care. Available from: https://www.ahrq.gov/policymakers/chipra/demoeval/what-we-learned/implementation-guides/implementation-guide1/index.html.
23. Jeffery N. Stakeholder engagement: a road map to meaningful engagement. Doughty Centre for Corporate Responsibility. Cranfield University School of Management. 2009. Available from: http://www.som.cranfield.ac.uk/som/dinamic-content/media/CR%20Stakeholder.pdf.
24. Preskill H, Jones N. A practical guide for engaging stakeholders in developing evaluation questions. 2009. Available from: http://www.rwjf.org/content/dam/farm/toolkits/toolkits/2009/rwjf48595.

Educational Policy Consequences from Mastery Learning

20

Marianne M. Green, Aashish K. Didwania, Diane B. Wayne, and William C. McGaghie

The "excellence for all" goal of mastery learning which is expressed throughout this book is a lofty objective. Most health professions educators agree that high achievement among learners with little or no measured outcome variation is a difficult but worthy ambition. We learn from Chap. 7, Implementing and Managing a Mastery Learning Program, that putting a mastery learning curriculum in place and managing its details can be daunting—just like the hard work of implementing and managing a traditional health professions curriculum. The mastery learning message of Chap. 7 is to start small, learn from experience and data, grow curricula at a pace that makes sense locally, and focus on mastery learning policies and practices that are within reach. We acknowledge, of course, that small and large mastery learning programs are grounded in education policies that differ from ordinary health professions education principles. The direction and scope of these education policy differences warrant close attention.

Webster's Ninth New Collegiate Dictionary defines policy as "2*a:* a definite course or method of action selected from among alternatives and in light of given conditions to guide and determine present and future decisions; *b:* a high-level overall plan embracing general goals and acceptable procedures…" Practical expressions of guiding policies across health professions education are seen in such actions as student selection; early didactic and simulation experiences and clinical rotations; formative and summative assessment practices; learner

M. M. Green (✉) · D. B. Wayne
Northwestern University Feinberg School of Medicine,
Departments of Medicine and Medical Education, Chicago, IL, USA
e-mail: m-green@northwestern.edu; dwayne@northwestern.edu

A. K. Didwania
Northwestern University Feinberg School of Medicine, Departments of Medicine and Medical Education, Chicago, IL, USA

W. C. McGaghie
Northwestern University Feinberg School of Medicine, Departments of Medical Education and Preventive Medicine, Chicago, IL, USA

W. C. McGaghie et al. (eds.), *Comprehensive Healthcare Simulation: Mastery Learning in Health Professions Education*, Comprehensive Healthcare Simulation, https://doi.org/10.1007/978-3-030-34811-3_20

advancement and graduation; faculty development; and many other large and small procedures. Implementation and management of mastery learning programs calls for recognition of education policies that diverge from standard methods of operation. This chapter aims to set forth and clarify the education policies that govern mastery learning and lay out the everyday consequences that result from this approach.

The Josiah Macy Jr. Foundation sponsored a 2017 conference on the theme, "Achieving Competency-Based, Time-Variable Health Professions Education" [1]. The conference theme is a synonym for mastery learning. The conference included scholars and thought leaders from a variety of health professions including nursing, medicine, and pharmacy. A co-author of this chapter (DBW) was a conference participant. The Macy Foundation conference report articulates education policies, principles, and actions that closely approximate the mastery learning model described in earlier chapters of this book. The Macy Foundation report states, "… educational innovations targeting the achievement of a fully competency-based, time-variable system are constrained not only by traditional views of education but also by existing structures and systems, such as university registrar systems, licensing requirements, board certification standards, and accreditation systems that rely on credit hours and fixed durations of training as evidence of sufficient academic achievement" [1]. These are all expressions of health professions education inertia as pointed out in Chap. 1.

The Macy Foundation report continues to discuss education policies that underlie mastery learning programs. "Full implementation of a competency-based, time-variable educational strategy will require health professions schools and training sites to develop a strategy to manage such a major change. All stakeholders (learners, faculty, administrators, staff, regulators, and committees served) must be included in the process. Much attention needs to be paid to faculty who will need to take on new roles and acquire new skills" [1].

The Macy Foundation conference report articulates five key policy recommendations to advance competency-based, time-variable health professions education [1]:

1. *System Redesign:* "Curricula, learning environments, and faculty development require systematic redesign to achieve a successful competency-based, time-variable health professions education system." Chapters 3 and 9 cover many of these matters.
2. *Creating a Continuum of Education, Training, and Practice:* "The benefits of competency-based education can only be realized when transitions between phases are based on attainment of competencies rather than time" (Chaps. 3, 17, and 18).
3. *Implement a Robust Program of Assessment:* "Leaders in health professions schools and their health care system partners should champion, develop, and implement a program of assessment that supports competency-based, time-variable training and explicitly links educational programs to improved health outcomes" (Chaps. 5, 16, and 18).

4. *Enabling Technologies:* "Health professions education and health care delivery institutions should develop and use enabling technologies in the implementation of competency-based, time-variable education throughout the professional education continuum of the practitioner."
5. *Outcomes Evaluation:* "Competency-based, time-variable health professions education is a transformational approach to both education and health care. With relentless focus on achieving desired care outcomes, each stage of a health care professional's education, training, and career is linked by a set of competencies aligned across the continuum" (Chaps. 5, 16, and 18).

The five educational policy recommendations expressed by the 2018 Macy Foundation conference report are reinforced and amplified by a 2018 journal article in *Academic Medicine* published by Jennifer Kogan and colleagues titled, "What regulatory requirements and existing structures must change if competency-based, time-variable training (CBTVT) is introduced into the continuum of medical education in the United States?" [2] This article lists eight education policy "Next steps to align regulatory requirements and existing structures to support a CBTVT continuum:"

1. "The LCME [Liaison Committee on Medical Education] should review and revise their accreditation standards using the lens of CBTVT. New standards that promote assessment and documentation of learner competence... should be developed."
2. "Medical schools should explore, study, and report different models of establishing tuition and managing cost of attendance."
3. "Medical schools should revise graduation requirements to describe how student competence, rather than required courses and rotations, is used to determine eligibility for graduation."
4. "Graduate medical education (GME) funding should be reformed so that payments are not tied to the initial residency period and length of training."
5. "Educational leaders and health care delivery institutions will need to partner to identify strategies to make predictable clinical scheduling and CBTVT more compatible."
6. "Accrediting, licensing, and certifying bodies should work together to discuss how to revise requirements for eligibility to sit for licensing and certifying examinations that are competency based rather than time focused."
7. "Educational leaders will need to reduce the silos across the medical education continuum. This might be accomplished by having a single set of developmental milestones that better link Undergraduate Medical Education (UME) and GME programs."
8. "It will be necessary to establish how to communicate learner competence across transitions using letters of evaluation, such as the MSPE [Medical Student Performance Evaluation], and letters of recommendation. In particular, accepted definitions about when a period of extended training represents an acceptable variation in competency acquisition and when it signifies a potential problem will be needed."

The Macy Foundation conference report [1] and the Kogan et al. journal article [2] leave the impression that sweeping changes in education policies and practices are needed to plan and implement CBTVT into health professions education. We aim to dispel this notion. In everyday practice, adoption of a mastery learning curriculum is a matter of scale and ambition. While newcomers to mastery learning should be aware of "big picture" education policy issues [1, 2], experience teaches that real-world programs should begin with simple and focused learning goals, recognize that health professions curricula represent only a sample of professional practice (Chaps. 3 and 5), learn from experience, and grow in ways that make local sense.

The rest of this chapter is organized as two main sections that cover the education policy consequences from mastery learning concerning its (a) benefits and (b) challenges. Within each of the two sections, the education policy discussion addresses four stakeholder categories: (a) learners, (b) education programs, (c) sponsoring organizations, and (d) governing bodies and the healthcare system (Table 20.1). The four stakeholder categories are separated for clarity and convenience. However, they are not mutually exclusive and have much overlap. The chapter concludes with a brief coda.

Benefits

Many benefits come from mastery learning education programs in health professions education. The benefits derive from mastery learning policies and practices described specifically in Chap. 2 and in many other locations throughout this book. Table 20.1 shows that the stakeholders range from specific individual learners to more general education programs, sponsoring organizations, and governing bodies and the healthcare system.

Learners

The most important benefits from mastery learning education programs in the health professions affect learners. There is no doubt that mastery learning of clinical reasoning and clinical skill boosts learner readiness to provide clinical care for patients. Many mastery learning skill acquisition studies in nursing, medicine, and several other health professions, summarized in five recent reviews [3–7], underscore this statement (see also Chap. 16).

Learner benefits from mastery learning programs in health professions education are plentiful. They include lifelong improvement, objective measurement, feedback, increased self-efficacy, and involvement in a clinical culture of constant improvement. Two examples are telling: (a) the utility of mastery learning to improve central line maintenance skills among experienced Intensive Care Unit (ICU) nurses and (b) mastery learning training to improve forceps-assisted vaginal delivery of newborns and to reduce rates of perineal trauma.

Table 20.1 Education policy consequences of mastery learning

	Learners	Education programs	Sponsoring organizations	Governing bodies and healthcare system
Benefits	Learner centered, e.g., mastery learning for central line maintenance Lifelong improvement, e.g., periodic booster sessions within a particular skill training program Objective measurement Individualized feedback Increased self-efficacy Culture of constant improvement	Accreditation Board certification success Faculty-learner engagement	Public accountability Efficiency Budgeting Culture of constant improvement	Public accountability Enhanced workforce skills Improved patient safety Better patient outcomes
Challenges	Evaluation apprehension Impression management	Learner selection and matching (all levels) Database security Schedule constraints Faculty resources, staffing, and training Enabling technology Credible assessment measures Learner advancement (standards) Inertia and local customs (risk aversion) Individual mastery plan for learners on different paths in the same program, e.g., women's health, respiratory care Communicate learner competence across transitions	Database security Schedule constraints Workforce improvement Faculty time and resources Accreditation requirements Inertia and local customs (risk aversion) Perceived higher cost due to increased time for mastery training	Ongoing workforce improvement Accreditation and governance (e.g., ACGME, ABMS, FSMB, NBME, NCSBN, APTA, ABIM, et al.)* Faculty oversight of assessments Time-based funding Inertia and local customs (risk aversion)

Notes

1. A challenging task is creating curricula and policies to address complex cognitive skills like clinical reasoning absent a "gold standard."
2. Can use milestones (Chap. 17) as an example of ACGME's foray into mastery learning.
3. Some key training topics right now are wellness (anxiety, depression, imposter syndrome, resilience) and workforce diversity. Can the mastery model address such topics?

**ACGME* Accreditation Council for Graduate Medical Education; *ABMS* American Board of Medical Specialties; *FSMB* Federation of State Medical Boards; *NBME* National Board of Medical Examiners; *NCSBN* National Council of State Board of Nursing; *APTA* American Physical Therapy Association; *ABIM* American Board of Internal Medicine

A team of ICU nurses and nurse educators collaborated with physician Jeffrey Barsuk to design and deliver a simulation-based mastery learning (SBML) curriculum on central line maintenance and care [8]. The central line maintenance curriculum intervention based on the mastery learning bundle addressed five tasks: (a) medication administration, (b) injection cap—needleless connector—changes, (c) tubing changes, (d) blood drawing, and (e) dressing changes. Project results show that task pretest scores ranged from a median of 0.0% to 73.1.% All posttest scores rose to a median of 100.% Nursing experience had a significant negative correlation with medication administration pretest performance. The multidisciplinary mastery learning team concluded, "[experienced] ICU nurses displayed wide variability in their ability to perform central line maintenance tasks. After SBML, there was significant improvement, and all nurses reached a [high and] predetermined level of competency" [8].

Obstetrician Dana Gossett and her colleagues created and implemented a mastery learning curriculum to better educate residents about forceps-assisted vaginal delivery of newborns [9]. The curriculum goals were to improve vaginal delivery efficiency and to reduce the rate of maternal perineal trauma. In brief, the results of the mastery learning education intervention reveal, "… a 22% reduction in severe perineal laceration … among women delivered by residents who had completed [mastery learning] forceps simulation training compared with women delivered by residents who had not. After adjusting for known maternal and delivery risk factors for perineal laceration, the magnitude of the reduction increased to 26% …" [9].

These two studies provide strong evidence that nurses and physicians providing high-acuity clinical care receive powerful professional benefits from engaging in education programs grounded in mastery learning policies. Downstream, translational benefits regarding improved patient care practices and patient outcomes are also plain from these powerful education interventions [3].

Education Programs

We anticipate that health professions education programs will benefit from curricula informed by mastery learning education policies. This view is shaped by the 2017 Macy Conference report cited previously [1] and the 2018 Kogan et al. journal article on the "regulatory requirements and existing structures [that] must change if competency-based, time-variable training is introduced into the continuum of medical education …" [2]. Experience and common sense also inform our point of view.

At least three facets of health professions education programs will be affected by policies that underlie the mastery learning bundle. The three facets are (a) accreditation, (b) certification examination success, and (c) faculty-learner engagement.

Accreditation is a key because health professions education programs cannot operate unless they fulfill basic accreditation requirements. Health professions education accreditation program requirements leave some room for variation, but core criteria usually include faculty and financial resources; physical space and equipment; curriculum quality, integrity, and conformity with state-of-the-art expectations; student selection and retention policies; faculty development; institutional commitment; and many others. The grinding gears of health professions education program regulatory requirements and innovative features of mastery learning curriculum interventions will no doubt produce "growing pains" and "fault lines" as education programs adjust to changing accreditation systems [10]. These and related issues are addressed in several cited sources [1, 2] and in Chaps. 18 and 19 of this volume. Spread of the mastery model within research programs that are sustained and cumulative will continue to build the evidence base that mastery learning and CBTVT approaches yield improved education as well as downstream patient care outcomes. Data from these reports will continue to impact and change accreditation requirements until they too have outcomes rather than process-based approachs to clinical education.

Health professions education program directors acknowledge frequently that a key index of academic success is the passing rate of their students on board certification examinations. Why accept and educate a student if that person's likelihood of passing a professional certification examination such as the U.S. Nursing National Council Licensure Examination or the National Physical Therapy Examination for physical therapy is low?

For example, U.S. medical education survey research published in 2009 shows that postgraduate residency program directors rank United States Medical Licensing Examination Step 1 scores second only to grades in required clerkships as a resident selection criterion. This finding applies to all medical specialties [11]. Survey research published in 2018 shows that residency program directors are even more reliant on USMLE Step 1 scores for resident selection, using the measure as the most important selection criterion [12]. Undergraduate health professions education programs using mastery learning models allow additional time for practice beyond the standard curriculum. This flexibility insists that all learners acquire basic and clinical science knowledge to rigorous mastery standards and will likely increase the probability that learners earn passing scores on board certification examinations.

Faculty-learner engagement in education events, exercises, simulations, and activities is a cornerstone of mastery learning curricula (Chap. 4). This principle is reinforced by a report issued recently by the Stanford University Graduate School of Education which asserts, "The students who benefit most from college [and professional education] are those who are most engaged in their academics … taking advantage of the opportunities and resources their particular institution provides. Engagement is the key" [13]. High engagement measured by course satisfaction surveys has been a uniform finding throughout our greater than 15-year experience with mastery learning programs in health professions education. Learners frequently state that clinical mastery learning experiences should be mandatory [14].

Sponsoring Organizations

Health professions education sponsoring organizations such a community and 4-year colleges, hospitals, universities, professional schools, continuing professional education providers, and many others also benefit from mastery learning education policies. The benefits include public accountability about graduates' readiness for unsupervised professional practice; goal-directed and efficient education program operations; mission-based budgeting; and formation of a culture of constant improvement. Former policies that believe a wide distribution of measured outcomes among health professions learners is "good enough" are no longer good enough. Education policies that expect all learners to achieve at a high mastery standard become the new normal. We express this as "excellence for all."

Governing Bodies and the Healthcare System

Bodies that govern health professions education such as accreditation organizations and the larger healthcare system also benefit from mastery learning education policies. The interests of governing bodies are advanced from assurance of greater public accountability about the measured and documented clinical fitness of the healthcare workforce. The healthcare system benefits from mastery learning education policies due to enhanced workforce skills, improved patient safety, and better patient outcomes. A recent scientific statement published under auspices of the American Heart Association (AHA) endorses this view with a focus on resuscitation education programs. The AHA scientific statement asserts that such programs should "Incorporate a mastery learning model for performance behaviors in which a minimum passing standard is required. Prioritization should be given to those behaviors that have a clear link to patient safety or clinical outcomes" [15]. Several Northwestern University studies have documented reduced healthcare costs as a result of mastery learning interventions (paracentesis, central line insertion, and laparoscopic surgery)—an important public health benefit (Chap. 19).

Challenges

When considering the challenges encountered from implementing a CBTVT with mastery learning curricula, we continue to acknowledge the impact on various stakeholders: learners, education programs, sponsoring organizations, and governing bodies and healthcare system.

Learners

For CBTVT to be successful in medicine, for example, learners need to embrace transparency and data sharing across the education continuum from UME to GME and into practice. Learners may experience discomfort with greater performance transparency that such a system expects. Learners who take more time to achieve competence than their peers may be reluctant to have that information shared in today's competitive environment. If a medical student takes longer to fulfill entrustable professional activity (EPA) requirements [16], she may worry that her competitiveness for residency will be affected. In a context where postgraduate medicine residency program directors are increasingly focused on objective data to sort a large pool of residency applications, will the learner who takes extra time to meet required EPAs be "screened out?" For CBTVT to work, such program directors will need to view the need for additional time to master competencies or EPAs as routine, not a weakness. The traditional culture where learners are apprehensive about evaluation and avoid asking for help to manage impressions about their competence among peers and supervisors must change [17]. Efforts to increase formative assessment that unites evaluation and education are increasing (Chap. 5). However, the mindset of seeking assessment and feedback toward the aim of continuous clinical improvement, rather than stigmatized remediation, must be accepted.

Not only do learners need to welcome constructive feedback as an opportunity to improve, they will also need skills in self-reflection and self-directed learning as training becomes individualized. Activated learners who can use assessment data to create learning goals and then seek additional education and assessment opportunities will be critical in a system that supports individual advancement. This is best done with a trusted mentor who has access to the learner's performance data and who provides feedback and guidance.

Education Programs

Training programs for medical students, residents, and fellows and learners in other health professions will need to endorse education where trainees progress at variable rates and where requirements are met by demonstrating competence rather than getting through a fixed curriculum time period such as a clinical rotation block. Additional resources for assessment, especially workplace-based assessment, are critical [18]. As students and residents progress through a curriculum at different training stages and with different learning styles, faculty need to be trained and flexible to meet the needs of these variable learners. Furthermore, time must be allotted for faculty to observe learners in the workplace more frequently to make valid decisions about competency achievement [18]. This will take additional financial support while clinical demands on faculty are increasing. Assessment programs need to be developed that use measurement tools which yield reliable data—longitudinal quantitative and qualitative evidence—that permit valid decisions about learner achievement (Chap. 5). Collection and use of large bodies of assessment data will require enhanced technology systems that can be shared across the education continuum and that can be easily accessed when decisions need to be made about a learner. Data security and stewardship will also need attention.

Programs will also face administrative challenges when learners progress through the curriculum at different rates. There will be logistic challenges in scheduling and tracking students who progress differently. Programs should consider how to manage learners' variable progression toward EPA, milestone, and other achievements and communicate learner competence across transitions. We must also consider individual trainee interests and provide achievement milestones corresponding to their goals. Examples include women's health tracks and physician scientist training programs. Administrative technologies should ease these changes.

An even greater challenge beyond individual programs' internal scheduling issues are training transitions. The advantages of CBTVT are limited if there is only one time annually when trainees graduate or advance to postgraduate programs. Residency and fellowship programs need to accommodate trainees throughout the year, and the National Residency Match Program (NRMP) in the U.S. and Canada will need revision to accept these changes. Scholars suggest that identifying several fixed times for transition (every 3–6 months) may make more sense [2].

Transcripts must change from documenting course credits to achievement of competencies expressed as EPAs, postgraduate education milestones, or other competency-based metrics (Chap. 17).

Sponsoring Organizations

Sponsoring organizations, hospitals, and health professions schools need to adjust to accommodate time-variable, mastery focused learning. Not only will resources like enhanced technology, faculty development, and protected faculty time be required, but institutions will also need to develop solutions to deal with workforce improvement. For example, in U.S. medical settings, residents and fellows now provide much clinical care. An additional shift of focus from "service" to "learning" will be needed and may be helped by nurse practitioners, physician assistants, or other personnel to provide consistent care.

As Kogan and colleagues point out, the current financial models of tuition payment and GME funding need change. Tuition and registration at health professions schools are based on time to degree. Schools may receive less tuition money if students progress through education programs at faster rates. Alternatively, if tuition is based on degree achievement, students who take more time may stress institution financial resources [2]. Similarly, the current U.S. Medicare funding model for GME presents challenges. Medicare-supported postgraduate medical residency slots are capped for each program and are based on historic numbers of medical residents in hospitals. In addition, Medicare only pays for the minimum accredited length of training for the first program where a resident matches. Later payment for more training is reduced by one-half. Money to the program may be at risk if trainees progress at faster rates. There may also be incentives to push residents to meet learning outcomes sooner if funding is reduced when training time is extended.

Governing Bodies and Healthcare System

Regulatory bodies also drive change. Today's accreditation requirements, board certification, and licensure policies are all time and process based. The LCME, the body that accredits U.S. and Canadian medical schools, requires schools to identify expected student outcomes. However, the LCME does not expect schools to document mastery of key clinical skills. Furthermore, the LCME continues to mandate "at least 130 weeks of instruction" for all students [2].

A review of the Federation of State Medical Boards website reveals time-based requirements for licensure in nearly all U.S. states [19]. Similarly, board certification also specifies time spent in clinical settings and other process measures like number of completed clinical procedures to sit for an initial certification examination. A new combination of time, process, and outcomes measures for board certification will improve program innovation. U.S. medical specialty boards like the American Board of Internal Medicine are advancing such innovative pilot projects using EPAs, curriculum milestones, and increased workplace-based assessment [20]. Similarly, The ACGME has implemented the Next Accreditation System that gives GME programs room to innovate if they measure and record successful outcomes. New pilot programs must be approved through the ACGME's Advancing Innovation in Residency Education program [21]. While promising, these programs incorporate small numbers of trainees and to date lack the rigorous assessment features of mastery learning. More rigor is needed to demonstrate that these new models of clinical training are not just more efficient but fulfill the true aims of CBTVT and mastery learning by producing highly skilled and effective physicians.

Despite the challenges we have outlined, there is no question that progress is being made in the education of health professions trainees toward an outcomes-based approach where the units of progression are mastery of knowledge, skills, and professionalism attributes toward the goal of improving health among individuals and the public.

Coda

Education policies that govern the design and delivery of mastery learning curricula in the health professions are different from policies that have shaped, managed, and controlled health sciences education traditionally. Large and small education policy changes are needed that will guide administrative practices and learner advancement. Our practical advice to health professions curriculum developers and managers is to be aware of policy shifts, start small, attend to local relevance, evaluate programs with rigor, and advance in ways that make sense. Over time the benefits of mastery learning for learners, education programs, sponsoring organizations, and governing bodies and the healthcare system will become evident.

References

1. Lucey CR. Achieving competency-based, time-variable health professions education. Proceedings of a conference sponsored by the Josiah Macy Jr. Foundation in June 2017; New York: Josiah Macy Jr. Foundation; 2018. Available at: www.macyfoundation.org.

2. Kogan JR, Whelan AJ, Gruppen LD, et al. What regulatory requirements and existing structures must change if competency-based, time-variable training is introduced into the continuum of medical education in the United States? Acad Med. 2018;93(3, Suppl):S27–31.
3. McGaghie WC. Medical education research as translational science. Sci Trans Med. 2010;2:19cm8.
4. McGaghie WC, Issenberg SB, Cohen ER, et al. Translational educational research—a necessity of effective healthcare. Chest. 2012;142(5):1097–103.
5. McGaghie WC, Issenberg SB, Barsuk JH, Wayne DB. A critical review of simulation-based medical education with translational outcomes. Med Educ. 2014;48(4):375–85.
6. Griswold-Theodorson S, Ponnuru S, Dong C, et al. Beyond the simulation laboratory: a realist synthesis of clinical outcomes of simulation-based mastery learning. Acad Med. 2015;90(11):1553–60.
7. McGaghie WC, Kristopaitis T. Deliberate practice and mastery learning: origins of expert medical performance. In: Cleland J, Durning SJ, editors. Researching medical education. Oxford, UK: Wiley-Blackwell; 2015.
8. Barsuk JH, Seburn S, Cohen ER, et al. Simulation-based mastery learning improves central line maintenance skills of ICU nurses. J Nurs Adm. 2015;45(10):511–7.
9. Gossett DR, Gilchrist-Scott D, Wayne DB, Gerber SE. Simulation training for forceps-assisted vaginal delivery and rates of maternal perineal trauma. Obstet Gynecol. 2016;128(3):429–35.
10. Nasca TJ, Philibert I, Brigham T, Flynn TC. The next GME accreditation system—rationale and benefits. N Engl J Med. 2012;366(11):1051–6.
11. Green M, Jones P, Thomas JX. Selection criteria for residency: results of a national program directors survey. Acad Med. 2009;84(3):362–7.
12. National Resident Matching Program. Results of the 2018 NRMP program director survey. Available at: https://www.nrmp.org/wp-content/uploads/2018/07/NRMP-2018-Program-Director-Survey-for-www.pdf.
13. Challenge Success. A "fit" over rankings: why college engagement matters more than selectivity. Available at: http://www.challengesuccess.org/wp-content/uploads/2018/10/Challenge-Success-White-Paper-on-College-Admissions-October-2018.pdf.
14. Cohen ER, Barsuk JH, Moazed F, et al. Making July safer: simulation-based mastery learning during intern boot camp. Acad Med. 2013;88:233–9.
15. Cheng A, Nadkarni VM, Mancini MB, et al. Resuscitation education science: educational strategies to improve outcomes from cardiac arrest. A scientific statement from the American Heart Association. Circulation. 2018;138:e82–e122.
16. Englander R, Flynn T, Call S, et al. Toward defining the foundation of the MD degree: core entrustable professional activities for entering residency. Acad Med. 2016;91(10):1352–8.
17. McGaghie WC. Evaluation apprehension and impression management in clinical medical education. Acad Med. 2018;93(5):685–6.
18. Singh T, Norcini JJ. Workplace-based assessment. In: McGaghie WC, editor. International best practices for evaluation in the health professions. London: Radcliffe Publishing Ltd; 2013.
19. Federation of State Medical Boards. USMLE Step 3. Available at: https://www.fsmb.org/step3/.
20. American Board of Internal Medicine. Competency-based medical education pilot programs. Available at: https://www.abim.org/program-directors-administrators/competency-based-medical-education-pilot-programs.aspx.
21. Accreditation Council for Graduate Medical Education. Advancing Innovation in Residency Education (AIRES). Available at: https://www.acgme.org/What-We-Do/Accreditation/Advancing-Innovation-in-Residency-Education-AIRE.

Mastery Learning: Opportunities and Challenges

21

William C. McGaghie, Jeffrey H. Barsuk, David H. Salzman, Mark Adler, Joe Feinglass, and Diane B. Wayne

This concluding chapter of *Mastery Learning in Health Professions Education* aims to chart new pathways for health sciences education and evaluation research. Unlike the first chapter in this volume, "Clinical education: origins and outcomes," which presents a detailed critique of the signature pedagogy of clinical education in the health professions, this chapter sets forth an optimistic agenda about twenty-first century education and evaluation research.

We begin by presenting six education and education research *opportunities* in health professions education. The six education and research opportunities include the following: (a) expand mastery learning curricula to include a broader range of

W. C. McGaghie (✉)
Northwestern University Feinberg School of Medicine, Departments of Medical Education and Preventive Medicine, Chicago, IL, USA
e-mail: wcmc@northwestern.edu

J. H. Barsuk · D. B. Wayne
Northwestern University Feinberg School of Medicine, Departments of Medicine and Medical Education, Chicago, IL, USA
e-mail: dwayne@northwestern.edu

D. H. Salzman
Northwestern University Feinberg School of Medicine, Departments of Emergency Medicine and Medical Education, Chicago, IL, USA

M. Adler
Northwestern University Feinberg School of Medicine, Departments of Pediatrics and Medical Education, Chicago, IL, USA

J. Feinglass
Northwestern University Feinberg School of Medicine, Departments of Medicine and Preventive Medicine, Chicago, IL, USA

W. C. McGaghie et al. (eds.), *Comprehensive Healthcare Simulation: Mastery Learning in Health Professions Education*, Comprehensive Healthcare Simulation, https://doi.org/10.1007/978-3-030-34811-3_21

skills training in medicine, nursing, and other health professions; (b) spread mastery learning curricula into patient education and education for family members and patient caregivers; (c) develop and test mastery learning curricula to better address training of clinical team skills; (d) widen education models where one's peers and other professionals serve as teachers and assessors; (e) enlarge mastery learning domains to cover a much wider range of non-technical clinical skills in addition to breaking bad news and difficult conversations; and (f) improve the quality and reporting of mastery learning research to ensure that future *research programs* are thematic, sustained, and cumulative and address translational science goals.

There are also many *challenges* on the mastery learning education and research horizon. We choose to name and amplify seven challenges that are now prominent: (a) assessment of complex clinical problems as a mastery learning base; (b) achievement of adaptive competencies in patient care; (c) the limits of mastery learning; (d) evaluation apprehension; (e) cultural and organizational questions; (f) mastery learning in the context of new and emerging technologies; and (g) in the USA, a lack of federal funding for mastery learning health professions education research.

Opportunities

Expand Mastery Learning Curricula

Current use of the mastery learning model in health professions education has focused chiefly on preparing physicians and nurses to perform invasive clinical procedures (Chaps. 12, 13, and 14). Mastery learning education and research has also been conducted on improving physicians' communication skills, especially breaking bad news and having end-of-life conversations with patients and families (Chap. 10). There is now an acute need to expand mastery learning curricula to a much broader range of clinical skills and a larger sample of health professions beyond medicine and nursing. Clinical curriculum development, faculty training, and creation of assessment programs that yield reliable data for learner advancement and entrustment decisions are needed to extend mastery learning across the health professions continuum.

Patient, Family, and Caregiver Education

Rigorous patient, family, and caregiver education is needed to boost patient quality of life, reduce morbidity and mortality, and lower patients' hospital length of stay and readmission rates. Mastery learning holds promise to address each of these healthcare goals.

To illustrate, physician Jeffrey Barsuk leads an interdisciplinary team of advanced heart failure physicians, nurses, and health services researchers at Northwestern Memorial Hospital (NMH) in Chicago. This team uses simulation-based mastery learning (SBML) to educate patients with advanced heart failure and their [usually family] caregivers who rely on ventricular assist devices (VADs) for survival while awaiting a heart transplant. Barsuk and colleagues report, "VADs are mechanical heart pumps that are implanted into a patient's left and/or right ventricle. An electrical cord (driveline) exits from the pump through the abdomen and is attached to a small computerized controller (that controls the actions of the pump) which is connected to a power source. VAD self-care . . . requires a high level of knowledge and meticulous skill performance by patients and caregivers. Adverse events related to VADs include driveline infections . . . and strokes that lead to a high readmission rate. Patients and their caregivers must be able to change the dressing at the driveline exit site using a sterile technique, change the controller if it malfunctions, change power sources . . . learn new medications, troubleshoot controller alarms, and, overall, adjust to a new daily lifestyle to help prevent those adverse events" [1].

This ambitious VAD mastery learning curriculum was developed as an education program for advanced heart failure patients and their caregivers to reduce complications associated with VAD. Educational rigor is important because under usual conditions preventable driveline infections occur at a rate of 1.31 per patient month after implant placement. Also, the overall mortality of patients with a VAD is 19% at 1 year [2]. Early results from the NMH mastery learning curriculum for VAD patients and their caregivers from a randomized trial are encouraging. Expressed in translational science terms (Chap. 16), T1 education results in the controlled simulation education laboratory and T2 clinical care results due to reduced bedside complications show that a powerful simulation-based mastery learning (SBML) education intervention ". . . provided superior VAD self-care skills learning outcomes compared to usual training. This study has important implications for patients due to the morbidity and mortality associated with improper VAD self-care" [3].

This early work with VAD heart failure patients and their caregivers suggests that the mastery learning model can be used to address many other patient education problems in a variety of healthcare settings. Other potential targets for patient mastery learning education include outcomes that healthcare educators want patients to acquire to minimize the risk of morbidity and mortality. Potential topics include self-administered peritoneal dialysis; home central venous catheter (CVC) management; wound, ostomy, and drain care; and taking complex medication regimens including intravenous infusions such as antibiotics, total parenteral nutrition, and injectable medications such as insulin, epinephrine, and anticoagulants.

Mastery Learning for Clinical Team Training

Chapter 11 of this book makes a strong case that in the health professions no one works alone anymore. In nearly all settings, today's healthcare is delivered by professional teams, not by individual providers working in isolation. This practical situation underscores the importance of developing and testing mastery learning curricula for health professions team training. Team training means that the focus of education and assessment practices must shift from persons to groups. Team training and assessment also means that mastery learning curricula will need to address team composition including teams with consistent members versus those that are interchangeable as in the US Army trauma training teams (Chap. 11). Team assessment will require minimum passing standards (MPSs) set for individual learners that are applicable to team-based mastery learning. Our multi-year experience with advanced cardiac life support (ACLS) team responses shows us that this work is substantially different than mastery learning for an individual clinical skill [4].

Peer Teaching and Assessment

Management and delivery of mastery learning curricula in the health professions can be labor intensive (Chap. 7). Learners engage in focused, deliberate practice to improve clinical skills and knowledge representations. The faculty workload is also intense because instructors need to set learning and practice conditions, document interrater reliability, monitor learner progress, provide feedback and debriefing, coach for learner improvement, and assess learners for professional entrustment decisions. The education workload in mastery learning is substantial for everyone.

There are many opportunities in health professions mastery learning curricula to engage learner peers as instructors and assessors. Peers are defined broadly and may include professional school classmates or other healthcare providers. For example, the concept of "near-peer teaching" has gained traction as an instructional strategy in health professions education. This approach uses senior learners, usually several years ahead of learners in the same health profession, to serve as facilitators for junior learners. Near-peer teaching is effective because junior student learners and senior student teachers share a common language, knowledge base, and social role [5]. The technique has been used in problem-based learning, clinical education, simulation, and other small group medical education sessions. Near peer teaching is valued by students because senior learners can leverage their recent educational experiences and add clinical context for younger peers [6].

Professional school classmates can contribute to peer teaching as a result of formative assessments within instructional units. Learners who meet or exceed the MPS quickly can work as peer coaches to help others who need more deliberate practice time to reach the goal (Chap. 2). This assumes, of course, that the education environment is governed by a spirit of cooperation and psychological safety among learners and faculty (Chap. 8).

Health professions educators should also consider the contribution that healthcare providers who have a different healthcare role than learners may add to education experiences. One successful example is the key contribution that respiratory therapists made during education of nurses and physicians in ACLS (Chaps. 3 and 4).

Non-technical Clinical Skills

Mastery learning curricula in health professions education have a strong record of helping learners acquire such procedural skills as endoscopic surgery, lumbar puncture (LP), CVC insertion and maintenance, thoracentesis, paracentesis, and other invasive maneuvers (Chaps. 12 and 13). Team-based clinical skills including ACLS can also be taught and learned to mastery standards (Chaps. 3 and 11). Evaluation research also shows that non-technical clinical skills such as communication (breaking bad news and end-of-life discussions with patients and families), situation awareness, and task allocation can also be addressed effectively using the mastery learning model (Chap. 10).

The opportunity to expand the mastery learning model to a broader range of non-technical clinical skills including patient handoffs [7], interprofessional communication, team leadership, resource management, and elements of clinical reasoning depends on educators' ability to assess outcomes reliably [8]. Creating mastery learning curricula is relatively easy for what Ericsson and Pool call a "highly developed field" where educational outcomes can be measured objectively and where there is professional consensus about correct answers [9] (Chap. 4). However, non-technical mastery learning curricula are much harder to develop because these professional practice behaviors do not fit the Ericsson and Pool definition. Progress toward developing and testing non-technical clinical skill mastery learning curricula will be slowed until consensual outcome assessment programs are created and tested (Chap. 5).

Mastery Learning Research

The mastery learning *bundle* is a set of seven complementary elements: (a) baseline, or diagnostic testing; (b) clear learning objectives, sequenced as units usually in increasing difficulty; (c) engagement in educational activities, e.g., deliberate skills practice, calculations, reading, etc.; (d) set MPSs for each educational unit; (e) formative assessment; (f) advancement to the next educational unit given achievement at or above the MPS; and (g) continued practice or study on an educational unit until the mastery standard is reached [10] (Chap. 2). The power of mastery learning resides in use of the complete package, the inseparable seven element *bundle*. However, each of the seven mastery learning pieces warrants research study and refinement.

To illustrate, Coughlan and colleagues performed a study involving Gaelic football [soccer] players that dissected, "How experts practice: a novel test of deliberate practice theory" [11]. These investigators found that experts "practiced the skill they were weaker at and improved its performance across pre-, post- and retention tests." "In contrast, . . . participants in the [comparison] group predominately practiced the skill they were stronger at . . ." [11]. Coughlan and colleagues conclude, "Findings provide support for deliberate practice theory and give some insight into how experts practice and improve their performance beyond its current level" [11]. The Coughlan et al. study is a research example about how to understand and improve one of the seven features of the mastery learning *bundle*. Research studies addressing the other six mastery learning bundle features are needed.

Longitudinal mastery learning research is needed at all levels across the health professions to better understand the sources and timing of clinical skill decay [12] and why clinical experience is not a proxy for quality of healthcare [13]. Early results are encouraging. A mastery learning study of clinical skill acquisition and maintenance shows that ACLS skills acquired to a mastery standard are retained without decay for up to 12 months [14]. Mastery learning of invasive clinical procedures such as central venous catheter insertion [15] and critical care skills (e.g., ventilator and hemodynamic parameter management and treating septic shock) [16] shows that these skills are resistant to decay over at least 12 months. More research is clearly needed, especially studies that compare mastery learning education interventions to other training methods, to determine if these early skill retention results can be replicated.

Beyond individual research studies, the utility and impact of mastery learning curricula in health professions education will be advanced by evaluation research *programs* that are thematic, sustained, and cumulative [17]. A prominent example of such a mastery learning clinical education and research program is the systematic series of CVC insertion and maintenance studies led by Jeffrey Barsuk with an interdisciplinary Northwestern team. The T1 to T4 (Chap. 16) studies are a series of CVC education and research reports that address mastery learning of (a) CVC skill acquisition in a medical simulation laboratory (T1) [18], (b) systematic setting of a CVC MPS by an expert faculty panel [19], (c) a demonstration that patients receiving CVC care from mastery trained medical residents experience fewer complications than patients cared for by residents trained traditionally (T2) [20], and that (d) mastery learning of CVC skills is responsible for an 85% reduction in central line-associated bloodstream infections (CLABSIs) in a medical ICU (T3) [21]. Collateral (T4) effects from this mastery learning CVC education and research program include (e) a demonstration of long-term retention of CVC skills [22]; (f) cost savings expressed as a 7:1 return on financial investment [23]; (g) unexpected yet welcome systemic educational improvement [24] that prompted a MPS increase [25]; (h) successful dissemination of the mastery learning CVC program from a tertiary care medical center to an academic community hospital [26]; and (i) educating attending physicians and ICU nurses in CVC patient care to mastery learning standards [27, 28].

One-off, stand-alone mastery learning education and evaluation research studies will have little impact unless they are connected to other thematic investigations that demonstrate translational, downstream patient outcomes (Chap. 16). Research connections contribute to a sustained and cumulative body of work that will enrich, improve, and extend the boundaries of the current mastery learning model in health professions education.

Uniform reporting of mastery learning evaluation research studies according to standardized reporting conventions is another opportunity to advance scholarship [29]. Standardized research reporting conventions shape and inform mastery learning curriculum development and research in all phases beginning with design, intervention character and intensity, deliberate practice features, pretest and posttest development, timing, data reliability estimation, and program management. Uniform research reporting contributes to clear understanding of procedures and results, continuity of data sets, opportunities for research synthesis, and the general progress of mastery learning in health professions education [29].

Challenges

Complex Assessment

Patient care delivered by health professional individuals and teams is a complex enterprise with many moving parts. Diagnosis, patient management, teamwork, procedural skill, medication reconciliation, image and diagnostic test interpretation, communication with the healthcare team and families, patient handoffs, navigating an electronic medical record (EMR), responding to crises, perceiving and responding to ethical issues, addressing ethnic and cultural matters, and a host of other competencies are all potential mastery learning targets in health professions education. However, as pointed out in Chaps. 4 and 5 on Instruction and Assessment in Mastery Learning, educators simply cannot teach and assess the complete universe of eligible knowledge, skill, and professionalism attributes. Instead, health professions educators teach and assess carefully selected *samples* of professional behavior shaped by accreditation requirements, professional practice guidelines, local preferences, habit, restricted time schedules, and many other influences.

Decades of behavioral science research on expert performance, summarized by Anders Ericsson and Robert Pool in their book, *Peak: Secrets from the New Science of Expertise*, are distilled in a key statement, ". . . a crucial fact about expert performance in general [is]: there is no such thing as developing a general skill" [9]. This indicates that attempts to measure and assess such general clinical attributes as "medical decision making," "cultural competence," and "interpersonal skill" will fail without clear operational definitions of their key elements.

The professional education and assessment needed to address complex clinical situation present a real challenge. Medical conditions of patients and families change rapidly, management of health problems may have more than one correct answer, and experts often disagree about the best course(s) of clinical action. How can health professions educators create and manage a mastery learning curriculum to prepare physicians, nurses, and other providers to manage complex clinical and social problems?

The answer, we believe, is to break down the complex clinical situation into a smaller set of education and assessment operational units—for example, a curriculum—on mastery learning in, say, geriatric care. The units will serve as an approximation to a "highly developed field" where outcome assessment is objective, "or at least semiobjective," that permit formative and summative decisions about learner progress and entrustment [9]. The set of operational units will cover knowledge and skill facets of geriatric care that are teachable and testable to mastery standards yet will never represent a census of the competencies needed to address all complex clinical cases. Such a deliberate sampling approach encourages health professions educators to develop curricula; teach, measure, and assess key features of complex clinical cases very well; learn from the experience; and find ways to improve continually. These smaller units can then be united as parts of a larger curriculum to assess overall care performance for multiple healthcare professionals.

This problem with complex clinical assessment is highlighted by the teaching message of surgeon Atul Gawande in his book, *The Checklist Manifesto*. Gawande states, "There are . . . all kinds of steps that checklists do not specify. They are not comprehensive how-to guides. They are quick and simple tools aimed to buttress the skills of expert professionals" [30].

Adaptive Competencies

Adaptive competence is a hallmark of professional practice. Cognitive psychologist Keith Holyoak asserts a professional with adaptive competence is one . . . "who can make an appropriate response to a situation that contains a degree of unpredictability." This contrasts with "routine experts who are able to solve familiar types of problems quickly and accurately" [31].

Intra-operative decision-making and procedural adjustment by a surgeon is one example of adaptive competence. To illustrate, if a colon cancer surgeon observes that a tumor not seen on imaging has invaded a patient's liver she may have to modify the operation. Adaptive competence is seen among health professionals every day in complex and simple situations: a pediatrician who changes an epileptic patient's seizure medicine due to an unexpected side-effect; the family physician who refers an elderly cancer patient to hospice rather than more aggressive chemotherapy; a nurse who needs to decide whether to call a stroke code or an on-call physician when a patient becomes slightly altered with slurred speech; a psychiatrist who prioritizes cognitive behavior therapy as an adjunct to medications to care for a patient with depression. Adaptive competence is a cornerstone of expertise in the health professions. How can educators increase the probability that their learners will acquire adaptive competencies and use the competencies effectively in patient care?

Health professions education clinical learning objectives change—sometimes quickly—due to time, setting, patient acuity, disease severity, advancing technology, and many other personal and interpersonal variables. Fluid clinical conditions prompt educators to prepare learners to expect the unexpected, respond to uncertainty, and develop adaptive competence. Ericsson and Pool present strong evidence that attests to the highly adaptive capacities of the human species [9]. These scientists point out that after much deliberate practice with continuous refinement of mental representations, "When an actual surgery diverges from the surgeon's mental representation, he or she knows to slow down, rethink the options, and, if necessary, formulate a new plan in response to the new information" [9].

A recent example from the aviation profession is a case study about the importance of adaptive competence and the training needed to reach that goal. Captain Chesley "Sully" Sullenberger, the pilot who performed the "Miracle on the Hudson" by safely landing a commercial airplane on the Hudson River in 2009 with no loss of life, testified recently before a US congressional panel. The panel was investigating simulation training for flight safety. Sullenberger stated, "We must make sure that everyone who occupies a pilot seat is fully armed with the information, knowledge, training, skill, and judgment to be able to be the absolute **master** of the aircraft and all its component systems and of the situations simultaneously and continuously throughout the flight" (emphasis added). "Pilots need physical, firsthand [simulation] experience to be prepared for emergencies." Sullenberger concluded his testimony with the statement, "Reading about it on an iPad is not even close to sufficient" [32]. The congruence of Captain Sullenberger's congressional testimony and principles of mastery learning with deliberate practice is evident.

Ericsson and Pool suggest that general adaptive clinical competence cannot be taught and assessed [9]. However, a sample of the component parts of clinical adaptive competence for specific situations or conditions can be operationalized and become the foundation of a mastery learning curriculum.

Limits of Mastery Learning

Health professions educators need to acknowledge that despite its utility in many training curricula, mastery learning is not a panacea. Mastery learning is not a cure-all for educational problems in the health professions. A "one size fits all" or "just add water" mentality simply cannot drive the use of mastery learning in health professions education.

We believe that mastery learning is most useful to help health professions learners acquire and maintain core or essential clinical skills that really matter in everyday clinical practice (Chap. 3). We also believe that curriculum developers, teachers, and assessors can *never* educate health professionals about all of the complex clinical conditions they will encounter in their careers, especially as healthcare changes and technology improves. Thus mastery learning should focus on carefully selected *samples* of clinical skills, reasoning, communication, and other learning outcomes (Chap. 5) that connect directly to patient care practices and patient outcomes (Chap. 16). After more than a decade of experience we identify several additional benefits of the mastery learning approach. These include high satisfaction among learners, receptivity to feedback, and the idea that additional deliberate practice is a necessary part of education and not a penalty. These features not only develop expertise but also imprint learners with the knowledge that lifelong skill development and assessment is necessary to practice at the highest level [33].

Evaluation Apprehension

Evaluation apprehension is ubiquitous throughout the health professions. The term refers to the widespread fear among health professionals in training and practice to be revealed as having an insufficient fund of knowledge or poor clinical skills. Evaluation apprehension produces a variety of dysfunctional behaviors including failure to ask for help with uncertain clinical problems and impression management, defending one's professional image in clinical and professional settings at all costs [34, 35].

Rosenbaum writes, "… the perceived need for impression management to protect one's professional image is extremely high in medicine." Rosenbaum also describes the "tacit calculus" common in clinical environments, "balancing the need to seek help against the likelihood of looking stupid" [35]. McGaghie contributes to the discussion, "… much of everyday clinical education and learner evaluation is an intricate kabuki play involving a fear of failure, impression management, the importance of portraying an image of competence, face saving, the power of subjective evaluations, and the value of establishing and maintaining one's clinical reputation. Objective, reliable data have no role in these performances" [34].

Evaluation apprehension is a powerful source of resistance to the development and implementation of mastery learning curricula in health professions education. Mastery learning pretests, for example, are specifically designed to detect learning and clinical deficiencies. The measured deficiencies, in turn, are used to give learners specific, actionable feedback; provide focus for deliberate practice; guide formative assessment toward the MPS; and finally inform summative entrustment decisions once the MPS is met or surpassed. This can only happen in mastery learning settings that are psychologically safe, when assessment data are used as a tool, not as a weapon—and everyone understands and lives by the rules.

There is a clear need to devise mechanisms to reduce evaluation apprehension in health professions mastery learning settings. Health professions educators who endorse mastery learning must engineer and operate safe and supportive learning environments that mitigate its influence, such as presimulation briefing [36]. In addition, early evidence suggests that learners who undergo successful mastery learning experiences simply "get over it." Successful mastery learning experiences boost student self confidence, lower anxiety, and increase motivation for more skill and knowledge acquisition. The learners grow accustomed to mastery learning curricula so steps of baseline assessment, deliberate practice, feedback, regular formative assessment, and more practice to reach a mastery standard become a new normal for education [33].

Cultural and Organizational Questions

The culture of health professions education has historically judged the learning and performance of students and healthcare providers as norm-referenced accomplishments. Competitive student selection, progress through basic science education, acquisition of clinical skills, and professional certification and licensure have all been judged in comparison to other learners, usually on a normal distribution of performance metrics. Academic achievement and clinical performance are judged by "grading on the curve" rather than in comparison to a MPS expected for all learners (Chaps. 5 and 6). The common result of this widespread cultural policy is uneven knowledge and clinical skill acquisition among nurses, doctors, physical therapists, pharmacists, midwives, and other health professionals (Chap. 1). A growing body of evidence shows that uneven skill sets among health professionals is a key source of substandard patient care (Chap. 16).

The idea that learning and professional practice in the health professions is "good enough" based on norm-referenced performance is no longer good enough. Health professions educators and certification and licensure bodies need to expect more from students and practicing professionals to ensure patient safety. Setting high education achievement and professional practice standards, and enforcing the high standards via accountability, represents a cultural paradigm shift in health professions education.

Another cultural and organizational challenge (also an opportunity) in the health professions concerns the introduction of mastery learning into continuing professional education (CPE) and maintenance of certification (MOC) programs (Chap. 18). There are two key barriers to the use of mastery learning in CPE and MOC. The first is an abiding ideology within the health professions about the value and utility of internal self-regulation; self and peer assessment; and stiff resistance to limits on post-certification scope of practice and income opportunities. Rigorous MOC requirements frequently meet opposition. This ideology has deep historical roots [37] and contemporary expression in what Susskind and Susskind term, "status quo bias," a preference for continuing to do things as they are done today [38]. A recent example of status quo bias is the report of a 2020 Task Force of the American Board of Internal Medicine which after 2 years of MOC deliberation recommended only modest changes in the focus and frequency of multiple-choice tests for MOC in that specialty [39]. This is troublesome for at least two reasons. First, continued reliance on multiple-choice examinations to certify and license healthcare professionals as competent to practice covers a very small sample of professional behavior. Psychometrician Brian Clauser and colleagues state, ". . . a passing score on a licensing examination may be seen as a *prerequisite* for acceptable practice but not a *guarantee* of acceptable practice" [40]. Second, issues of great importance to the public including clinical skill assessment, adaptation of new technology into practice, interprofessional collaboration, and team science have not yet been adequately addressed over the lifespan of continuing health professions education, certification, and licensure [38].

The second key barrier to introducing mastery learning into health professions MOC is the evaluation apprehension problem, discussed in the previous section. Clinical skill, knowledge, and professionalism attributes simply cannot be improved without reliable baseline assessment and feedback (Chap. 5). A climate of psychological safety and assurance that assessment data will be used as a tool, not a weapon, are essential to address this cultural and organizational barrier [34–36].

New and Emerging Technologies

The EMR; automated reading of digital MRI and dermatology images; personal, automated monitoring of such physiological metrics as blood pressure, hemoglobin A1c, and kidney function; robotic surgery; point-of-care ultrasound; educational simulations; genomic testing; DNA manipulations, and a host of other new and emerging technologies will challenge health professionals and the systems that govern their behavior throughout the future. Technological advancements in biology, computer science, nanotechnology, and other fields are advancing at a breathtaking pace. This not only means that most health professionals will likely narrow their scope of practice but also that patients will assume independent responsibility for more of their own healthcare. Cardiologist Eric Topol anticipates in his 2015 book, *The Patient will See You Now*, ". . . [we] are embarking on a time when each individual will have all their own medical data and the computing power to process it . . . from womb to tomb . . . even to prevent an illness before it happens" [41].

We find it ironic that in this day of rapid and continuing changes in all aspects of healthcare that the methods of educating and assessing health professionals have changed very little in the past century (Chap. 1). As the chapter authors of this volume have pointed out in many locations, we simply must improve health professions education practices to keep current and deliver quality patient care. New and emerging technologies will always challenge health professions educators to keep pace and to use the advancements intelligently. Mastery learning is only one educational approach to reach this goal.

Federal Funding

Healthcare research in the USA is funded chiefly through federal agencies including the National Institutes of Health (NIH) [42] and the Agency for Healthcare Research and Quality [43]. These agencies have a long historical record of financially supporting excellent basic and applied biomedical research to advance bioscience and inform healthcare clinical practice. However, funding for research in health professions education has been deficient or absent [44–47], despite strong evidence that financial support is linked directly to the quality of medical education research [48].

This circumstance prompted several members of our health professions education research group to criticize federal funding research priorities and call for reform. The research group asserts, "[NIH and AHRQ] statements about [research funding] policies and priorities focus on biomedical research, education of biomedical scientists, and conventional treatment options. They do not address the value of a skilled workforce in the clinical medical and health professions and the importance of rigorous clinical education for the delivery of effective healthcare. We assert that human capital, embodied in competent physicians and other health professionals, is an essential feature of [clinical science] even though NIH, Institute of Medicine, and AHRQ policies and priorities are silent about the contribution of clinical medical education to health-care delivery" [49].

We continue to endorse this statement because a growing body of research evidence shows that powerful health professions education grounded in mastery learning with rigorous assessment has direct effects on improved patient care practices and patient outcomes (Chap. 16). Financial support from US federal agencies will boost the health professions education research agenda and improve healthcare for the patients we serve.

Coda

The challenges we have outlined are real. However, we have learned that mastery learning can be a vital component of health professions education. Mastery learning is an invaluable tool to tackle the challenges of individual and healthcare team clinical competence and excellent patient care.

Despite mastery learning being in its infancy within health professions education, there are already many successful examples across a spectrum of translational outcomes from improved bedside performance to better patient outcomes (Chap. 16). We are responsible to build on these early successes while addressing new opportunities and challenges in health professions education. This will take sustained hard work. The good news is that long-run integration of mastery learning into health professions education will ensure that all learners achieve a high and uniform level of performance that leads to improving the care and outcomes for all of our patients.

References

1. Barsuk JH, Harap RS, Cohen ER, et al. The effect of judge selection on standard setting using the Mastery Angoff method during development of a ventricular assist device self-care curriculum. Clin Simul Nursing. 2019;27:39–47.
2. Kirklin JK, Pagani FD, Kormos RL, et al. Eighth annual INTERMACS report: special focus on framing the impact of adverse events. J Heart Lung Transpl. 2017;36:1080–6.
3. Barsuk JH, Wilcox JE, Cohen ER, et al. Simulation-based mastery learning improves patient and caregiver ventricular assist device self-care skills: a randomized pilot trial. Circ: Cardiovas Qual Outcomes. 2019;12(10):e005794. https://doi.org/10.1161/CIRCOUTCOMES.119.005794. Epub 2019 Oct 11.
4. Barsuk JH, Cohen ER, Wayne DB, et al. Developing a simulation-based mastery learning curriculum: lessons from 11 years of advanced cardiac life support. Sim Healthc. 2016;11(1):52–9.
5. Lockspeiser TM, O'Sullivan P, Teherani A, Muller J. Understanding the experience of being taught by peers: the value of social and cognitive congruence. Adv Health Sci Educ. 2008;13:361–72.
6. Bulte C, Betts A, Garner K, Durning S. Student teaching: views of student near-peer teachers and learners. Med Teach. 2007;29:583–90.
7. Didwania A, Kries M, Cohen ER, et al. Internal medicine postgraduate training and assessment of patient hand off skills. J Grad Med Educ. 2013;5(3):394–8.
8. Higham H, Greig PR, Rutherford J, et al. Observer-based tools for non-technical skills assessment in simulated and real clinical environments in healthcare: a systematic review. BMJ Qual Saf. 2019; 28: 672–86.
9. Ericsson A, Pool R. Peak: secrets from the new science of expertise. Boston: Houghton Mifflin Harcourt; 2016.
10. McGaghie WC. Mastery learning: it is time for medical education to join the 21st century. Acad Med. 2015;90(11):1438–41.
11. Coughlan EK, Williams AM, McRobert AP, Ford PR. How experts practice: a novel test of deliberate practice theory. J Exp Psychol: Learn Mem Cog. 2014;40(2):449–58.
12. Arthur W Jr, Bennett W Jr, Stanosh PL, McNelly TL. Factors that influence skill decay and retention: a quantitative review and analysis. Hum Perform. 1998;11(1):57–101.

13. Choudry NK, Fletcher RH, Soumerai SB. Systematic review: the relationship between clinical experience and quality of health care. Ann Intern Med. 2005;142:260–73.
14. Didwania A, McGaghie WC, Cohen ER, et al. Progress toward improving the quality of cardiac arrest medical team responses at an academic teaching hospital. J Grad Med Educ. 2011;3:211–6.
15. Barsuk JH, Cohen ER, McGaghie WC, et al. Long-term retention of central venous catheter insertion skills after simulation-based mastery learning. Acad Med. 2010;85(10, Suppl):S9–S12.
16. Moazed F, Cohen ER, Furiasse N, et al. Retention of critical care skills after simulaton-based mastery learning. J Grad Med Educ. 2013;5:458–63.
17. McGaghie WC, Issenberg SB, Barsuk JH, Wayne DB. A critical review of simulation-based mastery learning with translational outcomes. Med Educ. 2014;48:375–85.
18. Barsuk JH, McGaghie WC, Cohen ER, et al. Use of simulation-based mastery learning to improve the quality of central venous catheter placement in a medical intensive care unit. J Hosp Med. 2009;4(7):397–403.
19. Wayne DB, Barsuk JH, Cohen ER, McGaghie WC. Do baseline data influence standard setting for a clinical skills examination? Acad Med. 2007;82(10, Suppl):S105–8.
20. Barsuk JH, McGaghie WC, Cohen ER, et al. Simulation-based mastery learning reduces complications during central venous catheter insertion in a medical intensive care unit. Crit Care Med. 2009;37(10):2697–701.
21. Barsuk JH, Cohen ER, Feinglass J, et al. Use of simulation-based education to reduce catheter-related bloodstream infections. Arch Intern Med. 2009;169(15):1420–3.
22. Barsuk JH, Cohen ER, McGaghie WC, Wayne DB. Long-term retention of central venous catheter insertion sills after simulation-based mastery learning. Acad Med. 2010;85(10, Suppl):S9–S12.
23. Cohen ER, Feinglass J, Barsuk JH, et al. Cost savings from reduced catheter-related bloodstream infection after simulation-based education for residents in a medical intensive care unit. Simul Healthc. 2010;5(2):98–102.
24. Barsuk JH, Cohen ER, Feinglass J, et al. Unexpected collateral effects of simulation-based medical education. Acad Med. 2011;86(12):1513–7.
25. Cohen ER, Barsuk JH, McGaghie WC, Wayne DB. Raising the bar: reassessing standards for procedural competence. Teach Learn Med. 2013;25(1):6–9.
26. Barsuk JH, Cohen ER, Potts S, et al. Dissemination of a simulation-based mastery learning intervention reduces central line-associated bloodstream infections. BMJ Qual Saf. 2014;23(9):749–56.
27. Barsuk JH, Cohen ER, Nguyen D, et al. Attending physician adherence to a 29-component central venous catheter bundle checklist during simulated procedures. Crit Care Med. 2016;44(10):1871–81.
28. Barsuk JH, Seburn S, Cohen ER, Slade M, Mikolajczak A, Wayne DB. Simulation-based mastery learning improves central line maintenance skills of ICU nurses. J Nurs Admin. 2015;45(10):511–7.
29. Cohen ER, McGaghie WC, Wayne DB, et al. Recommendations for reporting mastery education research in medicine (ReMERM). Acad Med. 2015;90(11):1509–14.
30. Gawande A. The checklist manifesto: how to get things right. New York: Picador; 2009.
31. Holyoak KJ. Symbolic connectionism: toward third-generation theories of expertise. In: Ericsson KA, Smith J, editors. Toward a general theory of expertise: prospects and limits. Cambridge: Cambridge University Press; 1991.
32. Cole D. Sullenberger's experience in a 737 MAX simulator made him see how pilots ran out of time. Available at: https://www.cnn.com/2019/06/19/politics/chesley-sullenberger-boeing-737-max-scenario/.
33. Cohen ER, Barsuk JH, Moazed F, et al. Making July safer: simulation-based mastery learning during intern boot camp. Acad Med. 2013;88:233–9.

34. McGaghie WC. Evaluation apprehension and impression management in medical education. Acad Med. 2018;93(5):685–6.
35. Rosenbaum L. Cursed by knowledge—building a culture of psychological safety. N Engl J Med. 2019;380(8):786–90.
36. Rudolph JW, Raemer DB, Simon R. Establishing a safe container for learning in simulation: the role of presimulation briefing. Simul Healthc. 2014;9(6):339–49.
37. Friedson E. Profession of medicine: a study of the sociology of applied knowledge. New York: Dodd, Mead & Company; 1973.
38. Susskind R, Susskind D. The future of the professions: how technology will transform the work of human efforts. Oxford, UK: Oxford University Press; 2015.
39. American Board of Internal Medicine Assessment 2020 Task Force. A vision for certification in internal medicine in 2020. Philadelphia: American Board of Internal Medicine; 2015.
40. Clauser BE, Margolis MJ, Case SM. Testing for licensure and certification in the professions. In: Brennan RL, editor. Educational measurement. 4th ed. Westport: American Council on Education and Praeger Publishers; 2006.
41. Topol E. The patient will see you now: the future of medicine is in your hands. New York: Basic Books; 2015.
42. National Institutes of Health. NIH-wide strategic plan fiscal years 2016–2020. Available at: http://www.nih.gov/sites/default/files/about-nih/strategic-plan-fy2016-2020-508.pdf.
43. Agency for Healthcare Research and Quality. AHRQ research funding priorities & special emphasis notices, February 2019. Available at: https://www.ahrq.gov/funding/priorities-contacts/special-emphasis-notices/index.html.
44. Carline JD. Funding medical education research: opportunities and issues. Acad Med. 2004;79(10):918–24.
45. Reed DA, Kern DE, Levine RB, Wright SM. Costs and funding for published medical education research. JAMA. 2005;294(9):1052–7.
46. Archer J, McManus C, Woolf K, et al. Without proper research funding, how can medical education be evidence based? BMJ. 2015;350:h3445. https://doi.org/10.1136/bmj.h3445.
47. Gruppen LD, Durning SJ. Needles and haystacks: finding funding for medical education research. Acad Med. 2016;91(4):480–4.
48. Reed DA, Cook DA, Beckman TJ, et al. Association between funding and quality of published medical education research. JAMA. 2007;298(9):1002–9.
49. McGaghie WC, Issenberg SB, Cohen ER, et al. Translational educational research: a necessity for effective health-care improvement. Chest. 2012;142(5):1097–103.

Index

W. C. McGaghie et al. (eds.), *Comprehensive Healthcare Simulation: Mastery Learning in Health Professions Education*, Comprehensive Healthcare Simulation, https://doi.org/10.1007/978-3-030-34811-3